CANCER COMBAT

W9-AOA-935

BANTAM BOOKS

New York   Toronto

London   Sydney

Auckland

CANCER COMBAT

Cancer Survivors Share Their Guerrilla Tactics to Help You Win the Fight of Your Life

Dean King, Jessica King
&
Jonathan Pearlroth

With a Foreword by Samuel Waxman, M.D., and an Afterword by Walter Lawrence, Jr., M.D.

Cover photo: A triumphant Jeanne Clair, two months after undergoing a bone marrow transplant for non-Hodgkin's lymphoma, photographed after a two-and-a-half-hour trek to the top of a mountain in Darby, Montana. Photo credited to Bernard Clair. Life credited to Joseph R. Bertino, M.D.

Back cover photos (clockwise from bottom left):
Leigh Abruscato, holding her daughter, Lucy, on Christmas Day, 1996.
Marc Biundo, in New York City's Central Park.
Jeff Berman finishing his first New York City Marathon in 1992.
Dean, Jessica, Hazel, and Grace King celebrating Hazel's second birthday
in New York City's Riverside Park, June 1996 (Photo by Rachel Cobb).
Sheri Sobrato waterskiing at Princess Louisa Inlet, Chatterbox Falls, British Columbia.
Kathleen Crowley lifting her spirits on the Aran Islands, off the coast of Ireland, in 1996.
Jonathan Pearlroth in a moment of reflection, as the evening is spread out against the sky in
Westhampton Beach, New York.

CANCER COMBAT
A Bantam Book / January 1998

All rights reserved.
Copyright © 1998 by Dean King, Jessica King, and Jonathan Pearlroth
Foreword copyright © 1998 by Samuel Waxman, M.D.
Afterword copyright © 1998 by Walter Lawrence, Jr., M.D.

BOOK DESIGN BY GLEN M. EDELSTEIN

No part of this book may be reproduced or transmitted in any
form or by any means, electronic or mechanical, including
photocopying, recording, or by any information storage and
retrieval system, without permission in writing from the publisher.
For information address: Bantam Books.

Library of Congress Cataloging-in-Publication Data
Cancer combat : cancer survivors share their guerrilla tactics to help
you win the fight of your life / [edited by] Dean King, Jessica King
& Jonathan Pearlroth : foreword by Samuel Waxman : afterword by
Walter Lawrence.
p.   cm.
Includes bibliographical references and index.
ISBN 0-553-37845-7
1. Cancer—popular works.   2. Cancer—Psychological aspects.
I. King, Dean.   II. King, Jessica.   III. Pearlroth, Jonathan.
RC263.C2923   1998
616.99'4—dc21   97-44801   CIP

Published simultaneously in the United States and Canada

Bantam Books are published by Bantam Books, a division of Bantam
Doubleday Dell Publishing Group, Inc. Its trademark, consisting of the words
"Bantam Books" and the portrayal of a rooster, is Registered in U.S. Patent
and Trademark Office and in other countries. Marca Registrada. Bantam
Books, 1540 Broadway, New York, New York 10036.

PRINTED IN THE UNITED STATES OF AMERICA

FFG   10   9   8   7   6   5   4

With love and courage,
from those of us who have been before,
to those who are now battling cancer

CONTENTS

Foreword: Picking a Path to Recovery That Satisfies Your
           Personality, Your Needs, and Your Desires   ix
     by Samuel Waxman, M.D.

Introduction: Make *Cancer Combat* A Part of Your Team   1
     by Dean King

Acknowledgments   7

Your Fellow Guerrillas   8

PART ONE: THE FIRST FEW DAYS   37

Chapter 1:   Dealing with Discovery   39

Chapter 2:   Breaking the News   65

Chapter 3:   How to Be Brave When What You Feel Is Fear   77

Chapter 4:   Getting the Most from Your Medical Team   90

Chapter 5:   Testing, Testing, 1-2-3   106

Chapter 6:   Taking the Information Search into Your
            Own Hands   117

Chapter 7:   It's a Man's Job: Visiting the Sperm Bank   128

PART TWO: GOING TO WAR   135

Chapter 8:   Courage in the Face of Chemo   137

Chapter 9:   Radiation: Taking the Heat   158

Chapter 10: Hospital Strategies   169

Chapter 11: Coping with Surgery   179

Chapter 12: The Big Guns: Bone Marrow Transplant   197

Chapter 13: Battling Breast Cancer   207

Chapter 14: Bad Hair Days   220

Chapter 15: Damn the Torpedoes: Life Doesn't Stop During
            Treatment   233

Chapter 16: Complementary Treatments, Conventional and
            Otherwise   249

Chapter 17: Pushing the Envelope: Dealing with Recurrence,
            Chronic Cancer, Loss of a Limb, and Bad Days in
            the Hospital   269

PART THREE: ALLIES AND OTHER WARTIME
            MATTERS   281

Chapter 18: Eating to Win   283

Chapter 19: Family to the Front   293

Chapter 20: Companions in Arms: Making Friends Your Allies   312

Chapter 21: Psychological Support and Support Groups   326

Chapter 22: Getting Spiritual   339

Chapter 23: Hell's Bills   347

PART FOUR: AFTER THE WAR   359

Chapter 24: Rebounding and Rebuilding   361

Chapter 25: Making Peace: Transcendental Moments,
            New Perspectives, Volunteering   378

Afterword: The Importance of Teamwork   391
            by Walter Lawrence, Jr., M.D.

Resources   395

Books That Helped Us   399

Index   403

About the Authors   417

Picking a Path to Recovery That Satisfies Your Personality, Your Needs, and Your Desires

In my twenty-five years as an oncologist, treating cancer in almost every form, I continue to be humbled by this disease, which spares no age group and often strikes with no clear cause. But I have also been impressed and profoundly inspired by the tremendous strength demonstrated by positively focused cancer patients. These individuals are able to rebound from the initial loss of control that comes with a cancer diagnosis and obtain the strength not only to battle the disease on a personal basis but at the same time to inspire those around them in a team effort. The successful journey from despair to gaining control is not only reassuring to the patient but also creates a sense of urgency in the attending doctors and nurses and encourages families and friends to rally around the patient.

What is it that gives these patients the willpower and dignity to wage a successful battle against cancer? That's what this book is all about. It is about how to take control, how to gain momentum from each small victory, and how to rebound from the setbacks. It is about how to become—with the help of your chosen support team—mentally, physically, and often spiritually stronger in standing up to this life-threatening disease.

Cancer Combat is ultimately about gaining a useful and practical perspective in this determined fight for health. Its message is delivered in short, useful anecdotes that make the experience less lonely, less painful, and more positive. The advice of these cancer survivors covers everything from where they sought second opinions and spiritual strength to how they made hospital stays and chemotherapy less unpleasant—and thus more productive.

The insights of these cancer veterans were gained through personal experience. In that sense, they are the experts. Their suggestions—useful to both patients and professionals dealing with this disease—range from little things you can do to counteract the side effects of treatment, like using a plastic spoon instead of a metal one when chemotherapy has given you a metallic taste in your mouth, to ways to motivate yourself to keep up the fight, like figuring out how to maintain your sex life while you're in the hospital in order to remind yourself of some of the reasons why life is worth living in the first place. The stories told here reveal just how remarkably resilient and resourceful people can be.

During the battle against cancer—no matter who you are—there will be times of confusion, uncertainty, fear, and anger, which must be weathered with the best spirit you can muster. *Cancer Combat* can function as a back-pocket support group to help you take control. If you are facing a certain difficulty, find out how the contributors—normal people just like you—bridged that valley. Their stories may be able to help you navigate the valleys and peaks of the cancer experience and allow you to sustain a more predictable life during treatment. Sure enough, following a tough period, a time of rest and a glimmer of optimism may return to propel you forward.

The book's message is clear, powerful: Not only can you survive cancer, you can emerge stronger and wiser than before. Accept the fact that you have cancer. Make treating cancer a part of your life, but do not let it dominate you. Remain confident and maintain your personal strength and will to fight. Have a sense of humor about it when you can. These are the approaches that stand out in people who are successful.

There is no right or wrong way to carry on this battle. Only your way. The information in this book can serve as a road map to finding your way. Take strength in—and heed the advice of—those who have traveled the routes before you, but pick your own path, one that satisfies your personality, your needs, and your desires. And remember, doctors and hospitals can treat cancer, and mitigate the pain of treatment, better today than ever before. Armed with this knowledge and the insights available to you in *Cancer Combat*, make your experience as life-affirming as possible.

—*Samuel Waxman, M.D.,*
Zena and Michael A. Wiener Professor of Medicine,
Director, Rochelle Belfer Chemotherapy Foundation Laboratory and
Samuel Waxman Cancer Research Foundation,
Mount Sinai Medical Center,
New York, New York

Make Cancer Combat *a Part of Your Team*

Cold room. Hot lights. Surgeon stitching up an incision in my chest. The phone rings. The nurse tells him it's the lab for him. He wipes his hand, takes the phone. "Unhunh, okay." He hangs up and returns to his sewing. "You have lymphoma," he says flatly.

"What's that?" I ask groggily. After a year of shivering spells, bed sweats, midnight back blitzkriegs, and, finally, bulging, angry lymph nodes in my neck and chest, I am so ready for a diagnosis. Ready for a diagnosis, but—at the age of twenty-seven—not this one.

"Cancer of the lymph nodes," he says.

His job done, the surgeon exits.

I am lowered into a wheelchair and told that someone will come get me. Muddled and helpless, I wait for half an hour as the staff works around me, scrubbing down the OR for the next surgery. Still no one comes to get me. Finally, I pick up the surgeon's phone, dial nine, and call my wife at work. "You better meet me at home," I tell her voice mail.

Welcome to the world of cancer. It can be that bad—unprepared patients talking to doctors in too much of a hurry, or too hardened to their work, to realize the impact of their words and too used to the vocabulary of cancer to remember to explain. Even though I had suffered excruciatingly for more than a year, seeing my internist, various surgeons and physical therapists, no one had suggested I had cancer. In fact, one night I had simply lain on the couch shivering in pain and crying and thinking that—because no doctor could find anything wrong—maybe I was having a nervous breakdown.

My wife, Jessica, meets me at home. We call my parents, cry for a little while. We don't know what to do next. Finally, Jess and I walk down the street to a pie shop and order apple pie with ice cream. If *Cancer Combat* had been available at the time, I'd like to think we would have started reading it to each other then.

But it wasn't until later—after we had found out that I had a form of lymphoma known as Hodgkin's disease and was undergoing chemotherapy to treat it—that I realized there needed to be a book like *Cancer Combat,* one filled with the thoughts, advice, anecdotes, and perspectives of a new generation of cancer veterans.

The event that convinced me of that need occurred one sunny day just after I had received my intravenous dose of ABVD, one of the chemotherapy combinations. Instead of returning to our apartment where I'd sit on the couch and fade in and out of consciousness, emerging from my stupor only to vomit (this was before the wonderful antinausea drug Zofran became available), Jess and I decided to go to a nearby park. It was a weekday, and we sat in the empty outfield of a baseball field. To our happy surprise, the aftereffects of the chemo were greatly diminished by my simply being outside. I still vomited, but less, and I stayed much more alert.

My chemotherapist, Dr. Samuel Waxman, and I routinely had conversations before my treatments. He would shut the door to the examining room and no matter how often the nurses poked their heads in or how many times he was paged for a phone call, we would talk, about me—about how I felt mentally, about how my job was going—about how Jessica was holding up under the strain, and about other subjects of mutual interest, like my tribulations with the HMO I belonged to. Unlike many other doctors, Dr. Waxman listened. So I told him about my experience at the baseball field.

His response was, "You should write a book. There's a need for a new book from cancer patients, helping other cancer patients get through this experience."

So I went out and did the homework.

Was there a source for this kind of information, the kind that doctors don't necessarily tell you? From a new generation of cancer veterans and not one person's cancer story? And not a book by a doctor or specific to one type of cancer? The answer was No. In this age when the incidence of cancer is higher than ever, the ever-increasing number of cancer veterans needed a forum to share their wisdom about dealing with cancer—from the shock of being diagnosed and the initial state of denial, to easing the pain of surgery and chemotherapy (sometimes by means not officially sanctioned by the medical world), to the prospects for a future after cancer, a topic that should be brought up from the start but is too frequently overlooked.

To construct just such a book, Jessica and I recruited Jonathan Pearlroth, a young attorney who had battled non-Hodgkin's lymphoma and a recurrence and who had undergone several major surgeries and a bone marrow transplant. Jonathan agreed there was a need for such a book. He often laughs about his introduction to the world of cancer at the age of twenty-five. After the doctor said he had non-Hodgkin's lymphoma, he breathed a sigh of relief in the mistaken belief that lymphoma was "something bad," but "at least it wasn't cancer." Now a volunteer at Memorial Sloan-Kettering Cancer Center and at Gilda's Club, Jonathan has made helping others get through the trials of cancer therapy a major part of his life after cancer.

Our experiences complemented each other well. After I went into remission, Jess and I spent several more years in the medical system trying to have children by in vitro fertilization using my frozen sperm. In all, Jessica, Jonathan, and I have undergone a large spectrum of cancer experience, a good leaping-off point for talking to the many cancer veterans and cancer professionals we interviewed to assemble the practical advice and lessons that make up *Cancer Combat.*

Our goal was to bring together a community of cancer

survivors—real people who have battled and, in some cases, continue to battle cancer—to advise and support you, whether you are fighting cancer yourself or helping a friend or loved one in the fight. And we are very pleased with the result. We think it offers both hope and help.

The science and art of cancer therapy are making strides. According to the National Cancer Institute, in the first two years of the nineties, for the first time since records have been kept, death rates from cancer have dropped in the United States. More people are being diagnosed with cancer, but more are living longer with it or beating it.

The attitude we want to reflect in this book is a new one: Never say die, even when the diagnosis is cancer, no matter how bad. This isn't the once-hopeless cancer experience of decades past, when patients and their families often asked the doctor not to even tell them if they had cancer.

"I think our generation, in general, is different from generations gone by in that we don't just take what doctors tell us and blindly say, 'That's the best medicine and the only alternative,'" Peggy Schmidt, of Minnesota, told me one day, catching the spirit of this book. "We got three opinions on my husband's diagnosis of multiple myeloma. That was important. They were affirmations that, yes, this was the diagnosis, but they all brought us something different."

The Schmidts not only sought out the best of traditional medical care, they reached beyond that: "We've taken the holistic, or natural, approach. We've opted for some experimental treatment, and in addition to that, we have focused on prayer. I think as a family we would not have been satisfied with just one strategy." A growing body of evidence attests to the idea that anyone attempting to beat cancer benefits from this multi-targeted approach. Thus *Cancer Combat* not only covers ways to enhance traditional Western methods of battling cancer, but explores complementary approaches as well.

What to Do with What You Read
in Cancer Combat

The editors of this book feel strongly that everyone's cancer experience is a unique and personal journey. In most instances, there are not rights and wrongs, but personal choices that must be made to form the path of that journey. These decisions must be made based on a combination of factors: among them are the type and extent of your cancer; your level of fitness; your attitudes toward medicine, surgery, and complementary therapy; your family needs; and your spiritual faith. But this doesn't mean that your situation is so unique that your decisions must be made in a void.

On the contrary, as cancer veterans, we have faced many of the same situations and choices. What we offer here is a wide spectrum of experiences from which you can learn before making your own decisions. Quite frequently, in fact, you will find presented side by side in *Cancer Combat* two opposing opinions or different ways of dealing with situations. You may agree with one or the other, or you may want to borrow from both. An additional element in each chapter is the advice from medical and other health professionals, spiritual advisers, and others whom we found valuable to us. Seize what's here or use it as a springboard for searching out the kind of support you need.

That's what *Cancer Combat* is all about.

It's a presentation of possibilities and practical advice.

It's the things we found that helped, things we wished we'd known, things we left undone and later regretted. Of course, during your battle against cancer, you should make all final decisions with the help of whoever constitutes your own team of personal, spiritual, and medical advisers. We hope that *Cancer Combat* becomes a part of that team, providing a group of empathetic voices—a friendly community of veterans of the cancer experience—with wise and hopeful suggestions, and, yes, even a sense of humor when you might need it most.

—Dean King

Please note: *Cancer Combat* does not endorse or recommend any specific doctors, institutions, or treatment plans. The purpose of the book is to add to the insight patients and their family members can bring to the many discussions, situations, and choices they face in battling cancer and in improving life during and after cancer. The editors recommend that all decisions regarding cancer therapy and quality-of-life issues be made in consultation with doctors, other appropriate professionals, and family members and be based on the individual's needs and inclinations.

ACKNOWLEDGMENTS

The editors would like to thank Dr. Samuel Waxman, Dr. Walter Lawrence, Jr., Dr. Ed Clement, Dr. John Shelton Horsley, Jr., and the many other outstanding health-care professionals who contributed to *Cancer Combat*. Our highest esteem and gratitude go to our fellow guerrillas, the many cancer veterans who personally contributed to this book. Their selfless gift of time, energy, and eloquence will help many cancer patients, their families, and their support teams during the battle against cancer and afterward.

We also wish to thank Elizabeth Aquino, Ariana Pearlroth, Ilana Rein, and Logan Ward for their invaluable and tireless help. Special thanks to Katie Hall and Jody Rein for their wisdom and enthusiasm and for helping us present this group of voices in the most helpful way.

YOUR FELLOW GUERRILLAS

Meet the contributors to *Cancer Combat*. Here are our hobbies and professions, loves and locations, and our greatest achievements since kicking cancer. Note: Elizabeth Martin, Bill Thomas, and Charlotte Wells are fictitious names for contributors who wished to remain anonymous.

The thirty-year-old mother of a newborn daughter, **Leigh Abruscato** had just moved to El Paso, Texas, with her husband in 1994 when she discovered a stage-two malignant tumor in her left breast. Her husband, newly employed by International Paper, arranged for a transfer to the couple's hometown of Mobile, Alabama, so that they could be with Leigh's family during her treatment. Leigh scrapped her first treatment plan—a lumpectomy, radiation, and chemotherapy—and, because of a family history of cancer, opted for a more aggressive treatment, a bilateral mastectomy with six months of chemotherapy, half of which was the new drug Taxol. She followed up with reconstructive breast surgery. Her treatment took place at the Mobile Infirmary Medical Center. A stay-at-home mom, Leigh enjoys walking, reading, and cooking.

Patty Aicher's aunt, Catherine Matus, was diagnosed with ovarian cancer in 1984 and underwent surgery and chemotherapy treatment at Long Beach Hospital in California. Patty spent many hours in her aunt's hospital room and says, "I tried to put myself in her position and treat her the way I would want to be treated. I talked to her directly and in the same voice I had always used with her—not with that exaggerated voice people often use with the ill. I didn't baby her. I kept her informed about events taking place in the world and in our family." Patty lives in New York City, where she does voice-overs and works as a fitness instructor and personal trainer. She enjoys running, boxing, and going to the theater.

An oncology nurse educator at the University of Minnesota Hospital and Clinic in Minneapolis, **Lorraine Anderson** was diagnosed with breast cancer in January of 1995 at the age of forty-six. She was treated with lumpectomy, chemotherapy, and radiation. At the time she was diagnosed, Lorraine's job was to educate nurses on oncology and bone marrow transplants. "All the stuff I was going through I was teaching," she says. Lorraine is married. She enjoys gardening, golfing, and reading mysteries.

Katherine Arthur, who lives in Wayne, Pennsylvania, was forty-three in 1985 when she discovered a lump in her breast that turned out to be malignant. Her kids were ten, twelve, and fourteen at the time, but she says she never really felt afraid because of her belief that God would guide her. Five years later, she was back in Pennsylvania Hospital for surgery after a spot was discovered on her lungs. The spot wasn't malignant, but her recovery from lung surgery was slow. With her husband, Bob, Katherine is currently raising money for the Timothy School, a low-cost private school for inner-city children in North Philadelphia. Katherine plays the piano and has attended the same Wednesday Bible study group for thirty years.

At age forty-eight, **Rick Asselta** was diagnosed with cancer of the esophagus. In 1992, he had his esophagus removed at Yale–New Haven Hospital. A Danbury, Connecticut, high school teacher and guidance counselor, Rick runs marathons and enjoys involving the students at his school in camping, outdoor adventure, and ecological studies. He is married and has a daughter and a son.

Donna Avacato was twenty years old when she was diagnosed with osteosarcoma, the most common form of bone cancer occurring in teenagers. She was treated at Lenox Hill Hospital in New York City in 1979. Her left knee and femur were replaced, and she was put on a year's regimen of Adriamycin chemotherapy. She now lives in the Bronx and enjoys writing poetry, listening to rock and classical music, and playing chess.

Born and raised in Boston, **Tim Batchelder** was diagnosed with Hodgkin's disease in 1994 at age twenty-five. Treated at Boston's Brigham and Women's Hospital, he underwent four weeks of radiation. Tim is currently a freelance health writer and graduate student in medical anthropology at the City University of New York in Manhattan. A wilderness enthusiast who has canoed in northern Canada and biked across Colorado and Utah, Tim has spent many weekends since his illness hiking in the mountains of New England.

In 1990, at the age of thirty-two, **Jeff Berman** was diagnosed with chronic lymphocytic leukemia, a disease usually found in people over sixty-five. Because it is slow-moving, he didn't begin treatment until 1993. "Among people under fifty, it's extremely rare," he says. "They don't know much about how it acts in younger people. For most people with cancer, you hit it as hard as you can and try to get rid of it. But for me, it's ongoing." Jeff lives in New York City and is being treated at the Kaplan Cancer Center at NYU Medical Center. He is the president of the nonprofit Cancer Support Services, an organization that helps him and others cope with cancer and offers exercise programs for cancer patients in New York City.

When **Mark Biundo** was diagnosed with sarcoma in 1993 at the age of twenty-nine, his doctor bluntly told him that he might have to lose his leg in order to keep his life. He was treated at Memorial Sloan-Kettering Cancer Center with surgery and a form of radiation called brachytherapy, in which the radioactive substance is sealed in a container and placed on the surface of the body near the tumor. Fortunately, he has both his life and his leg today. A customer-service representative for Bell Atlantic, Mark lives in Glen Head, New York. He sails, rides horses, and gardens.

At age eighteen, **Katie Brant** was diagnosed with a malignant brain tumor. In June and July of 1989, she underwent surgeries to remove the tumor. She then had cranial radiation for six weeks and thirteen months of aggressive chemotherapy. In October 1995 and May 1996 she had relapses and was operated on again, for a total of four brain surgeries. The last was followed by two stem cell transplants. While undergoing radiation and chemotherapy, Katie attended the University of Pennsylvania as a General Honors student. She graduated cum laude with her class. Now twenty-seven, Katie is the Cause-Related Marketing Specialist for Time Inc. in New York City, creating marketing partnerships between Time Inc.'s magazines and nonprofit organizations.

New York–based journalist **Richard Brookhiser** was thirty-seven years old in 1992, when he first noticed the pain in his stomach that turned out to be testicular cancer. Born with only one testicle, Richard developed a tumor in the speck of testicle that never matured. Doctors removed a grapefruit-sized malignancy, leaving his healthy testicle intact. At New York University Medical Center, he underwent four months of chemotherapy, one five-day session each month. Richard is a columnist for *The New York Observer* and a senior editor of *National Review* magazine. His books include *Rules of Civility, Founding Father: Rediscovering George Washington,* and *The Way of the WASP.* In the summer, he and his wife like to travel "to exotic places where you can't drink the water."

In 1990, when she was fifty-eight years old, **Kay Chenoweth** was diagnosed with pancreatic cancer. Treated in Lafayette, Louisiana, she began by having the Whipple procedure—extensive surgery to remove half of the pancreas, half of the stomach, some of the small intestine, and the gallbladder. She followed up with six weeks of five-day-a-week radiation and a year of chemotherapy, once every three weeks. Kay enjoys reading, especially the fiction of Madeleine L'Engle. An avid traveler, she has visited China, Egypt, and the Galápagos Islands and has led antiquing trips to England.

A securities trader and investment adviser who lives with his wife in New Canaan, Connecticut, **Maurice Chesney** was diagnosed with lung cancer in 1991 at the age of forty-six. Maurice was treated at New York Hospital and Memorial Sloan-Kettering for about eight months with both chemotherapy and a pneumonectomy. After first being told that his cancer was incurable, he believes the second opinion he received saved his life. A father of four, Maurice spends time volunteering, playing tennis and golf, and reading.

After helping her sister battle Hodgkin's disease as a teenager, **Jeanne Clair** was diagnosed with non-Hodgkin's lymphoma in 1991 at the age of thirty-five. She was treated with chemotherapy, radiation, and a bone marrow transplant at Memorial Sloan-Kettering in 1992. Jeanne's first career was in real estate, but in 1996, she received her master's in social work and currently works with children in New York City's East Harlem. She likes to read memoirs and nonfiction and is an active runner, swimmer, skater, and scuba diver.

Lower back and intestinal pain and trouble digesting food were the first manifestations of **George Clark**'s testicular cancer. "The doctors first thought I had some kind of digestive tract problem," he says. That was in 1987, when George was twenty-nine years old. After surgery to remove the testicle and three months of chemotherapy, the cancer returned. George had another operation to remove abdominal tumors and more chemotherapy. He relapsed again, had part of his lung removed, and received another round of chemo, followed by a week at the Livingston Foundation Medical Center in San Diego. A computer consultant, George enjoys skiing, mountain biking, and sailing his thirty-six-foot sloop, *Miss Conduct,* in San Francisco Bay. He has been cancer-free since 1989.

Jim Clement was thirty years old and working as an insurance sales agent in Greenville, North Carolina, in 1989, when he was diagnosed with testicular cancer. He had an orchiectomy to remove his right testicle and an aortic lymph node dissection, which rid him of cancer and its threat. Today, Jim, who golfs, hunts game birds, and fishes the nearby Pamlico River, runs his own company, Fickling and Clement Insurance. His daughter, Louise Mann, who is three years old, is his favorite achievement since he beat cancer.

An Olympic marathoner in 1988, **Mark Conover** was thirty-three years old when he was diagnosed with Hodgkin's disease in 1994. He received chemotherapy every two weeks for six months in San Luis Obispo, California, and went on to compete in the 1996 Olympic marathon trials. A magazine editor and freelance writer whose articles appear in a variety of running publications, Mark also coaches runners. In addition to running, Mark enjoys fishing and water sports.

Born in 1939, **Estelle Cooper** worked as a health care administrator in New York City. After being diagnosed with lung cancer, she underwent surgery, radiation, and chemotherapy. Although the treatment was successful, Estelle died of causes unrelated to her cancer before the publication of this book. A dedicated volunteer at Memorial Sloan-Kettering, she often helped set up a welcoming tea service for patients and their families on Sunday afternoons.

Scott Cox, who lives in Earlysville, Virginia, was twenty-one when he was diagnosed with colon cancer in 1990. He had surgery to remove a golf ball–sized tumor, and then doctors determined that two out of twenty-seven neighboring lymph nodes were malignant, which led to a year of once-a-week chemotherapy. A police officer in the Albemarle County area, Scott remains friends with his oncologist, who lives down the road. Scott likes to hunt and fish and says his finest achievement since beating cancer was marrying his wife, Amy. "We were dating at the time of my illness, and she really helped me," he says. "She stood by my side."

Kathleen Crowley was twenty-three years old in 1985 when she was diagnosed with acute lymphoblastic leukemia. She was treated at Clara Maass Medical Center in New Jersey and Memorial Sloan-Kettering, where she received chemotherapy, total body radiation, and an allogeneic bone marrow transplant (one in which the healthy marrow comes from a family member other than an identical twin or from an unrelated donor). Kathleen has eight brothers and sisters, but only her sister Mary Pat was a perfect match as a donor. Every May, Kathleen sends Mary Pat a Mother's Day card to thank her for giving her a second shot at life. A traveler and dancer of everything from the Irish jig to salsa, Kathleen celebrated the tenth anniversary of her bone marrow transplant in the sky—in a hot-air balloon. She is currently a social worker at several northern New Jersey hospitals where she counsels people with cancer, especially those who need bone marrow transplants.

Tony Dalo was born in Queens, New York, and raised on Long Island. He was forty-six years old when he was diagnosed with cancer of the larynx. He was treated with surgery at Memorial Sloan-Kettering Cancer Center in New York in 1990. Tony was a social worker for a time and is currently a cabinetmaker. He is married, and his full-time hobby is his seventeen-month-old daughter.

A violinist and music teacher in Greenville, North Carolina, **Candace "Mamie" Dixon** was thirty-six in 1989 when she learned she had Hodgkin's disease. She began her treatment with twelve months of chemotherapy. After doctors discovered polyps in her abdomen, she underwent exploratory surgery, followed by three months of radiation therapy. Mamie enjoys "gigging," working out, gardening, and skiing, primarily at Snowshoe Mountain in West Virginia. Her favorite achievement since she beat cancer is her "wonderful" new attitude. "It's infectious, and as a teacher, I feel I can infect my students in a positive way."

June Dressler was twenty-eight when she was diagnosed with carcinoma of the uterus in 1977. Treated at Jackson Memorial Hospital in Miami, she underwent a radical hysterectomy and the removal of fifty lymph nodes. June lives in Hollywood, Florida, where she is a counselor for deaf students and teaches sex education in the Dade County public schools.

Abby Drucker, who works in institutional sales on Wall Street, helped her mother in her battle against cancer of the uterus, including two and a half months of radiation at Memorial Sloan-Kettering in 1993. Abby, now twenty-eight years old, spends her free time combing flea markets in upstate New York for good deals on antiques, especially Art Nouveau pieces, and attending Off-Broadway plays. She volunteers at Gilda's Club. A former Brooklyn schoolteacher, her mother now owns an antiques business.

"I was fifteen when I found a lump on my leg that ended up being a soft-tissue sarcoma," says **Frederick Duckworth, Jr.,** who is now thirty-eight and a gastroenterologist in Richmond, Virginia. "I had initial surgery, which is basically just an incisional biopsy, and I had my leg amputated a few months later. After that, I took chemotherapy for two years." Frederick is married and has two children. He enjoys golf, fishing, and other outdoor activities.

An intellectual-property attorney in New York City, **Jerry Dunne** was forty years old when he was diagnosed with non-Hodgkin's lymphoma in its early stages. "I felt a lump in my groin area, and my girlfriend said, 'Go check it out,' " says Jerry. "The doctor said I had a hernia, so I had hernia surgery. During the surgery they found that the lymph node was enlarged. They clipped it out, and it was cancerous. So because of that hernia, the lymphoma was discovered very early." Jerry had surgery to remove two affected lymph nodes, then eight weeks of radiation treatment at Mount Sinai Medical Center during the summer of 1989. Since his bout with lymphoma, he has taken up sailing and brewing beer.

Diagnosed with throat cancer in 1987 at age sixty-one, **Betty Marx Dwin** was treated with surgery at Mount Sinai Hospital in New York, where she also underwent rehabilitation, learning how to use her speaking apparatus. Betty lives in New York City and is president of Betty Marx, a company that manufactures laryngectomy neckwear. She speaks to young people on the hazards of smoking.

Born in New Brunswick, Canada, **Laura Eastman** has spent most of her life in New York City. In 1986, at the age of fifty-nine, she was diagnosed with cancer of the oropharynx, the part of the pharynx that extends from the base of the tongue to the back of the throat. She was treated with surgery and six weeks of radiation therapy at Memorial Sloan-Kettering. A devout Episcopalian, Laura collects rare books, rides horses, and attends the opera and symphony.

Kathleen Eldrid may be the only adult in the country who has lived more than four years with a primitive neuroectodermal tumor, an extremely rare bone/soft-tissue cancer that normally affects children. In 1992, she had surgery to remove the malignancy on her back at Maine Medical Center in Portland and followed up with holistic treatments. An advocate for alternative medicine and its inclusion in health insurance coverage, she conducts workshops for adults and high school students. In 1995, she spoke at the Center for Advancement in Cancer Education's annual conference. Today, she continues the battle against her cancer, taking herbal treatments and enjoying time with her two daughters and new grandchild.

An operations employee at a New York financial-services firm, **Susan Fischer** was diagnosed with breast cancer in 1988, when she was forty-one years old. She underwent surgery and six weeks of radiation at Memorial Sloan-Kettering, where she later became a volunteer. That led to a new career and her current position as a vice president at Health Care Chaplaincy, an ecumenical organization that trains and provides clergy to work with hospital patients.

At the age of twenty-seven, **Michele Fox,** of Lorton, Virginia, was diagnosed with acute monocytic leukemia and began treatment at Alexandria Hospital and Georgetown University Hospital. A physical therapist assistant, Michele enjoys exercising, especially hiking, and playing with her yellow Lab, Murphy.

In 1984, when **Jacqueline Frank** was thirty, she was diagnosed with Hodgkin's disease. Her treatment at New York University Hospital lasted ten months and included a surgical procedure called a laparotomy (in which her spleen was removed and other organs biopsied), eight months of chemotherapy, and six weeks of radiation therapy. A film producer, Jacqueline's interests include theater, opera, skiing, horseback riding, and triathlons—swimming a half mile, running four, and biking eighteen. She grew up in New Jersey and currently lives in New York City.

President of Graphography, Inc., a direct-mail company, **Jerry Freundlich** was forty-seven when doctors told him he had non-Hodgkin's lymphoma. Beginning in 1991, he underwent eight months of chemotherapy and radiation therapy at Memorial Sloan-Kettering in New York. Born in the Bronx, he currently lives in Manhattan with his wife and two children. His interests include golf, running, and listening to jazz and classical music. In

1993, Jerry and his wife started the Cure for Lymphoma Foundation, which raises money for cancer research.

A former career pilot, **Bill Goss** has flown navy planes, built underground and underwater mines, been hit by a car and by cancer, and still he keeps plugging away. In 1993 at the age of thirty-eight, Bill was diagnosed with melanoma of the ear. Doctors removed the malignancy during a twelve-hour operation at the Navy Hospital in Jacksonville, Florida. Since then, Bill has taken several alternative treatments, including a daily shot glass of a Canadian Indian herbal tea called essiac; an odorless capsule (or one-half clove) of garlic; and one hundred milligrams of DHEA, an adrenal hormone. Over a period of eighteen months, he had a series of reconstructive surgeries to rebuild his ear. Happily married and the father of twin eight-year-olds, Bill teaches self-defense to battered women, boxes, and wrestles. He lives in Orange Park, Florida.

A New York fashion model, **Ivy! Gunter** was in her twenties when she was diagnosed with bone cancer in 1980. After her right leg was amputated above the knee, Ivy! underwent a year of chemotherapy at Memorial Sloan-Kettering and Piedmont Hospital in Atlanta, losing her hair in the process. Rather than give up as a model, she used her differences to her advantage by creating an image of bald purity. The author of *On the Ragged Edge . . . of Drop Dead Gorgeous,* Ivy! has appeared on many television shows, including *Heroes: Made in the USA.* She is an aerobics instructor, has her own exercise video for pediatric amputees, and has won several medals in the Disabled Sports USA competitions. In 1996, she helped kick off the Summer Olympics in Atlanta as an official torchbearer.

Attorney **John Hall** was diagnosed with Hodgkin's disease in 1986 at the age of forty-nine. "Actually, it was a split decision," he says. "It's a little unusual for someone in their forties to have Hodgkin's disease. My pathologist, who thought it was non-Hodgkin's lymphoma, sent samples to the National Institutes of

Health. They said it was Hodgkin's." Treated at Baylor Hospital in Dallas, John had his enlarged spleen and a few lymph nodes removed and underwent six months of chemotherapy. John swims, plays tennis, and enjoys pursuing good food and wine.

A former family therapist and public health administrator, **Enid Handler,** who now lives in Chapel Hill, North Carolina, used her experience in working with nonprofit organizations and in the health field to help her son Evan battle leukemia. When asked how she came up with so many creative and dynamic ways to solve the logistical problems she faced, Enid replied, "I think some of this comes from my background, and the rest of it is what you pull up from inside yourself."

Evan Handler was twenty-four years old and working on Broadway when he was diagnosed in 1985 with acute myelogenous leukemia (AML), a disease in which abnormal, immature white blood cells produced in the bone marrow accumulate in the bloodstream and marrow. Over the course of six months, Evan had three rounds of conventional chemotherapy. After a two-year remission, he had a recurrence of the leukemia and was treated again at Memorial Sloan-Kettering. He had an autologous bone marrow transplant at Johns Hopkins Hospital in Baltimore and has been cancer-free ever since. Evan has played leading roles in seven Broadway shows, including *Brighton Beach Memoirs, Broadway Bound, I Hate Hamlet,* and *Six Degrees of Separation,* and has appeared in the films *Ransom, Taps, Sweet Lorraine,* and *Natural Born Killers.* His much-praised one-man performance and book *Time on Fire: My Comedy of Terrors* (Little Brown, 1996; Henry Holt, 1997) deals with his illness.

In 1989, **Tali Havazelet,** then thirty years old, was diagnosed with ovarian cancer. Treated at Mount Sinai Medical Center in New York, she underwent a radical hysterectomy and ten months of chemotherapy. Tali has cut her seven-day work week at a New York City law firm down to a more manageable three. She records readings for the blind and dyslexic and volunteers in the kitchen at God's Love We Deliver, which feeds homebound people with AIDS. She also makes ceramics and weaves.

A former high school English teacher and mother of one, **Ginnie Higginbotham** of Florence, Alabama, discovered she had ovarian cancer in 1993 at the age of fifty-three. She had a hysterectomy in Birmingham at Baptist-Montclaire Hospital and eight months of chemotherapy at Northwest Alabama Cancer Center as prescribed by M.D. Anderson Cancer Center in Houston. An amateur actor, Ginnie courageously opened in *Love Letters* on the night of her second chemotherapy treatment. For eleven years she served as director of the American Heart Association's Northwest Alabama Region.

A former high school state champion runner from Mobile, Alabama, **Lisa Eubanks Hollingsworth** developed leukemia in 1983, when she was a nineteen-year-old student at Louisiana State University. She underwent three weeks of radiation therapy and a rigorous chemotherapy regimen—one session per week for two years—that she compares to the grueling two-mile race, once her forte. "The worst part of the two-mile race is the end, because you're hurting so bad," she says. "The closer I got to the end of the two-year treatment, the more I wanted to quit." In 1985, doctors deemed her cancer-free. Lisa lives with her husband and two children in Mobile, where she works as an information specialist for a group of cardiothoracic and vascular surgeons. As a member of the Coalition for a Tobacco-Free Mobile, she speaks to schoolchildren about the dangers of smoking. Lisa is also a volunteer for the American Cancer Society's speakers bureau.

Living in Pikeville, Kentucky, **Danny Johnson** was twenty-one years old in 1972 when he was diagnosed with synovial sarcoma, a cancer of the soft tissue around his knee. The tumor was discovered while he was undergoing knee surgery after a basketball injury. He was treated at St. Jude's Children's Hospital in Memphis because the disease occurs most frequently in children. Johnson, who has a master's degree in education and guidance counseling, is a guidance counselor, basketball coach, and radio sports announcer. Despite his leg amputation, he is currently planning to walk the Appalachian Trail from Georgia to Maine.

A club kid living on the edge of dawn, **Leslie Kaul** was twenty-one when she was diagnosed with Hodgkin's disease in 1981. She was treated with radiation, had a recurrence in 1984, and was treated with chemotherapy, both times at Memorial Sloan-Kettering. Later, she decided on a career in cooking. She apprenticed at a variety of New York's top restaurants, including Union Square Cafe, Lespinasse, and Gramercy Tavern, and is now a chef working for a company called Daily Soup. Her favorite achievement since being cured is quitting drinking. Her sister, Rachel, is also a contributor to *Cancer Combat*.

Rachel Kaul was diagnosed with cervical cancer in 1995 at the age of twenty-eight and twice underwent surgical conization, a procedure in which a portion of the cervix is removed. Rachel, who lives in Ann Arbor, Michigan, is a social worker in the health-care field. She enjoys skiing, reading contemporary American fiction, and watching independent and foreign films. She volunteers at the Gilda's Club chapter in Royal Oak, Michigan. Her sister, Leslie, is also a contributor to *Cancer Combat*.

In 1990 at the age of twenty-seven, **Dean King,** a free-lance writer and editor, was diagnosed with Hodgkin's disease. He was treated at Mount Sinai Medical Center with chemotherapy by Dr. Samuel Waxman, who later suggested he create this book, and with radiation at Cabrini Medical Center. His wife, **Jessica King,** also a writer and editor, accompanied him to every treatment.

Since beating cancer, they have had three "miracle babies," Hazel, now three, Grace, now two, and Willa, born just before this book went to press. The Kings recently moved to Dean's hometown, Richmond, Virginia, after ten years in New York City. Both Dean and Jessica are graduates of the University of North Carolina at Chapel Hill. They have served on the associate board of the Samuel Waxman Cancer Research Foundation since

1991. Their hobby is cross-country walking; together they have trekked the Na Pali coast in Hawaii, the Pilgrim's Way in England, and the Tour de Mont Blanc in Europe.

Dean is also the author of *A Sea of Words* and *Harbors and High Seas,* companion books to Patrick O'Brian's Aubrey-Maturin novels. He is the editor of the book series Heart of Oak Sea Classics, published by Henry Holt. In her infrequent spare time, Jessica, who attended the Ecole des Beaux-Arts in Paris, is a painter.

In 1991 at age twenty-five, **Monica Ko** was diagnosed with non-Hodgkin's lymphoma. She was treated at Sloan-Kettering for over a year with chemotherapy, radiation, and a bone marrow transplant. Born and raised in New York City's Chinatown, where she still lives, Monica works as an employment specialist. Her interests are sports, the outdoors, travel, and the theater. She volunteers at Sloan-Kettering, where she counsels patients going through bone marrow transplants.

In 1981, **Joe Kogel** was twenty-five and living in Ashland, Oregon, when a mole on his left shoulder was diagnosed as metastatic melanoma. Treated at the Rogue Valley Medical Center in Medford, Oregon, and later at Memorial Sloan-Kettering, he had surgery to remove the tumor and an axillary dissection, the removal of his left armpit's lymph nodes. He followed up with a macrobiotic diet. Later that year, he relapsed and had the new cancer removed. He has been in remission since 1982 and now lives in Providence, Rhode Island, where he is a storyteller and writer of autobiographical articles.

At age thirty-three, **John Kruk** was diagnosed with testicular cancer. He had a testicle removed and received radiation therapy. "I guess it had a good side," says John, an all-star first baseman for the Philadelphia Phillies at the time. "I think a lot of men who have a lump are afraid to have it checked. But doctors have said that since I went public with this type of cancer, more men in Philadelphia are getting treated." After a nine-and-a-half-year career in major league baseball, John now runs a two-hundred-and-fifty-acre farm in Keyser, West Virginia, with his wife, Jamie. When he's not mowing grass and baling hay, John likes to play golf.

In 1985, when **Susan Laggner** was thirty years old and pregnant with her fourth child, she became extremely sick. After the birth, doctors discovered the cause—medulloblastoma, a rare brain tumor usually found in infants. Surgery to remove the tumor was followed by three months of radiation therapy. Now living with her family in Williamstown, Vermont, Susan works as a receptionist in an orthodontist's office. She likes to walk, ski, read to her children, and sew quilts.

Married and strongly desiring motherhood, **Madeleine LaPorte** was told she had ovarian cancer when she was twenty-eight years old. Despite doctors' recommendations to remove both ovaries—even though only one was affected—she insisted on keeping one in order to have children. In 1974, she had her right ovary removed at Sacré Coeur Hospital in Montreal, Canada. A few years later, she gave birth to a son. Eighteen months later, she had a girl. Still cancer-free, Madeleine lives in Montreal with her teenage children, Stephane and Genevieve.

In 1991, when she was thirty years old, **Karen Lawrence** was diagnosed with breast cancer. When doctors told her the news, she says she felt as if a truck had hit her, but she quickly began the business of getting cured. She had a lumpectomy and received six months of chemotherapy and six weeks of radiation therapy at Memorial Sloan-Kettering. Karen lives in New York City and works as a sales manager at a wine and spirits company. She plays tennis, paints, and is an actor with the Pulse Ensemble Theatre.

In 1994, **Jodi Levy,** twenty-eight years old, was diagnosed with non-Hodgkin's lymphoma. She moved from Washington, D.C., her home for six years, back to her hometown, Morris Plains, New Jersey, for treatment—six months of chemotherapy, and three weeks of daily radiation therapy. "My family was always very close, but I think this kind of thing pulls you together even more," she says. Now, three years later, her positive attitude has renewed her enthusiasm for biking, camping, traveling, and visiting museums. She also enjoys attending the ballet, theater, and symphony. Currently a medical student in New York, Jodi has considered oncology as a possible specialty and hopes to bring her patients the same kind of extraordinary, compassionate care that she received from her doctors during her illness.

Josh Malen was diagnosed with Hodgkin's disease in 1995 when he was twenty-four years old. He was treated with chemotherapy and radiation at New York Hospital and with monoclonal antibodies at Deaconess Hospital in Boston. In 1996, at St. Agnes Hospital in Westchester County, New York, he had two bone marrow transplants. Before his illness, Josh worked for the International Rescue Committee in the former Yugoslavia. He enjoys playing guitar, following international affairs, and building miniature military models.

A student at the University of Michigan, **Karen Manheimer** was twenty-four when she was diagnosed with non-Hodgkin's lymphoma in 1991. A native New Yorker, she was treated at both the University of Michigan Hospital and Mount Sinai in New York with surgery and chemotherapy. She travels, cooks, collects fossils, and makes quilts.

Elizabeth Martin was forty-six when she discovered she had breast cancer in 1980. She was treated with a mastectomy and six months of chemotherapy. Elizabeth has four children, the youngest of whom was in high school at the time. "He handled my cancer pretty well," she says. "In fact, at one point he offered to get me some marijuana to try. I said, 'Don't you dare.'"

In 1994, a month after having a mammogram that revealed nothing out of the ordinary, **Kristina Matsch** discovered a lump in her right breast that turned out to be malignant. She was thirty-five, married, and working as an administrator in a Delaware secondary school. At New York's Beth Israel Medical Center, she underwent a modified radical mastectomy and had thirty-one lymph nodes removed, ten of which were positive. She then had six months of chemotherapy at the University of Pennsylvania Medical Center in Philadelphia and five weeks of radiation therapy at Paoli Memorial Hospital. In between the chemo and the radiation, she had an autologous bone marrow transplant, and she is currently taking tamoxifen. Kristina and her husband now live in Denver, Colorado. She likes to play tennis and participates in Races for the Cure around the country. Recently she spoke to Presence France—the first French cancer support group, started by her cousin, who lives in Paris—about her experience and maintaining quality of life after cancer. "I'm back to doing everything I've always done," she says.

A stay-at-home mom, **Karla McConnell,** who is currently finishing up a degree in education and plans to teach, was diagnosed in 1995 with acute myelogenous leukemia (AML) and began treatment the same day at Indiana University Medical Center. At the time, she was thirty-two years old, married with three children, ages eight, ten, and eleven. Karla enjoys gardening, singing, church activities, and directing kids' musicals. Her sister, Lou Ann Sabatier, is also a contributor to *Cancer Combat.*

In 1980, when **Melanie McElhinney** was fifteen years old, she was diagnosed with osteogenic sarcoma and had her leg and hip amputated at the Medical College of Virginia in Richmond. Melanie speaks professionally, sometimes for the American Cancer Society. "I think there's a mainstream message here," she says. "We all go through adversity, different types of adversity, but it's universal. How we handle that adversity is what's important."

Melanie recently married and started her own public relations and consulting business in Richmond. She sings (she's sung the national anthem at Richmond Braves baseball games), snow skis with wrist outriggers, and is learning how to water-ski. She was one of President Bush's "thousand points of light."

At age thirty-five, **Tim McLaurin,** a writer and a veteran of the Marine Corps and the Peace Corps, was diagnosed with multiple myeloma (multiple plasma cell tumors), a disease most common in people in their fifties. He received chemotherapy at the University of North Carolina Hospital in Chapel Hill for six months and went into remission. Four months later, he had a bone marrow transplant at the Veterans Hospital in Seattle, Washington. Tim's children, Christopher and Megan, were four and six at the time, and, spurred by his illness, Tim wrote a book for them called *The Keeper of the Moon.* His latest books are *The Last Great Snake Show* and *Lola,* a novel in free verse. Now forty-two years old, Tim teaches at North Carolina State University. His lifetime hobby is keeping snakes and other poisonous reptiles, a topic about which he often speaks professionally.

In 1989, when she was forty-six years old, **Marcia Moosnick,** a native Virginian, was diagnosed with breast cancer. Treated at Mount Sinai Medical Center in New York City, where she now lives, and at New York Medical College in Valhalla, New York, she had a lumpectomy, followed by chemotherapy and radiation. The mother of two daughters, ages twenty-three and twenty-six, Marcia is a special-occasions photographer. She enjoys listening to jazz and classical music, singing in her temple choir, walking, and playing tennis.

Diagnosed with Hodgkin's disease in 1980, when he was forty years old, **Frank Narcisco** underwent chemotherapy and radiation at Memorial Sloan-Kettering, beginning a decade-long battle that involved four relapses. In 1990, after his last recurrence—in his lungs and liver—Frank was told he was too old for a much-needed bone marrow transplant. However, he convinced his doctor to let him be the oldest patient ever to receive the transplant, which not only paved the way for other people over fifty but also put him into sustained remission. President of Dun-Rite Movers, Frank lives in the Bronx, New York, with his wife and children. He is a motorcycle enthusiast.

An all-American and academic all-American football player at Iowa State, **Karl Nelson,** originally from DeKalb, Illinois, was drafted to play in the National Football League by the New York Giants in 1983. He started as an offensive lineman in fifty-five straight games from 1984 through 1986, ending with the Giants' victory at Super Bowl XXI. In 1987, at the age of twenty-seven, Karl was diagnosed with and treated for Hodgkin's disease. He returned to the Giants as a starter in 1988. At the end of 1988, he had a recurrence of Hodgkin's and underwent chemotherapy. He formally retired from the Giants in 1989 and broadcasted games on the radio through 1994. He also wrote a book called *Life on the Line,* which deals with his battle against Hodgkin's disease. He currently lives with his wife and two daughters in Montvale, New Jersey, and works as a 401(k) specialist.

Claire Noonan was twenty-nine years old when she discovered she had breast cancer in 1993. She was treated at Memorial Sloan-Kettering, where she had nearly thirty lymph nodes removed. "I felt very, very lucky, and that was so hard to explain to people," says Claire. "You're thirty years old, you're losing your breast, and you feel lucky? I felt fortunate to be at Memorial with wonderful doctors and a great staff." She started reconstruction surgery at the time of the mastectomy. She had six months of chemotherapy and three surgeries. Claire has since moved from New Jersey to Pasadena, California, where she works for a retail division of the Walt Disney Company. She has two dogs and enjoys photography, skiing, and scuba diving.

When ovarian cancer struck **Diane Noyes** in 1986 at the age of forty-one, she was working in the northwestern part of the country as an independent beauty-and-fashion sales rep. After her treatment—a hysterectomy and seven months of what she calls "industrial strength" chemotherapy at Seattle's University of Washington Hospital—Diane did not let cancer end her career. Instead, she integrated the two, working on beauty for cancer patients. She wrote a book called *Beauty and Cancer* and founded the nationwide Beauty and Cancer seminars (based on tips from her book). An avid gardener, she lives in Washington State with her husband.

A licensed practical nurse specializing in geriatric care, **Cathy Owen** was diagnosed with a brain tumor when she was twenty-five and the mother of an infant son. She had brain surgery and received radiation treatment in Portsmouth, Virginia. Now thirty-six and with a clean bill of health, Cathy lives in Chesapeake, Virginia, with her husband, Ross, and sons Cameron (twelve) and Tyler (eight).

In 1985, at age twenty-five, **Jonathan Pearlroth,** a native New Yorker, was diagnosed with non-Hodgkin's lymphoma while he was attending law school at the University of Virginia. He was treated with several major surgeries and chemotherapy. A relapse resulted in total body radiation, more chemo, and a bone marrow transplant. After his treatment, he left a job on Wall Street to spend a year on the beaches of Rio de Janeiro to write about his cancer experience. Currently, Jonathan is practicing at an international law firm and volunteering with people who have cancer at Memorial Sloan-Kettering and Gilda's Club in New York. Looking back on his cancer experience, he believes his life philosophy can be summed up in four words: "If not now, when?"

A mechanical engineer for a manufacturer of spacecraft and space science instruments in Boulder, Colorado, **Damon Phinney** was diagnosed with metastatic prostate cancer in 1989, at age fifty-nine. He worked full-time for six years while battling cancer and then retired but continues part-time as a consultant. Early on he used strenuous bike riding to help offset the side effects of his cancer treatment, and in 1996 he completed his goal of riding forty thousand miles within ten years of diagnosis. The father of Olympic cycling medalist and professional cyclist Davis Phinney, Damon himself has been pedaling since 1952. He especially enjoys biking in the Alps and the Rockies.

Having grown up in China and the United States and risen to the position of assistant secretary of commerce in the Carter administration, **Elsa Porter** saw breast cancer as just another challenge. Diagnosed in 1974 at the age of forty-five, she had two modified radical mastectomies, which cured her. Refusing to let the cancer slow her down, Elsa continues to work, hike, and swim. She lives with her husband in Oregon, where she also likes to garden, read, and watch birds. She is the proud mother of five children and grandmother of eight.

In 1986, at age twenty-two, Canadian **David Rakoff** was working in Tokyo as a translator for a publishing company, when he noticed a lump in his neck. After Japanese doctors told him the lump might be malignant, he returned to Canada, where he was diagnosed with stage-one Hodgkin's lymphoma. Treated at the Princess Margaret Hospital in Toronto, David received three months of radiation therapy. The cancer later resurfaced, spread, and progressed to stage three. He then underwent nine months of chemotherapy, which cured him. Now thirty-two, David lives in New York, where he is the Communications Manager at Harper-Collins Publishers. In his spare time, he writes fiction, paints, and acts in Off-Off-Broadway plays.

Genya Zelkowitz Ravan was born in Poland and grew up on Manhattan's Lower East Side. In 1992 she was diagnosed with non-small-cell lung cancer and was treated for four months at Sloan-Kettering. She is now fifty-six and is an artist and a singer currently living on the Upper West Side in New York City. Her résumé includes recordings with major record companies, live performances at Carnegie Hall, the Atlanta and Miami Pop

Festivals, and Madison Square Garden, as well as appearances on the Johnny Carson, Mike Douglas, and Dick Cavett shows.

In 1985, when she was thirty-one years old, **Blythe Ritchfield** was diagnosed with squamous cell cancer of the sphincter muscle. Over a three-month period, she was treated with radiation therapy and chemotherapy at UCLA. Raised in California, Blythe currently lives in Santa Fe, New Mexico, where she is the executive director of the Life Center for Youth and Adults, which provides programs for at-risk youth and counseling for anyone battling chronic or catastrophic illness. A nature buff, Blythe also enjoys creative writing and conceptual sculpting.

Lou Ann Sabatier's husband Mike was thirty-six years old when he was diagnosed with throat cancer in 1993. Her sister, Karla McConnell, who is also a contributor to *Cancer Combat,* was thirty-two when she was diagnosed with leukemia in 1995. Lou Ann helped them both, one from nearby, the other from afar, weather the storm. A magazine consultant, Lou Ann lives in Falls Church, Virginia, and has one child, Grant, who is twelve. She enjoys sports, music, and antiquing.

In 1980, at age forty-one, **Ruth St. John** discovered that a large mole on her shoulder blade was melanoma. She had it removed surgically at St. Joseph's Hospital in Atlanta. "They told me that I might never be able to play tennis again," Ruth says. "I worked and worked just to be able to hit the ball. After a year, when I was finally able to raise my arm high enough to serve correctly, I felt I had beaten it." Ruth lives in Atlanta with her husband, Richard. They have two grown children and a grandchild. She owns a small antiques shop, and swims, golfs, and paints.

In 1995, **Brian Schmidt,** a thirty-nine-year-old CPA living in Shoreview, Minnesota, was diagnosed with multiple myeloma. He has received treatments at the University of Arkansas–Little Rock, the Mayo Clinic, and the Sarasota Medical Hospital in

Florida. A bone marrow transplant in 1996 put Brian into remission, but because myeloma tends to return, he is currently in an experimental vaccine program conducted through the University of Arkansas–Little Rock and the National Institutes of Health.

A financial headhunter, **Peggy Schmidt,** Brian's wife, says, "We have focused on the positive. When I look forward or backward, I get scared. But if I live in the present, I'm in great shape. Brian is a very optimistic, inspirational individual, and I think to a large extent that's why he's doing as well as he is today." Peggy and Brian have two sons, ages six and nine. They enjoy water sports, skiing, bike rides, and church.

A former Roman Catholic monk and a high school teacher and administrator in New York, **Frank Sheridan** was fifty-five years old when he was diagnosed with non-Hodgkin's lymphoma in 1992. He began treatment at Columbia-Presbyterian Medical Center that year and completed two regimens of chemotherapy in ten months. At night he also worked as a hospital social worker. Known as Francis X. Sheridan to the Marist Brothers of the Schools, his former order, Frank says: "Having cancer was a very spiritual experience. I felt I was ready for the challenge, for the big questions about death and the afterlife." Since going into remission, Frank has walked the New York Marathon three times.

Kevin Shulman was twenty-four and living in New Jersey when he was diagnosed with testicular cancer. Treated at New York Hospital and Memorial Sloan-Kettering for six months starting in 1980, he had an orchiectomy—the removal of a testicle (on the way to surgery, he pinned a note to his gown that read "Remember! It's the right one")—bilateral lymph node dissection, and chemotherapy. A sales trainer who bikes and plays tennis, Kevin lives in Marlboro, New Jersey, where he and his wife volunteer occasionally as short-term foster parents for children waiting to be reunited with their parents.

In 1971, when she was forty-one years old, **Rhoda Silverman** of Queens, New York, was diagnosed with breast cancer. She was treated at Sloan-Kettering, where she underwent a modified radical mastectomy. A mother of three children and grandmother of seven, Rhoda is a former office manager. She volunteers as a patient and family liaison at Mercy Hospital on Long Island.

A thirty-eight-year-old free-lance bookkeeper and triathlete, **Charlene Sloane** was diagnosed with breast cancer in 1991. She had a radical mastectomy and reconstructive surgery at New York University Hospital. Three years later, the cancer returned in her other breast. "It was more aggressive this time," she says. "The treatment was another radical mastectomy and six months of chemotherapy. After each chemo session, I gave myself about five days off, and then I'd be back in the water swimming. I did two one-hundred-mile bicycle rides while on chemo. The athletics really kept me going." A resident of Long Island and the mother of a twenty-two-year-old son, Charlene enjoys yoga, quilting, knitting, running, biking, and weight training.

In 1987, at age twenty-four, **Sheri Sobrato** was diagnosed as having a rare brain tumor called choroid plexus carcinoma. At the time, she was working in New York as a financial analyst. She returned to her hometown, Atherton, California, for treatment—surgery to remove the tumor, six weeks of daily radiation, a short regimen of chemotherapy administered to her central nervous system through a head shunt, and fourteen months of systemic chemotherapy. Today, Sheri, who lives in Atherton, is training to be a psychotherapist for at-risk youths and families facing illness. She volunteers at the Packard Children's Hospital at Stanford and the National Brain Tumor Foundation in San Francisco, and she is helping establish a support network for young adults with cancer for the San Jose American Cancer Society. An avid traveler and adventure-sports enthusiast, Sheri has explored parts of Africa and Scandinavia, trekked in Nepal, and completed a NOLS (National Outdoor Leadership School) course in Wyoming since going into remission. She has also taken up windsurfing, mountain biking, rollerblading, yoga, and backpacking.

Elsie Stone was diagnosed with non-Hodgkin's follicular nodular lymphoma in 1985 at the age of forty. She was treated with surgery, three months of radiation therapy, and seven months of chemotherapy at Porter Hospital in Denver, Colorado. After an additional two weeks of chemo, she had a bone marrow transplant, and then a peripheral stem-cell transplant. Throughout the ordeal, Elsie relied on her faith in God and on her husband Bill's medical research. Together, they made an unbeatable team. Elsie and Bill live in Aurora, Colorado. She is also grateful for the support of her children, her church community, and other friends.

In 1991, at age thirty, **Bill Thomas** was diagnosed with Hodgkin's disease in the neck and chest. "I was in the shower one day, soaping up, and I noticed a soft lump on my throat. I just monitored it for the next few weeks," he says. "It got bigger and harder, so I went to see my internist. He thought it was nothing to worry about. I saw a couple of ear, nose, and throat guys, and they told me all sorts of strange stories—one thought one of my ribs had pushed up a fatty deposit." Bill was treated with radiation at Stanford University. Bill lives in California and plays tennis, hikes, and swims.

Janice Thomas, an Oklahoman who now lives in Midland, Texas, learned she had acute lymphatic leukemia in 1993. Forty-one years old, she was told she would live only two weeks if she did not pursue treatment. A doctor at M.D. Anderson in Houston prescribed a new six-month chemotherapy protocol, which included sixteen treatments through a four-inch shunt in her head. Zofran, the antinausea drug, was the "miracle," as Janice calls it, because it accelerates treatment from a two-year to a six-month period by reducing nausea and, thus, raising the patient's tolerance. She followed up this treatment with six months of rehabilitation for nerve damage in her leg. Today, she bikes, reads fiction, listens to classical music, and volunteers at a YMCA, a hospice, and the American Cancer Society. She is the mother of two children, ages six and nine.

A senior at Virginia Commonwealth University, **Dale Totty** was twenty-one when he was diagnosed with fibrous histiocytoma of the shoulder in 1981. His right arm, shoulder, and collarbone were amputated during an eight-hour operation by surgeons at the Medical College of Virginia in Richmond. That was followed by radiation therapy for about six months. Originally right-handed, Dale had to start over again with his left hand. Now thirty-eight, Dale is a father of two, a professional real estate appraiser, and an award-winning wildlife artist. He hunts and fishes.

A comedian, ex-housewife, mother, and husband-calling-contest winner, **Clara Trusty** remained strong and funny throughout her cancer experience, using humor to get through the rough times. Diagnosed with acute leukemia in 1991 at the age of fifty-three, she underwent eleven months of chemotherapy at Community East Hospital in Indianapolis, Indiana. Now healthy, Clara lives in Fountaintown, Indiana, where she continues to perform stand-up comedy at conventions and banquets. She also likes to garden and weave baskets. She is married, and has four children and five grandchildren.

Judy Weiner was a fifty-three-year-old high school principal in Miami, Florida, when she was diagnosed with acute myelogenous leukemia in 1993. Facing two years of chemotherapy, she requested a less demanding position at the school. Once her treatments were completed, Judy, who is married and has three children and two grandchildren, retired early to pursue her interests in art, reading, volunteering, and traveling.

When diagnosed with cancer in one breast at the age of thirty-four, **Charlotte Wells** opted for a double mastectomy because her family had a history of breast cancer and she had two young children. "Being able to see my children at the end of the day helped get me through it," she says. "Having to get up to do something with them kept me positive throughout the treatment. People offered to take them, but I really wanted them home and needed them home, emotionally and physically." She also underwent six weeks of chemotherapy.

Sue Winard is a doctor who lives in Rego Park, New York. Her mother was diagnosed with ovarian cancer in 1995 and was treated with surgery and chemotherapy. Now seventy-eight and a great-grandmother, her mother volunteers at New Rochelle Hospital in New York.

In 1988, following a trip to Spain, **Bev Yaffe,** at age fifty-one, was diagnosed with islet cell carcinoma, a rare form of pancreatic cancer. It later spread to her liver. After surgery at Long Island Jewish Medical Center, she was treated with chemotherapy in New York City. A housewife and hospital volunteer, she enjoys life, golf, travel, reading, biking, walking, and spending time with her husband, three sons, two daughters-in-law, two granddaughters, and dear friends.

The assistant principal violinist of the Metropolitan Opera Orchestra in New York City, **Toni Rapport Zavistovski** was thirty-nine when she was diagnosed with breast cancer in 1981. She had a lumpectomy and eight weeks of radiation therapy. Four years later, she had a recurrence, which led to a mastectomy, the removal of seven lymph nodes (five of which were malignant), and thirteen months of aggressive chemotherapy. Toni says, "Music-making is a reflection of what one's soul is all about, and because I was profoundly affected by having cancer, it had an effect on my music. If one's own experiences are more profound, I think the expression becomes more profound." Toni is the mother of three daughters and a son.

PART ONE

The First Few Days

CHAPTER ONE

Dealing with Discovery

No matter how long the symptoms have been going on, no matter how painful they have been, no matter how well prepared you are for the probability of having cancer, it is simply overwhelming to find out that you have what has long been perceived to be a terminal diagnosis. In some form or other, denial is a phase most people go through following diagnosis. But accepting that you have cancer is one of the steps you must take to defeat it.

Anger is also natural. "Why me? Why did it take so long to diagnose? Why was I misdiagnosed three times?" These are common frustrations. What follows in this chapter are some of our stories about discovering we had cancer. You'll probably see that you suffered from similar pains and anxiety in the prediscovery stages. Yes, there was some questionable sleuth work on the part of some of our doctors. That comes with the territory, especially when you are young. Nobody expects you to have cancer.

These are our war stories to help you put your own discovery in perspective, and we hope you'll find some effective approaches for dealing with your own diagnosis. You're not the only one whose doctor took too long to figure out the problem. And, although it might seem like it, you probably weren't selected by some evil god to endure unjustified punishment. Above all, you're not alone. Putting the recent past into context is one of the first steps on the road to recovery.

MY GYNECOLOGIST CALLED me at the school where I taught. "You have cancer," he said. "I would like to see you in my office as soon as possible." I remember dropping the phone and standing in the school office unable to move. A secretary took the phone and talked to the doctor as someone ushered me into the principal's office. I was twenty-seven years old and thought the word "cancer" was synonymous with death. I was angry that my doctor chose to tell me over the phone. And to call me at work and blurt out those dreadful words while I stood in a public place with office staff and strangers all around, no less.

Luckily, someone called my brother, and he picked me up from school since I was too distraught to drive. The ride to the doctor's office was long and scary. We didn't talk, but I was comforted by his presence. Having my brother with me was the best antidote to the most difficult moment of my life.

—*June Dressler*

I HAD JUST moved to New York. I was twenty-one and wild in the streets. I lived with people who were in bands, and we thought we were pretty fabulous. I worked as a waitress in a crappy restaurant. Life started at two in the afternoon and ended at six in the morning. One day I was dressing for work, and I noticed one shoulder was higher than the other. It looked two inches higher. It was very strange. But there was no pain, so I ignored it. About a month later somebody finally convinced me I should get it looked at. So I went to some clinic and was told I had bursitis. That seemed strange because my understanding of bursitis was that it takes years to develop, and it's an arthritic condition. So I ignored it for another month, and then I really began to not feel well. I had night sweats, and I felt discomfort in my shoulder. I couldn't raise my arm. Somebody else told me to go to a preventive medicine clinic, and I walked in.

The examining physician said, "Uh, I think a specialist should look at you." I found out later that the specialist was an expert in Hodgkin's disease. He knew exactly what it was. But nobody told me. They just said that maybe they should take a needle biopsy, so they had me lie down in the office and took a biopsy of the area, which was really shocking and frightening and painful. I was completely unprepared for it.

After a week, the doctor told me he thought it was a lymphatic tumor, but that they hadn't gotten enough tissue from the needle biopsy and I needed to have an incision biopsy at the hospital, none of which meant anything to me. I was a dumb kid out on my own in the brave new world. So I showed up like they told me to at "Memorial Hospital"—only it was Memorial Sloan-Kettering Cancer Center. The word "cancer" had not entered my mind until I saw it on the building. I thought, "What is this?"

The surgeon found out that I'd been taking aspirin because of the discomfort and told me he couldn't do the procedure that day because aspirin is an anticoagulant. At this point my parents were aware of the situation, so I said, "What am I supposed to tell my mother?" He said, "I'll call your parents. Give me their number." This was a long-distance phone call, and I got suspicious.

The surgeon asked me, "What did your doctor tell you?" Then he started telling me that ten years ago this diagnosis could have been the kiss of death, but now with chemotherapy . . .

I said, "Chemotherapy? Is it malignant?"

He said, "Huh. Well, it's not the end of the world."

I still didn't hear the words "Hodgkin's disease" at this point. We're talking about a four-month process during which I had been completely in the dark—partly because I had not been aggressive about finding anything out. Finally, on this day I reached the point where I realized what we were talking about. I left the hospital and went home, and as soon as I walked in the door, my parents phoned. They were both crying.

—*Leslie Kaul*

I'D BEEN A runner since high school. My running eventually got me to the Olympics in 1988. I won the Olympic trials marathon that year. After that, I battled injuries, but I was running pretty well again in 1991 and began training for the '92 Olympic marathon trials. But I started to get a lot of colds and flus. My immune system was just not up to snuff. I thought, "I'm over-trained. I'm going through a phase and I have to ride it out." I'd done that earlier in my running career.

I did start to come around before the trials, but I still felt like there was a problem because my energy level wasn't up to par. I ran the race and finished tenth. Considering my health problems, I thought that was pretty respectable, but everything continued to dwindle.

I was running with a doctor friend and wheezing quite a bit, and he said, "I think I know your problem: You have asthma." So I saw an asthma doctor, and he put me on all these different inhalers. But my energy still wasn't there. I couldn't work out hard like I used to. By October of 1993, I started to feel really worn down. I was being inducted into the Hall of Fame at my alma mater, Humboldt State, in northern California, and that weekend I took a turn for the worse. I started to have night sweats and fevers.

I went back to my asthma doctor when I got home, and I said, "There's really something wrong now." He felt around and noticed an enlarged lymph node on my neck and right away sent me to a pulmonary specialist. I had X rays taken of my lungs before I went to see the specialist. They let me take them to the doctor, and I read the X-ray person's report: "Possibility of lymphoma should not be ruled out."

I thought, "Lymphoma? What the heck is that?" I went to the library and researched it. I knew then what it was going to be. The next day I had the biopsy, and the diagnosis of Hodgkin's disease was made.

It's the ultimate humbling experience to hear the doctor tell you that your health has completely failed you. It makes you realize that you are but a speck in the universe and not here for a long time. It makes all the trivial things you've heard about or argued about and the games you've played with yourself and others seem stupid and insignificant. While I was in his office, he left for a while, and I cried. Everything around me started humming, and I went home and sat on the couch for a while and had to regroup and realize, "Here I am."

In a way, it was a relief to find out there was a severe problem. It had taken a year and a half to diagnose. I had noticed the lump in my neck at some point, and I should have questioned it more, but I'm a skinny guy. Things stick out a lot. They had X-rayed my lungs in August of 1993, and nothing had shown up. By October, it was clear that there were tumors there. It had spread from my shoulders down to my pelvis. Now, at least, I knew that the reason I wasn't running well or feeling well wasn't just in my head. When the diagnosis was made, I knew what I was dealing with and could get on with the battle. That's when I really was able to focus on getting well.

—Mark Conover

I HAD A seventeen-month-old baby, and I was run-down. I'd lost about ten pounds, and that should have been a tip-off, but I just thought, "Great, I'm losing weight." I started feeling tired and decided to see a doctor. Everybody led me to believe it was just in my mind and that my baby was the cause of it, the stress of having a baby. They said to just go home. I saw about seven doctors before I finally said, "Maybe I need a chest X ray. I have this cough, a very persistent cough. Maybe I have bronchitis, and you could prescribe some drugs."

The doctor was a good friend. This is a little town, so he was my neighbor. He took an X ray. Everybody was just laughing and having a good old time. Then all of a sudden they got real quiet. The nurses turned as white as a sheet, and I thought, "Hmm, this doesn't seem too good."

They showed me the X ray, and there was a huge tumor on top of my lungs. It looked like if you had that in your body, you would never recover. That's why they were so startled. They looked like they were thinking, "You're going to die tomorrow." They started all the tests that minute. The doctor said he had to send off to see what type of cancer it was and whether it was treatable. He said, "If we can treat this, you have a real good chance. We'll know within three months. But if we can't, you need to go ahead and be getting your affairs in order."

What? Get my affairs in order? I was shocked. He was saying,

"Make your will and make sure everything is right. You don't have long if it doesn't respond." I was just heartsick.

Luckily, it responded.

—*Mamie Dixon*

Minimizing the Sense of Loss

I've found that one of the biggest issues cancer patients struggle with is a sense of loss. You may feel:

- The loss of independence and control.
- The loss of your normal role as parent, spouse, sibling, coworker, or boss as you refocus priorities to battle cancer with everything you have.
- The loss of your salary or job or standard of living.
- The loss of innocence: The world no longer feels like a safe place.
- The loss of hopes and dreams for the future: You must now readjust plans and live in the present.
- The loss of good health and energy.
- The loss of good looks.
- The loss of cheerfulness and sociability.
- The loss of closeness with friends and family members who have a hard time dealing with illness.

Here are some ways to minimize the sense of loss:

- Identify the things you can control, such as your choice of doctor, your diet, the way you spend your time, the people you associate with.
- Try to retain a sense of yourself as a whole person, not just as a patient. Keep up with your regular activities as much as possible. Maintain family rituals.
- Talk to others who are going through the same thing. Realize you're not in it alone.

- Concentrate on getting better, on feeling gratitude for the things that you do have.
- Understand that it is normal to have mood swings and more intense emotions than before.
- Make yourself as physically comfortable as possible. Take some of your possessions to your hospital room and have someone bring you home-cooked meals when possible.
- Spend as much time as you can with those who care about you.
- Integrate your cancer experience into your life story. It's an important part of your life—but not the only part of your life.

—Linda Roberts,
Social Worker, Memorial Sloan-Kettering Cancer Center,
New York, New York

IT STARTED WITH sore muscles. My shoulders were achy. I used to like to train with weights, and it felt like I had been working out too hard, like I'd overdone it or tried to lift too much. It didn't go away, so I went to see my doctor. She diagnosed it as tension and gave me muscle relaxers. It developed into a headache that would not go away, and it was excruciating. It kept me in bed for a couple of days. I went back to see the same doctor, and again, she diagnosed it as tension. I'm a physical therapist's assistant, working with patients and their rehabilitation; it's not super high stress. My social lifestyle was normal. I had a boyfriend who I'd been with for three years. I was twenty-eight years old and very healthy. I ate well. I exercised daily. I don't know what caused her to diagnose me with tension.

This all took place over a span of about two weeks, and by then, I had pain in my hips, my knees, my shoulders. It felt like the pain was in my bones. I was at the point where I just couldn't walk. Finally, my parents took me to the emergency room at Alexandria Hospital. I was there for about eight hours and finally admitted because my white blood cell count was eighty thousand, which was dangerously high. I was in so much pain that they gave me morphine. That took the pain away immediately, and then the next day, the pain was gone. I don't know if that one shot of morphine did it, but it went away.

The next day I was diagnosed with acute monocytic leukemia.
                                                —*Michele Fox*

ONE SATURDAY MORNING at the beginning of my sophomore year at LSU, I woke up feeling really bad. I was nauseated, and I had dry heaves. One of my sorority sisters became concerned and stayed with me all day. That afternoon, I decided I was sick enough to warrant going to the hospital in Baton Rouge. She drove me to the emergency room, where I continued to dry-heave and have cold chills. They admitted me, but they didn't know what was wrong. I started throwing up green bile, and the doctors did all sorts of tests and finally decided to call my parents and have them pick me up. My parents drove me back to Mobile, where I stayed for about five days while nobody could figure out what was wrong with me. Eventually I felt better and went back to school.

I decided then and there to get back to my healthy ways. I had won state championships in cross-country and track in high school. It was time for me to get off the party wagon and put discipline back into my life, so I went to the track coach and told him I was interested in joining the team. I ended up working out with the swimming and track teams that fall and winter.

Around mid-March, I began to suffer what I thought were side effects of getting back into shape. I had tenderness and pain in my sternum area and around my kidneys. My back ached. I had trouble breathing while I was running, and my joints were sore. My gums were bleeding, and I had profuse night sweats. I would get up sometimes three times in the middle of the night to change not only my pajamas but the sheets because I was sweating so much. I discussed all of these things with my coach, and finally he told me to go home and let my family physician check me out.

So around the beginning of April, I went home, and my dad, who is an anesthesiologist, sent me to an ob/gyn, thinking all this was hormone-related and that maybe I had a kidney infection. The ob/gyn did a urinalysis and found out that I had a bladder infection, so she put me on erythromycin, which is an antibiotic, and sent me back to school.

I was in my car driving along I-65 toward Baton Rouge when I started feeling like I wasn't going to be able to finish the trip. I knew something was up. A friend of mine and another guy from

Mobile happened to drive up alongside me. They were waving at me, and I flagged them over and asked if one of them could drive me to Covington, Louisiana, where my ex-boyfriend's family lived. I was still very close to his family.

By the time I got there, I was having chills and feeling really weak, and all I wanted to do was get into bed. So Mrs. Morse put me to bed and fixed me some Wisconsin cheese soup (which I can barely eat today because I associate it with my diagnosis). The Morses called my parents, who came to Covington to pick me up.

The next day, my dad sent me over to the hospital for some blood tests. They did a peripheral blood smear and diagnosed me as having mono. They said I needed to go home and go to bed and after a few days' rest, I'd feel better. That was on Monday, and on Wednesday, it was obvious that I wasn't getting better, so my dad got me an appointment with a hematologist/oncologist, all the while denying that anything bad could be wrong. He and my mom were in the middle of setting up a new office for him over in Fair Hope, so I went to the doctor by myself.

In the back of my mind, I thought I might have leukemia. Being a zoology major and premed, I had studied all about the blood system and the lymph glands and the immune system. Also, in high school I had read a book called *Eric,* which was about people with leukemia. When I sat down in the doctor's office and described my symptoms—the night sweats, my head, sternum, and joints hurting, and my back aching—the doctor didn't say anything. He just made some notations and went out of the room to talk to his nurse. He told me that they were going to do a bone marrow biopsy. That made me think that my hunch was right.

When he extracted the marrow, it was so packed with white blood cells that instead of being red, as it should be, it was gray. It was very thick and hard to pull out. The nurse had big tears in her eyes, and later she told me that the last patient whose bone marrow had looked like that had not made it. I knew it was leukemia. I knew that the doctor had already told my parents because he was on the phone in the hall for a long time, and I could hear him trying to comfort my father. As an anesthesiologist, my dad works a lot with pain management, so he had already been through several deaths with cancer patients. I was in a state where I was more concerned with my parents and how they were going to take this than anything else.

The doctor came back in and said, "We're going to put you in the hospital tomorrow, but what you need to do right now is go home. Your mom and dad will be there shortly." He didn't want to tell me the diagnosis since I was there without my family and had to drive home by myself.

So I went home and dug through all my books to find *Eric* and then went for a long walk. I concentrated on just breathing and trying not to hyperventilate. Then I did some laundry. I focused my energies on folding the clothes, thinking, "I've got to get these clothes washed and folded so I can get back to school." That was my denial, trying to convince myself everything was normal. My parents finally rolled in about sunset, and Mom walked in the back door and went straight by me with her sunglasses on. I said, "Hey, Mom," and I heard this crack in her voice. I could tell she'd been crying. I said, "Where's Dad?"

She said, "He's outside. He'll be in in a minute."

I folded my last item and walked to the back door and poked my head into the garage. Dad wasn't anywhere to be seen, so I went outside. He was pacing back and forth. I said, "Dad, is everything all right?" He didn't say anything. I said, "Dad, is there something seriously wrong with me?" He just kind of looked at me, biting his lip, and I saw tears well up in his eyes.

He said, "What do you think you have?"

I said, "Do I have leukemia?" and he burst out crying. He grabbed me and drew me to him, and I just stood there. I was thinking, "How am I going to comfort him?" And my mom came out and hugged me, and she said, "We're going to beat this thing." All I could think of was that this was so corny, so Hollywood. What was I supposed to do? I was just at a loss. I was thinking, "I'm the child, they're the parents, they're losing it. What am I supposed to do?"

From that moment, I felt like my childhood was over. That sense of naïveté where you think you're going to live forever had gone, and at that moment when I knew my parents were truly scared, the fear hit me.

—Lisa Hollingsworth

I HAD A multitude of things going on. I was in my senior year of college and taking a heavy load of courses as well as working full-time. I had just gotten married the summer before and had a couple of job offers to choose from. That was probably the toughest thing, being uprooted from that schedule.

I'd been feeling pretty run-down—I had some lymph nodes under my arm that were swollen—so I went to the doctor and was treated for mononucleosis. Then they thought I had Hodgkin's disease, and I was treated for that. Then they decided that wasn't the case. They would give me antibiotics, and I'd feel a little bit better. But then I'd feel rough again—never anything really bad, just feeling not right and really tired.

Around the first of the year, I started noticing pain in my chest, actually behind my collarbone and down in my rib cage. A tumor finally showed up, but even then it took close to a month before they could diagnose what it was.

After my biopsy, the internist who was handling me called my wife while I was at work and told her that it was malignant but was nothing to worry about. The internist led her to believe that they'd just go in and take it out, and we'd get on down the road. But it didn't work out that way. Here we are, dumb about cancer in general, and the next thing you know, after a couple of tests, lo and behold, we're finding out you can lose your arm, and you might not even live. That was a real shock.

It was a fibrous histiocytoma, a type of sarcoma, of the shoulder, a fairly rare form of cancer. At that time, the treatment was very experimental, a trial-and-error situation. My surgeon was a pretty straightforward person, and I responded well to that. He said, "I'm gonna tell you when it's good and when it's bad, and this isn't good. But we're gonna do what we can." Prior to that, I feel like I got kind of jerked around, but I never held that against anybody. A lot of people said I should have sued and done all these different things. I didn't see anything being accomplished by that. I had other things to worry about.

—*Dale Totty*

I FELT A lump in my breast and thought it was just a cyst. But because there was a history of breast cancer in my family, I took it upon myself to get a mammogram. It was no big deal. I was thirty at the time. I got a phone call on a Friday from the receptionist at my gynecologist's office who said, "We just called to tell you that there are abnormalities in your mammogram, and you have to see a breast surgeon." My gynecologist never called.

I said, "Well, I'm thirty years old, and I don't have a breast surgeon." She gave me a name in New Jersey, and I called him and set up an appointment for the following Monday. I thought, "This can't be a big deal. Otherwise somebody would want to see me right now." On Monday, the breast surgeon did a needle aspiration and then scheduled a biopsy for the following Thursday. During the biopsy, he said, "Come back to my office tomorrow. Don't come alone."

Of course, I did, and that's when he told me that they believed I had breast cancer and would need a mastectomy and then six months of chemotherapy. It's my nature to deal with a crisis myself before I can share it with other people. I walked around the park for half an hour with my dog and cried the entire time. And that was it. That was my grieving period. I never went through a period of "Why me?" or anything like that. My only big concern was who was going to take care of Mickey, my dog, if anything happened to me.

Then I communicated the news to my family. My younger brother had friends from college working at Memorial Sloan-Kettering. At that point, everything was taken out of my hands. "You're going to Memorial, and these are the people you're going to see, and this is what is going to happen." I did get a second opinion to see if they could do some other form of treatment, but it was determined that the mastectomy and chemo were what I needed.

This was all going on around Memorial Day, and my breast surgeon said, "Okay, we'll put you in the hospital on Thursday and do the surgery on Friday." I still don't think it had hit me because I said that I had plans that weekend. She said, "This is a hospital, not a hotel."

The night I checked in, they didn't have any rooms on the breast floor. So I was put on the lung floor. My mother smokes three packs of cigarettes a day, and I just sat up there thinking, "I can't believe that these people are suffering so much, and Mom is still doing this." When I came back from surgery, they put me on the floor where all the other breast cancer patients were, and it was somewhat of a relief.

I never, ever, ever in my mind thought that I was going to die.

The severity of what I was up against never became an issue. It wasn't like I was blocking it. I just thought, "Okay, we're going to deal with this and be positive."

—*Claire Noonan*

I WAS BORN with a mole in the middle of my right shoulder blade. It was dark in color and about the size of a half-dollar, and over the years doctors would check it for changes in size or color. It wasn't until I was forty-one years old that the sleeping giant decided to surface. I had scratched it, and it began to change. However, knowing something could be happening and doing something about it was a war I fought with myself. I put antibiotics on it and wished it would go away. I stayed out of the sun (something, I must confess, that is very difficult for me), and I watched it carefully. I feared going to a doctor to hear a diagnosis and feared what I felt certain they would find. It was foolish of me to wait three months and give that speeding monster a chance to grow and spread.

When it began to ooze constantly, I knew I couldn't put it off. So off I went with hopes that it would be minor. The doctor immediately did a biopsy and told me then that he believed it was malignant. It was one of the most frightening days of my life.

Doctors determined that the mole was melanoma—the most malignant of all accessible cancers. It could quickly metastasize through both the lymphatic system and blood vessels to the lymph nodes and internal organs. Within two days, I was in the operating room.

—*Ruth St. John*

I'M ON THE Throgs Neck Volunteer Ambulance Corps in the Bronx, and as part of being an EMT, you're supposed to do abdominal palpations on patients. You put your hands over the four quadrants of the abdomen, and you palpate, and you get all kinds of data from it. So I woke up one Saturday morning, and I was lying in bed just resting and thinking about this, and I said, "I haven't done palpations in a long time on anybody's abdomen. I'll practice on myself." So I practiced on my own abdomen. A soft abdomen is called benign. You're supposed to find a benign abdomen. And I found, to my shock, that my abdomen was hard.

I had two jobs—the other one was in an emergency room—and while I was there I said to a friend, who was a resident and an oncologist, "Do me a favor. Check out my abdomen." So I lay down on the gurney and he palpated the four quadrants of my abdomen. His face turned white. He said, "You have something. Go find out what it is."

I went to my regular doctor, and he said, "You have something. Go get a CAT scan."

I went for a CAT scan where I work, Cabrini Medical Center, and the technician said, "I'm going to do an abdominal. I'll take twenty-five pictures, and then you can go home." So she took her twenty-five pictures, and she came back and said, "You know, these pictures are so good, I think I'll take some more."

I said to myself, "Bullshit, lady. You found more than you bargained for."

My private doctor told me, "You have an abdominal mass."

I went back to Cabrini, and the doctor looked at the CAT scan and said, "You have cancer, and it is very extensive."

I have two master's degrees, and I sat there like an idiot, saying, "What does 'extensive' mean?" Because sometimes you can't handle information when it's told to you.

The guy just said, "Lots and lots and lots."

At this point, my sister-in-law, who's an oncology nurse at Columbia-Presbyterian, got angry at me. She said, "You're not going anyplace but where I know the best muckamuck doctor is." At the time, I was vulnerable, but I'm very glad I took her advice.

I went to see a doctor at Columbia-Presbyterian. He said, "We have to do a biopsy." The lymphoma was all through my abdomen, and it was extensive. A high tumor load. There's one channel on the left side that goes from your abdomen through your diaphragm and bypasses your chest into your neck, and the cancer had spread up that channel to the lymph nodes in my neck. Actually the biopsy was from the lymph nodes in the neck. And they put a label on it—diffuse large-cell lymphoma. That was helpful because they really drove me crazy when they used all these conservative expressions—"you have a mass"—and didn't define them. Finally they put a label on it, and the guy said to me, "You have a lot of it, and it's a very aggressive disease."

I said, "Can you treat it aggressively?" That he did. He treated it very aggressively.

—*Frank Sheridan*

IN DECEMBER OF 1994, I went in for a routine Pap smear, and got a call from the doctor that it had come back with irregular cells. He said, "Don't worry about it. This happens a lot. We'll do a follow-up in five or six months. It's probably just an infection." So he calmed me down. I went on with my life and, prior to the follow-up, moved to Michigan to start a new job. I did not have a doctor there, so I scheduled an appointment for a Pap smear at Planned Parenthood, which was near where I worked.

A nurse practitioner did my second examination. This is a woman who had spent all of her time doing very simple exams of young women. I told her I'd had an irregular Pap. She had the same reaction: no big deal. But during my examination, she took a look at my cervix and literally gasped. She said, "Well, there's definitely something going on. I'm not going to do this Pap. I'm going to send you to a doctor." She came around to talk to me, and her glove was covered with blood.

They had a list of doctors at Planned Parenthood, and I chose one who was on my insurance plan. I went to see him, and it was one of the worst experiences of my life. He was very cold, didn't even shake my hand. I tried to explain to him the experience I'd had with the nurse practitioner, how she'd gasped, and I'd been bleeding, and I was really concerned. He looked at me and said, "Is she a member of the College of Gynecologists and Obstetricians?"

I said, "Well, no, but she's been doing this for twenty-five years at Planned Parenthood. You'd think she's seen a lot of cervixes."

He said, "Well, she's a nurse practitioner. I wouldn't put much stock in what she says." When I had first walked in, I had told him that I needed a colposcopy—that's what the nurse practitioner had told me—and I think that's what set him off. He felt it necessary to put me in my place, and he did.

He began the exam, and his tone changed. He said, "Well, yeah, there's something going on here. We're definitely going to need to do some tests." At that point he did the colposcopy. Basically the procedure involves looking at the cervix with a microscope and a light, and frequently a little biopsy is done during it. But he performed the biopsy without telling me. I was lying there on the table, and suddenly this uncomfortable and painful thing happened with no warning. To this day, I firmly believe he just wanted to hurt me. He was mad.

I left there and called my sister. I was hysterical and feeling like such an idiot—like I'd somehow treated this professional badly and brought this on myself. My sister was quick to correct me. She made sure I realized that this guy's treatment of me was out of the realm of the reasonable. I was so confused that it took me a long time to feel emotions like anger and the strength that comes from it. At this point, I decided to start the process of finding doctors I could trust.

On a coworker's recommendation, I went to see a doctor who was retiring but was willing to talk to me about the test results and to recommend other doctors. I liked her quite a bit. She was in her early sixties, and a throwback to the sixties, with a holistic approach to health. She was very cool and hip and basically thought the other doctor was an asshole. She said, "You did the right thing. When you don't feel comfortable with someone, you leave, and you find somebody you are comfortable with."

She went over my records with me and showed me that I not only had severe dysplasia but that it was possibly cancerous. She said, "You've got to take care of this. You need to ask questions and push. Get a file and carry your medical records around, and find somebody you like. If it means interviewing twenty people, then interview twenty people."

Starting up my own medical file and keeping copies of everything for myself was the best piece of advice I got the entire time. Then she referred me to a doctor to do a cone biopsy, where they take out a cone-shaped piece of your cervix. It's a way of seeing if you have cancer, but it also becomes a treatment in itself because they try to remove all the dysplasia. Older doctors tend to do it with a knife. Younger doctors prefer a laser.

She recommended I see an older doctor because the lab prefers to have it done with a knife. When you do it with a laser, there's a small amount of tissue that's burned in the process, and if any of those microscopic cells on the border are cancerous, they can't be read. She recommended that I switch doctors after the cone biopsy because the guy she was sending me to was not one I would want to see every month. He was grandfatherly and kind, but very old school—I'm the doctor, you're the patient.

When I went to see him, he downplayed everything. "This is no big deal. I don't expect there to be any problem. Don't spend another minute worrying about it."

I started getting frustrated. Why were people encouraging me not to get worried? I was feeling unsure and afraid, and it made me feel guilty and self-indulgent having these professionals tell me not to worry. I had no concept of how this would affect my life or how to find out because no one was encouraging me to do my own research—except for the one woman doctor. So I started buying books and talking to people. What I found out was that although a lot of women have dysplasia, most who have severe, cancerous dysplasia are older and haven't gone for regular Pap smears. It just isn't seen in healthy twenty-eight-year-old women. It was very difficult to find people who could help me understand what was happening.

I had the cone biopsy. It was uncomfortable and painful and worrying, but the doctor assured me that he'd gotten everything and that I'd be fine. And then I got a call from him. The lab results had come back, and there were no clear margins on the piece of tissue they'd taken out, which meant that the dysplasia extended even farther up into the uterus. That's when I decided the game was over. I was going to take control of the situation. I was going to be worried and demanding, and I was going to tell people to stop treating me like a hysterical person. I had my medical file, and I did some exploring and found a doctor who was considered one of the top five physicians in the state and who was the director of the teaching wings of three different hospitals. He was difficult to get in with—youngish, under fifty, very hot.

I went to see him for a consultation. I sat down and had my file and my paperwork and my planner and my suit on. I was ready. I told him I was very frustrated, and I needed somebody to help me find out what I needed to do at this point. I still had cancer and so far had not been able to feel concerned about it, because no one else seemed to be. He was the first person who looked at me and said, "I think you should be concerned, and I don't think you're crazy. I think you need a lot of questions answered."

We talked for about an hour. And now that I know how busy he is, I understand how amazing that was. He said, "What I'd like you to do is to go see these three doctors—another gynecologist, an obstetrician who deals with high-risk pregnancies, and an oncologist, and all of them are going to examine you and talk to you about the repercussions of having another cone biopsy and what happens if we don't get it all. All of those 'what if?' questions. So make a list of questions for each doctor, and go do it. And then we will decide what kind of treatment you want."

He also said, which I think was valid, that the doctor who had done my first cone was a good doctor. His style was different; he was a good doctor for people who want to put their trust in somebody else. Dr. Cash underscored the fact that it was okay for me to search for a doctor whose style I was comfortable with. That was as important a part of treatment as the treatment itself.

I saw the doctors that he recommended. The doctor for high-risk pregnancies examined me and talked to me. He told me what to expect, what to try, and how to think about it. That was helpful. At the time, I hadn't even thought about kids. All I was thinking was, "Get this cancer out of me." But Dr. Cash had said, "These are questions you're going to want answered."

Same thing with the oncologist. He said, "Okay. Here's what I think is going to happen: We're going to do the second cone, and you're going to be okay. I think that probably by the time you're forty or fifty, you're going to need a full hysterectomy because these cancers tend to come back. But they tend to be isolated to the area that they started in because it's a specific kind of cell that's really only in the female reproductive system." He said, "Am I telling you, 'Don't worry, you won't get another form of cancer'? No. Can this be an indicator that you're prone to certain kinds of cancer? Yes. But it doesn't have to be, and you don't have to approach it that way. If we do the second cone and find more trouble, here's what we're going to do . . ."

He went through everything with me, and I walked out of there thinking, "Okay. I know what I'm dealing with now." I felt very comfortable saying, "Let's get this done."

—*Rachel Kaul*

I WAS OVERSEAS in the Marshall Islands, in the Peace Corps from 1967 to 1969 and was exposed to a chemical, similar to Agent Orange, used to kill trees. I now understand that the stuff has a ten- to twenty-year span of creating problems. On this specific island lived the Ujelang people, and their home had been used for hydrogen-bomb testing. Other volunteers who were out there, as well as many of the island people, have also gotten cancer. In fact, a group of medical people goes out and checks the people regularly because the radiation has caused a substantial amount of cancer. I saw one of the island chiefs die of it.

Parasitic infections were also a problem there—parasites that get into the stomach lining and cause continuous acid buildup—so generally my internals were messed up. At any rate, what happened was my stomach lining and the thing that keeps the acid from getting up into your esophagus deteriorated. The internal turmoil had been going on for a long time, a couple of decades, but I ignored the pain. It kept getting worse and worse, and finally I went to see a good doctor in Danbury who said he thought we had the beginning of some changing of cells. For three years, he kept it as much under control as he could. We were waiting for a particular new operation to be perfected. When the cells started to go cancerous, however, they said, "That's it. Let's go." This cancer was particularly insidious.

So I went up to Yale in New Haven, and a surgeon performed an operation in which he removed the entire esophagus and took the stomach and moved it up to the neck, connected it to the stub that was left. Then I began the arduous procedure of adapting to it. Chances for survival from this particular procedure were pretty slim. Most of the people I talked to were not making it at that point.

But I had learned a valuable lesson from the Ujelang people. They were pretty ingenious. One time we got caught in a hurricane out on the ocean, and I thought we were going to die. I kept asking these guys, "Why are you so calm? We're going to die!" Their attitude was, "Rick, either we'll make it or we won't. The things you can do something about, you do, and those you can't, you accept." That got through to me, and that helped me through the cancer. I took the attitude: Here's what we've got, let's deal with it. I'll do what I can do, what I can't, I can't.

—*Rick Asselta*

I WAS A freshman in college having dizzy spells. The health clinic said that I was probably just eating poorly and drinking too much, which I was. They suggested that I eat peanut butter crackers in the morning. I was at Colgate University in upstate New York, and I usually saw my parents only on major holidays. So it wasn't until the summer after my freshman year on a vacation in Europe that they saw me have one of these dizzy episodes, and they said, "We're going to look into that when we get home."

We got home on a Sunday, and I had to go to the grocery store for—I still remember the three things I had to buy—oranges, dog food, and Dove. I always sensed the dizziness was coming right before it happened; it turns out it was an aura right before a seizure. This time, I had the feeling it was about to happen, and then nothing happened. Or so I thought. I was in the grocery line with my girlfriend, and I remember putting the things on the counter. The next thing I knew, I was getting in the car. My friend looked at me, and she was pissed. "What the hell were you doing back there?" she said.

I said, "What are you talking about?"

She said, "You thought you were funny?"

Then she described to me what had happened. The checkout woman told me how much it was, and I said, "Whose groceries are these?" Then I said, "These aren't my groceries; I don't have money for this." As she was recounting this, I got scared because I had no recollection of it at all. And I was *driving* as she was telling me.

That was on Sunday. I saw the doctor on Tuesday. He said it sounded like a petit mal seizure, like my mom had thought. On Wednesday I had an EEG to see if they were seizures. That night he called and said, "I'm really sorry, but you are epileptic." I had just finished my freshman year, and what that meant to me was that I was going to take medicine that wouldn't allow me to drink for the rest of my college years. Pretty upsetting at the time. Then he said we needed to see if there was scar tissue or anything else causing these seizures—possible, but highly improbable.

So I had my first MRI that Thursday, and that night my doctor called and said, "I'm sorry. You have a brain tumor, but it's a small one." Small or large, it was a tumor in my brain, and it was horribly shocking. I was an athlete and so strong. They called back the next day and said, "We're sorry, we had more people look at it, and it isn't just a small tumor; it's larger than your fist. You have to come in right away."

So on Friday I went with my parents to Children's Hospital in Philadelphia. I hadn't turned nineteen yet, so they recommended that I go there. They said, "Yeah, we've got to get this out." And I was on the table Monday morning. It all happened quickly, which was a great thing. Surgery went well, as far as we knew. We didn't know a thing about brain tumors. I recuperated quickly and was out of the hospital in about four days.

My parents and I sat down and talked about the next steps. They were recommending radiation therapy, and I had to sign a form saying that I understood all the possible side effects, which included brain hemorrhages, decreased IQ, new cancers, and it was all pretty horrendous. That's when we decided we needed a second opinion. We were referred to a guy at NYU who is all over the news: Fred Epstein, the miracle worker. He was on *Oprah*.

He took one look at it and said, "Don't do a thing. I'm going to take more out." So I had another surgery about a month after the first. After that, NYU and Children's Hospital in Philly couldn't agree on the pathology, but in the end they compromised and called it anaplastic astrocytoma in the right temporal lobe.

—Katie Brant

I HAD JUST had my first son, and I was having these spells where I blacked out. Nobody could figure out what it was. The first time it happened, they told me it was hypoglycemia. The second time, I was in the car with my son, who was ten days old, and had a seizure. They told me it was the trauma of birth. I'm a nurse, but I didn't know what was happening to me. I just had to go by what they told me.

Ten months later, I had another seizure. This time, they took me to the hospital. I don't know how they finally picked it up at this hospital, but they told me when I woke up in the emergency room that I had a brain tumor. I told them I needed to go home; I had a baby to take care of. After you have a seizure, you feel fine. You just wake up. You're drowsy, but you don't recall anything that happened. The doctor said, "No. There's something seriously wrong with you. We're keeping you overnight."

Even though I was a nurse, when the doctor sat down and told me about the tumor you could have knocked me off the bed with a feather. Brain tumors were just something I'd read about in books. To think that I had one was just so farfetched. I never had any other symptoms. That's why it took them so long to catch it. They said I'd probably had it most of my life, that it was a slow-growing tumor that finally grew to a size where it was affecting my functioning. They said that they needed to do tests and figure out how to approach it.

From the beginning, I never felt that I was going to die. I thought maybe I wouldn't be as normal as I am, but that's all. I took it one day at a time and was very calm. I had an excellent doctor who explained everything to me. Because I was a nurse, I was more aware of what they were doing to me and what was going on around me. So I probably wasn't quite as frightened by the whole situation as somebody not in the medical field.

—*Cathy Owen*

I'M A POLITICAL journalist, so I mark my life by election campaigns. I got married on the eve of Reagan's election, and I got cancer on the eve of Bill Clinton's. At the time, I was following candidates, and there was nothing dramatic, but I noticed that it was kind of painful buckling myself into seatbelts in airplanes, and I had sort of mild abdominal discomfort. I was also having to go to the bathroom a lot.

My internist thought it was a bladder problem, so he sent me to a urologist. This was on a Thursday. The urologist looked at it and said that there was nothing wrong with my bladder, but he wanted me to come back for an ultrasound test the next day. When he looked at the results, he said, "There's something in there. You've got to see a surgeon." I saw the surgeon on a Monday, and I checked into the hospital on Wednesday, and I had the operation on Friday. It was eight days; it was like going down a chute. Actually, that was probably good because the period of worry up front—when you don't know what you're dealing with—was very compressed. What they found was testicular cancer, which is pretty common in men under forty. But it was an uncommon form of it because it was undescended testicular tissue.

I've had only one testicle all my life. When I was a little boy, they did an operation to see if there was an undescended one because those are likely to become cancerous. They didn't find anything. Then several years before '92, my internist said, "Why don't you have an MRI just to see if there's something in there? It's a new technology. They didn't find anything in 1960, but maybe they'll find something now." But again they didn't find anything. Well, there was something there, and it grew to 3.7 pounds—the size of a great big grapefruit.

My favorite detail was that when testicular tissue metastasizes, it's got all your genetic information in it. That was science fiction—like male pregnancy. It was really a ghastly little detail, but it was so over the top it was kind of funny.

The operation was a success, and they got it all out. Unfortunately, it had already spread to my lungs, which they found through a CAT scan. That meant I had to have chemotherapy. The good thing about it is that the chemo for testicular cancer is very well understood. I didn't get into one of these situations where one doctor says you should do radiation and somebody else says no, no, no, you should do chemo. There wasn't any dispute among the doctors as to what to do with it. It was one kind of chemo. The bad side is that the major chemical is one called cisplatin, which is very rugged, the chemo of champions.

For four months I went to the hospital once a month. I'd go in for five days and have the stuff administered over that period. They were able to check the progress of what they were doing by taking blood samples because this cancer leaves markers in the blood. And fortunately, the markers did go consistently down.
—*Richard Brookhiser*

I WAS A first baseman for the Philadelphia Phillies. We were playing in Los Angeles. It was the ninth inning, and in L.A., there's always dew on the grass by that time of night. Well, I hit a little swinging bunt in front of the pitcher. He fielded the ball, rolled, and fired it to first. The ball skipped in that wet grass and hit me in my protective cup. The cup shattered, and I knew there was going to be some swelling.

The season continued, and I tried not to think about it too much. We were heading to the playoffs and the World Series, and

I had to keep playing. It was hurting, but I didn't want to have it checked out.

After the season, I had trouble getting up from a chair without it hurting real bad. It hurt to the point where it'd make me want to throw up. I knew there was something wrong, but I was being stubborn. My wife kept yelling at me, "You've got to go to the doctor. You've got to go to the doctor."

I said, "No, it'll go away." But it didn't. It kept getting worse, and then I noticed a big knot on my testicle. In February, during my physical before spring training, I mentioned it to the doctor. He checked it out and said it was just a hematoma and would go away. So I went on with spring training, but it kept getting bigger and more painful. They sent me to a doctor who did an ultrasound, and he said it was just a hematoma and that I should take anti-inflammatories, and it'd go away.

I said, "Okay, that's fine. I feel better about it now." But again it kept getting worse and hurting more. It got to the point where every time I bent over to play my position, I felt like I was going to throw up. The knot and the testicle were swollen and getting bigger. So I went back to the doctor for more tests and blood work.

Again, he said, "It doesn't look like anything. You're fine."

Well, it kept getting worse, but I didn't want to keep complaining about it. They'd think I just didn't want to play. Finally, we were playing in a game, and it was the second inning, and I went in and told them, "I'm done. I can't take this anymore. It's making me sick to my stomach."

So, of course, being baseball people, they said, "Okay, we'll send you to our doctors in Philadelphia and find out nothing's wrong with you, and then you can come back and play."

In Philadelphia, I went through a bunch of tests and then flew back to Clearwater for more spring training. The tests came back, and they said everything seemed fine. "It's just a blood clot that got hard, and that's all it is, and once the swelling goes down, you'll be fine." A couple of days later, it just wouldn't stop. Nothing was better. They sent me back to Philadelphia, and the doctor asked, "How long has this been hurting?"

I said, "For about five months now."

He said, "Oh, my God, I thought it had just started. Has the swelling subsided?"

I said, "No."

He said, "Well, there are two things we can do. We can re-move your testicle, and that will relieve your pain, or you can continue taking anti-inflammatories." I had been taking anti-inflammatories every day for three months, and I told him they weren't working.

He said, "If we remove your testicle, you'll be out for a week or so, and then you can start playing again."

I said, "That's fine. Let's do that."

He said, "You and your wife go have lunch and talk about it and then come back and let me know." So we went to lunch, we talked about it, and we agreed it was best to have it removed. I couldn't take the pain anymore. Every time I'd sit down or lie down and try to get up, I'd almost throw up. I wasn't going to live like this any longer.

I told the doctor, and he said we could do it right then. I said, "Fine, let's do it." So he did.

At about eleven o'clock, I woke up, and the doctor came into my room and said, "The operation went well. You just had a big knot on the side of your testicle, and everything is fine." We were relieved, naturally.

But the next morning a doctor came in about seven o'clock and said he had to do a lymphangiogram. I said, "What for?"

He said, "Well, didn't the doctor tell you last night? You have cancer."

I said, "Get the hell out of here."

He said, "Within a week we'll start radiation." Later they told me that the doctor told me everything was fine because I was still groggy, and they wanted to make sure that I knew what they were talking about.

How do you get mad when someone says, "We've discovered you have cancer"? They had run all the tests and everything. They were convinced that nothing was wrong because of the tests. The thing is, if I had waited, then who knows what would have happened? Fortunately, we chose to take the testicle off.

The hit I took didn't have anything to do with it, but it made me have it checked, which I never would have done. I had the athlete's mentality: Nothing can affect you, you're indestructible. I was stupid. A lot of people in Philadelphia blamed the pitcher,

Mitch Williams, for what I had. I had to explain to everyone that Mitch saved my life. If he hadn't hit me with the ball, I wouldn't have known anything was wrong. I guess I was lucky that I got hit in the balls by a ball. How many people can say that?

—*John Kruk*

CHAPTER TWO

Breaking the News

Telling other people that you have cancer is a very difficult thing to do. It is also a very personal and individual act. It could almost be said that there are as many ways to break the news as there are people with cancer multiplied by the number of people they need to tell.

Often, spouses, significant others, or parents are with us at the time of discovery. It's usually a very emotional moment that we share together, one that we will never forget. After that, it almost always helps to put a little time, whether a few minutes or a day or two, between the discovery and the calling of family and friends. The time buffer allows us to put on our game faces and to determine just how much we want to reveal and to whom. It also gives us time to figure out how these people can best help us in the initial stages of the treatment and recovery process.

In fact, one of the first acts of delegation you might want to make is to assign one or more close friends, work colleagues, or family members to tell other people. The act of telling can be very emotional and draining because while you might have dealt with your initial grief, now you have to deal with that of the people you tell. If you do choose to delegate the informing of your colleagues, friends, or family, be sure to have the person assigned explain that you weren't feeling ready to talk about your diagnosis yet. Later, you can explain that although you wanted to tell everyone personally, you needed to build your emotional reserves for the tasks ahead.

For those you do talk to, you probably want to set both a realistic and optimistic tone. It often helps to have a list of reasons you have for being optimistic. That way you can forestall morbid dwelling on your situation which you will probably find counter-productive.

Telling children is an even more delicate matter. For tips from a hospital counselor, see page 74.

WHEN I WAS first diagnosed with cancer, my reaction was: How can this be happening to me? It *can't* be happening to me. I've mistakenly stepped into somebody else's life! I just wanted to wake up and find my mother at my side, saying, "Now, now, sweetheart, everything's all right. It was just a bad dream."

But I knew that it wasn't a mistake and that I needed to get back home to New York from law school in Virginia as soon as possible. I called my father to tell him that I'd be on the evening plane to LaGuardia. But I decided not to tell him what had happened; I just couldn't break that kind of news on the telephone. I took a deep breath and tried to sound as nonchalant as possible as I gave him my flight number and arrival time. Inside my head, I was screaming for help, and I was almost overcome by sadness when he said he would hold off eating so that we could have dinner together at a favorite Italian restaurant near the airport. I couldn't tell him that I was coming home with a tumor in my belly and that Italian food wasn't going to do the trick.

I hung up the phone and dived into bed. I was exhausted, paralyzed by my secret, and after only a few sobs I drifted off to sleep.

When I woke up a short time later, my frame of mind had

changed. The nap seemed to have lifted the heavy cloud of grief. Something had been recharged in my head, and I began to think about gathering all the help I could get. Withholding the news from my father had been a mistake, for whatever struggles lay ahead of me, they would necessarily, and intimately, involve my parents. The sooner they knew, the better.

I picked up the phone and called my mother. She was somewhat surprised to get a call from me at her office, but she was no less ebullient as she sang out, "Hey, Jonny, when are you coming home? Is your father going to pick you up?"

I took a deep breath. "Mom," I began, "I have to tell you something." I tried to go on, but my voice cracked and I began to sob. It was at least thirty seconds before I could bring myself to speak. When I did, the words left my lips in an explosive burst. "Mom, I was just diagnosed as having cancer."

My mother was silent. I brooded on how much damage that short sentence must have done to her. But how should a son tell his mother he has cancer? I cursed myself for having made the call. I'd been right the first time: This was not something you did on the phone.

Then my mother spoke. "What did the doctor say?" she asked softly. "Tell me what he said."

"He told me that I have lymphoma." I read to her from the pathology report the doctor had given me: "Diffuse histiocytic lymphoma . . ."

I thought I heard a sob, but when my mother spoke, it was in the same even tone. She asked for the spelling of the disease and told me that she would call back as soon as possible.

When the phone rang ten minutes later, it was my stepfather, Hal. "Can you believe what's happening?" I blurted out. "Have you ever heard of anything so crazy?"

His response will remain forever etched in my brain. "Jonathan," he said firmly, "I just spoke with my doctor, and I want you to know that what you have is eminently curable." The word "eminently" jumped out at me. I didn't know if it meant my chances were fifty percent or ninety percent, but I did know that it was a fancy way of saying "highly," which meant that I had a fighting chance to lick it. His reassuring tone had the resonance of a guarantee, and it made me feel I had regained some power. At that moment, I began to relax and to sense the first glimmerings of hope rising in my chest, which, under the circumstances, felt like a rush of euphoria.

—*Jonathan Pearlroth*

MY FRIENDS, MY relatives from far away, everybody was calling, and they were nervous because they didn't know what to say to me. I was more comfortable on these phone calls than they were. Unfortunately, most people want to hear things like statistics. They want absolute facts, and there isn't a whole lot of factual data in this situation. Instead of focusing on the medical aspects of my illness, I tried to allay people's fears by telling them that my doctor said it was not only treatable but curable—that was an important word to hear.

I explained, "I don't really know what's ahead, but I plan to get through it. Thank you for being here, and I may need to talk to you again." To my closest friends and relatives, I said, "I'm going to need you, so please be there." Most people told me later that they felt much better after they talked to me. I guess they were relieved by my attitude or my explaining things or my not sounding weak and frail and depressed.

—*Jodi Levy*

THE WORD "CANCER" scares people. As the person with cancer, you can either cause panic or you can try to relieve that panic. The more you know about your situation, the more control you have. Take the time to sit with your doctor. Bring in a tape recorder, if necessary, and ask questions. Then, when people ask you, you can say, "This is the status. I don't know everything, but I do know this."

I was very honest and detailed with people. Being able to share knowledge about how many lymph nodes were taken out and what their status was alleviated people's worry. Of course, it was a very select group of people, and I didn't tell them everything. But it's helpful to give them some information, because they feel like they're part of the healing process by knowing the details.

—*Claire Noonan*

MY PARENTS KNEW I was sick because they had been with me the weekend that I started getting night sweats and fevers, and I had told them, "Boy, there's really something wrong." When I called and told them it was Hodgkin's disease, the first thing my mom said was, "Is it serious?" I started crying and said, "Mom, what do you think? I have cancer." Then she started crying, and they drove down here that night—a five-and-a-half-hour drive. They didn't know what to make of it at first until they heard me break down, and then it hit them too.

—*Mark Conover*

THE MOST DIFFICULT thing when you first tell people is the absolute shock. One of the best ways to handle it—this is a bit of advice that I wish I had been given and I think is really important—is to designate one person whom you are very close to and have that person give the news to everybody else. After you have told your closest friends and family, that person can be the filter for everyone else. Then if you want to talk to more people, you can pick up the phone and call them.

I didn't do that, but I wish I had. My phone rang off the hook—everybody was concerned—but at some point you need to rest. You need to get well. I come from a big family and was fortunate in keeping the group of people who knew very small, but you can still spend at least five hours on the phone talking to just a few people.

I didn't tell a lot of people at work either. Everything happened very quickly. I called my boss and had him meet me for breakfast the day before I was being admitted to the hospital. I told him what was going on, and he was great. He asked who he should tell, so I told him, and for six weeks while I was not at work, they absolutely kept that trust. That was great.

I wasn't embarrassed by getting cancer. It wasn't like I didn't want to say the C word, but at the time, I was working as a buyer for Linens 'N Things, where you have huge, huge vendor contracts and you're in charge of a big pencil. I just knew, the way things are in my industry, that I would have been embarrassed at the hospital because hundreds of vendors would have sent flowers. It's the one-upmanship of the industry. So I refused to let people know what was happening. It caused wonderful rumors:

She's off having the president's child; she's checked into . . . great rumors.

—*Claire Noonan*

I SHOUTED MY cancer diagnosis out to the world. I shared what was going on with anyone who cared to listen. The more I talked, the more I was able to connect with others and to develop a large cheering section. If you are open and honest about your situation, most people will extend their love to you, and that wonderful mass of support can give you strength to move forward with your treatment. By talking, I lightened my own burden and made my disease less scary. Each time I told somebody, I put my fears on their shoulders, which, of course, were a lot sturdier than mine.

—*Rhoda Silverman*

FOR TWO WEEKS after I was diagnosed with breast cancer, I wasn't able to tell anybody. I didn't tell my father or my boyfriend or any of my friends. I didn't know how to tell them. I was afraid that they wouldn't be able to handle it, or that maybe they'd abandon me. Finally, one night at dinner with my father and his girlfriend, I said the words, "I have cancer." I removed the armor that had kept the world at bay but that had also trapped the pain within, and I was relieved to hear their words of support. They were very helpful and determined to help me beat it. After that, I was able to tell everyone. I finally allowed myself to be human.

—*Karen Lawrence*

MY PARENTS DIDN'T tell me that my mother had uterine cancer until a year and a half after her diagnosis. What makes it more unbelievable is that I was (and still am) a physician practicing in radiation oncology. It's not that my parents are dumb, or incapable of navigating the medical world, or superstitious in an Old World sense. On the contrary, they are college-educated and intelligent. I believe that they didn't tell me because of a concept called denial. They thought that not talking about it meant that things were under control, that it would all just go away or, conversely, that talking about it would only give it more fuel to grow.

I also believe that by not telling me, they thought they were protecting me. But trying to protect others is often a roundabout way of protecting yourself. I guess they were afraid of my reaction and how that would make *them* feel. They knew that as a physician, I would take a hard look at the situation. And I *did* take a hard look at the situation. But their waiting so long to tell me created hard feelings.

You have to be sure that all communication is open and honest and that you don't try to spare a family member the news, because it always makes things worse. People who love you don't want to be excluded. Regardless of whether they are trained as doctors, nurses, or bricklayers, they love you, want to be a part of your life, and may even wind up having some input that could save it.

—*Sue Winard*

IT WAS VERY hard to tell my family because in the Chinese culture, cancer is taboo and the word is never mentioned. We never talked about it openly. They referred to me as being "sick" or having a "problem." Since I grew up in Chinatown in New York City, even telling my friends was difficult because they, too, were steeped in the Chinese superstition about cancer. To this day, only three of my closest friends know I had cancer. The one group I was able to tell was my coworkers. Their help and support made me realize the importance of talking about what you are going through. Luckily they understood that you can hate the illness without stigmatizing the person who is ill.

—*Monica Ko*

I BELIEVE THAT you "do cancer" the same way you "do life." In my case, I was twenty-five and in law school at the University of Virginia when I was first diagnosed. My biggest worry in the world had been whether I would become a corporate lawyer and make money or a public-interest lawyer and help people. When I was told I had lymphoma, I realized that I didn't care what kind of lawyer I was going to be. I just wanted to survive. I remember praying to a God that I wasn't even sure I believed in, asking Him or Her to cure me of the cancer. I remember thinking how happy I would be to scrub toilets for the rest of my life, if only I could get through the cancer treatment and live a full life. These aren't the everyday thoughts of a twenty-five-year-old. How in the world was I going to share all that with my classmates, my friends, my contemporaries, who were concerned mostly with getting a job and landing a date on Saturday night? But the converse to that question was, "How am I *not* going to share all that with others?" How can I keep people in the dark about such a life-shaping and shattering event? When you're diagnosed with cancer, all you can think about is that you have cancer. It simply overrides all of your other daily concerns.

With time, I learned to be honest with myself about how the cancer made me feel and to reach out to others in a balanced, appropriate way. I had to explain to the dean of my law school why I was leaving school abruptly. I needed to tell my boss at the law firm that had hired me for the summer that I would miss a couple of days each week to undergo chemotherapy treatments. If someone needed to be told about my cancer, then I told them matter-of-factly and without any shame. I didn't need to explain to everyone why I was bald. I didn't need to relate each detail of my daily treatment to everyone. It was crucial, however, for me to be able to tell my friends and family everything that was going on with me. I simply told them the straight, honest facts. The more I shared, the greater relief I felt. It would have been unbearably lonely to have kept the illness—even the details of my surgery, chemotherapy, radiation, and all of the side effects—to myself.

—*Jonathan Pearlroth*

Telling Your Children

MY DIAGNOSIS WAS a total shocker. I felt fantastic but had gone to the doctor just because I had some bruising on my arms that was not going away. They sent me right over to the hospital to a hematologist for blood work, and thirty minutes later, I was diagnosed with leukemia. I had very little time; they basically told me to go home, pack a suitcase, and get up to the med center.

The diagnosis was so unexpected that I had brought my kids—ages twelve, ten, and eight—with me. Luckily, they were in another room. My husband was not with me, but he knew something was up, because he had called the doctor's office and found out that they had sent me for blood work. So he was en route.

We went home. We sat the kids down. We had very little time, but we wanted to make sure we told them that word, "cancer." We didn't want them to hear it from someone else. That word is scary. They had usually heard it in the context of dying. They were pretty upset, but it was amazing how well they coped with everything.

—Karla McConnell

WHEN BRIAN WAS diagnosed, a social worker at the hospital gave us some advice regarding our children that has really helped us in discussing Brian's illness.

Number one, be honest. Tell the children from the beginning exactly what is going on. When she said that, I knew she was right, but I also knew that the impact of telling them their father had cancer would be phenomenal because my mother had died of cancer two years before, and we hadn't hidden my mother's cancer at all.

In fact, our children saw my mother the day before she died. She had been unconscious the whole day, and when I went home for dinner, our older son, who was six at the time, said, "I want to see Grandma before she dies." I had mixed feelings about it, but I took him.

We walked into the room, and she was awake. She said, "Anthony, my best friend." I was bawling. He sat up on her bed and ate a bowl of cereal, and then we left. He seemed fine during her funeral and her wake. But telling them about their father's diagnosis so soon after made me nervous.

The counselors also told us to be hopeful but not to make any promises. So we were honest with them from the beginning, but we did not dwell on the negative side of it. We told them that he was sick, and explained what he was going to do to get better and why he was going to be gone next week. And even though he would lose his hair, it would come back healthier. We told them that it was a treatable cancer—very different from their grandma's.

They understood that it was a different situation, and they've been able to accept it. The older one is busy and friends with the world, and except for the spiritual side—he asks God for us to be healthy—he tries to put it in the back of his mind. The younger one has taken it more upon himself to help Brian. He wants him to talk about it, about how he's going to get better, about what happened last week. He seems to remember just about everything.

So we've tried to be honest, but we don't tell them what could happen. There's no point in going into some of the grim stuff the doctors tell you—the odds they throw at you. We feel that with the type of cancer Brian has, we can be somewhat hopeful. It'll come back someday—we don't know when—but it's treatable.

—*Peggy Schmidt*

WE TOLD OUR older son, who was five, that I had something in my body that was making me sick and had to have it removed with surgery. We didn't want to go into too much medical detail since he was so young, but we talked to him about what the surgery would be like and told him that he needed to be careful physically with me for a while afterward. We made sure to explain to him that the reason I wouldn't be able to pick him up at first was because I would be weak from the surgery, not because of anything that he had done.

He was mature enough to understand everything we told him, and he responded very generously to it—by taking care of me and being very protective. He loved helping me and bringing me things on the days that I was in bed with chemo.

—*Charlotte Wells*

How to Tell Young Children You Have Cancer

How you tell children about a parent's illness depends on their age and developmental stage. Children under five are at a point developmentally where they're more focused on their own needs, so what's most important is to continually communicate that they are going to be cared for. Be explicit about how their needs are going to be met: "While Mommy's at the cancer center having treatment, Grandma's going to cook your breakfast, and Grandpa's going to take you to day care." Their equilibrium is thrown off if things aren't normal, so it's important to maintain their routine as much as possible.

Use words that a child understands. A young child may not understand the word "cancer" but may understand "Mommy doesn't feel well" and "Mommy needs medicine." Present the situation in a hopeful but not unrealistic way. You certainly don't want to lay a foundation of distrust with the child.

Children under the age of ten are very attuned to physical changes that a parent might go through. Explain before the changes occur what might happen: "Mommy's getting treatment and may lose her hair, but it's going to grow back." Some parents want to protect their children by not giving them details, but it ends up making it more difficult for the child when the changes occur.

I recommend that my patients bring their children to the cancer center at least once. I give them a tour, show them where their parent is going to get treatment, have them meet the nursing staff, and show them what an IV looks like. That takes the sense of mystery away. When children aren't given information, they have to use their imaginations, and in their minds, the situation is usually a lot worse.

—Karen Atkin, L.C.S.W.,
Oncology Social Worker, Arkansas Cancer Research Center,
Little Rock, Arkansas

TELLING KIDS CAN be a tricky business. We didn't tell the little ones—our two-year-old and four-year-old—that I had cancer. The two-year-old certainly wouldn't have known what we were talking about. When I went in for surgery, we said something like, "Mommy has to go to the hospital for a little operation, and she'll be back." We did tell our older daughters, who were thirteen and fifteen, that it was breast cancer. They came to the hospital to visit, but my husband and I felt that the little ones were so young at the time that it would be unsettling for them to see me in a hospital bed.

Even with the older ones, we felt that they were at such a vulnerable age that we put it in a very positive light for them. We said that the surgery and chemotherapy would take care of everything. I was terrified to terrify them. I wanted desperately for them to see that this really wasn't going to be so bad, and I think that I went a little bit overboard in trying to protect them.

I wanted them to ask me any questions that they had, but we didn't really talk much about it after our original discussion, and that was a big mistake. I didn't realize that it was important to communicate about what was going on from time to time—to keep the lines of communication open. It's not that I ever refused to talk about it, it's just that it became a nonissue. I made light of it too much. My daughters never indicated this to me until much later, but they had terrible concerns, being at that vulnerable age and being girls. They were concerned first of all about me but—considering the hereditary aspects of breast cancer—also about themselves since my mother had had it as well. I would definitely advise women not to dwell, but to talk about what they're going through. Daughters ought to be able to share their fright, their worries, their questions. It's not that our girls had questions that I refused to answer, and I'm not even sure that they were conscious at the time that they were burdened with all of this, but I didn't pave the way for them to consciously question what they were going through.

—*Toni Zavistovski*

CHAPTER THREE

How to Be Brave When What You Feel Is Fear

For many of us, post diagnosis—before the surgery, chemotherapy, or radiation even began—was emotionally the hardest time. While you're still going through the barrage of tests and meetings with doctors, the great unknown lies in front of you, and that is, frankly, scary. You and your closest advisers are analyzing the extent of your cancer, pulling together your medical team, and making the decisions that will set the course of your treatment and healing process. You will need to strike a balance between depending on your own vigilance and information-gathering and relying on the doctors you choose to work with.

At the same time, you need to focus on the present—how you feel right now and what you can do to feel physically and mentally better. Sure, you'll think back over the last six months or however long it's been, going over all the details—that's only natural—but you have to let that go. Hashing it out again and again won't help. If you have anger, recognize that, but deal with it and move on.

Take heart, you *will* be able to deal with the physical or mental stress of treatment for one simple reason: It's what makes you get better. Cancer treatment has made great strides over the last decade, and pain control even more so. Just as statistics often become dated as soon as they are printed, so, to a certain extent, do the war stories. For example, in the early nineties a new drug called Zofran became available that greatly reduced the nausea experienced with chemotherapy, and even more recently, for those who need a bone marrow transplant, the increased use of stem cells has made the process much less invasive. In the grand scheme of things, think of all the people who have defeated cancer before you with less refined techniques. Take strength in the fact that you are the beneficiary of their experiences.

But don't try to fight the battle all at once. You'll get gloomy. One of the most important mental tasks is to concentrate on taking things one step at a time. When you focus on each individual task, each time you take care of business—whether it's surviving two hours in a doctor's waiting room or having your first bone marrow test—you feel the satisfaction of accomplishing that chore, and you feel that much more in control.

Naturally, you have many questions that you're anxious to have answered, and chances are your doctors just can't satisfy all of them. Ask if they can refer you to a cancer veteran who has been through a similar treatment, or seek out a cancer vet through one of the many local or national cancer organizations (many of which are listed in the Resources section on page 395). Friends may suggest people too. If you find a conversation is making you feel uneasy, politely cut it off. If you sense that the person cannot focus on the details and advice that will help you to gain confidence and to succeed, find another person to talk to. And if you simply do not feel up to talking to someone else who has been through treatment before you, that's okay too.

But strongly consider having your spouse, relative, or close companion talk to a veteran. There is simply too much to be learned for you to ignore altogether the wisdom of those who have recently preceded you through the same treatment—and too much courage to gain from their victory stories.

I REMEMBER LYING on the table during my biopsy, and the surgeon must not have anesthetized one part of my neck because I felt a zing of pain. I jumped a little, and the doctor apologized and said he would give me some anesthesia. The nurse standing on the other side of me held my arm and said, "Sorry. Are you okay?" And I broke out crying. I'm usually a good patient. I can withstand pain, and I'm not a complainer. But it was such a crazy day—I had just found out a few hours before that I had lymphoma—and there was so much fear and emotion involved along with the physical pain that that one zing set me off.

I thought, "I can't cry convulsively on this table because this guy has a knife in my neck. Not a good idea." So I tried to collect myself and to not think about all the things going on. I knew I needed to be calm to get through the next few minutes, so I concentrated on slowing down all the functions of my body, really trying to relax everything and take deep breaths. I told myself that whatever was happening—however huge it was—I could get through the next couple of minutes just by doing this, and that was all I needed to do for right now. I gradually calmed myself down and was able to close my eyes. By the time the doctor was stitching me up, we were talking about his children playing lacrosse at their university, so obviously I had relaxed.

On the way out, I signed some papers and the doctor told me how to take care of the dressing, and I said, "I feel so lethargic. I just feel like a puddle. Did you give me a general anesthetic after that?"

He looked at me and smiled. "No, that was you," he said.

That was one of the most empowering things that happened in the beginning. It made me realize that my ability to mentally control some of my physical reactions was strong, a lot stronger than I would have expected. It made me realize that whatever pain or nausea was ahead of me, I had some—maybe not complete, but some—level of control over how I was going to respond to it.

—*Jodi Levy*

I'LL NEVER FORGET the day I found out my husband had cancer. It was the blackest day of my life. I remember waking up that night and being overwhelmed by a sense of emptiness. The room seemed darker than it had ever been. Miraculously enough, Dean was sleeping soundly, and the last thing I wanted to do was wake him up, but I felt so alone and scared. Then it occurred to me that the cliché about taking one day at a time was absolutely on target, and I began concentrating on just getting through this night. I started saying to myself in a singsong voice, "He's going to be okay. He's going to be okay. He's going to be okay." I kept repeating it and repeating it until I fell asleep. It became a mantra that I used throughout his illness to help me stay calm through the rough times.

—*Jessica King*

THE FACT THAT I had cancer seemed devastating, but the knowledge that other people had been through it before me and survived—had been through less refined treatments and had gone on to have families—gave me encouragement. This really hit home when I received a letter from a man I didn't even know. Grady Ballanger, a professor down in Louisiana and the uncle of a good friend of mine, felt compelled to write because he had been through the same thing. But he had been through it in the seventies. At the time, he'd been a guinea pig in the treatment of testicular cancer.

His letter made me realize that it was because of people like him that my outlook was so much better and the steps to positive results so much more predictable. The letter said to me, "Don't be alarmed. Others have gone through this before you." To hear that from someone I didn't even know, who cared enough to write, meant more to me than I can describe. I keep Grady's letter in a lockbox to this day.

—*Jim Clement*

WHEN I WAS diagnosed with breast cancer, the only women I knew who had had breast cancer had died within three years; therefore, no matter what the doctor told me, I believed that I, too, would die within three years. Then one day I met a woman who had been treated for breast cancer four and a half years before. Wow! It changed my entire view of things. I saw concrete, living proof that there were survivors beyond three years. After seeing her, I had hope.

—*Susan Fischer*

DURING MY CHEMOTHERAPY, I was in constant contact with a friend of mine from college who had had Hodgkin's disease and had been through chemo the year before. She gave me advice and told me what to expect. She prepared me for hair loss, mouth sores, and other side effects. It was helpful to call her and ask, "Did this happen to you? How long did it last? What did you do to make it better?" It was good to have someone to laugh with about having a bald head and getting stared at in the super-market, losing underarm and leg hair, going through a second puberty once chemo was over.

—Karen Manheimer

YOU NEED TO be careful about talking to other cancer patients and comparing diseases because they are often very different, even if they have the same name. The prognosis depends on the stage of the cancer and the type of treatment and medications. I spoke with one girl who also had ovarian cancer and later died, so I thought I was going to die. Instead, what you should compare and discuss is feelings: your feelings about your kids, your rela-tionships with your coworkers, and your feelings about losing your hair. These are the experiences you truly have in common.

—Diane Noyes

I WASN'T THE sweet type of patient. I allowed myself to show my anger, and I yelled and cursed through it all. My roommate in the hospital crossed herself every time I cursed. She must have blessed herself a dozen times a day. But I needed to get it out. I don't believe that passive people do well. You need to talk, scream, laugh, cry, and do whatever you have to do to get rid of what's inside you.

—Genya Ravan

The Stress of Stress

The diagnosis of cancer is very stressful. Many patients feel responsible for their recovery and do not allow themselves to experience any negative emotions because they are worried about the stress acting against their illness. They believe that if they don't keep up a happy, positive attitude, or if they don't put up a fight, they won't do well. I've found that it's helpful for cancer patients to express sadness, fear, depression, loneliness, anger, or whatever they happen to be feeling. It's important for them to admit that they feel tired or sick sometimes. Acknowledging your feelings does affect your health: It improves it.

—*Nancy Coady Lyons,*
Chief Nurse, Autologous Bone Marrow Transplant Unit,
Memorial Sloan-Kettering Hospital,
New York, New York

AFTER I WAS first diagnosed with Hodgkin's disease, I would dress in a coat and tie for doctors' appointments. I didn't know exactly why. One doctor even told me I should dress more comfortably when I went to his office. But for me it was somehow instinctual to dress up.

Later I was reading Patrick O'Brian's *The Fortunes of War,* a novel about Jack Aubrey, a British Navy commander during the War of 1812, and it suddenly became clear why I had chosen to dress for the appointments. In this passage from the novel, the enemy, an American frigate named *Chesapeake,* is in sight just off the coast of Boston, and the men on board the *Shannon* are waiting for the battle to start: "They walked on to the quarter-deck without speaking: all the officers were there, and all had changed their uniforms, some like Broke and his midshipmen, in the modern style of round hats and Hessian boots, some like Jack, in the traditional gold lace, white breeches and silk stockings; but all wore finer clothes than usual, as a mark of respect for the enemy and for the occasion."

—*Dean King*

FOR ME, IT was essential to retain control over my own treatment, to be involved in every aspect of my therapy and ultimate cure. It meant asking endless questions and reading all the medical literature I could get my hands on; it meant talking to other patients and staying alert to everything that was said and done around me; it meant never backing away from necessary diagnostic tests and therapeutic procedures, even though they might have been painful and disturbing.

In order to beat cancer, you have to fight. In order to fight, you have to learn everything you can about your enemy. This doesn't mean you don't feel fear. On the contrary, fear is normal and part of the process. What it means is that you need to have courage, and courage is not the absence of fear, but the ability to act in spite of fear.

—*Jonathan Pearlroth*

I HAD TEN days between my diagnosis and my surgery. Since I didn't know what the consequences of my surgery would be—including whether or not I would lose my leg—I decided to use those ten days to get all of my affairs in order for the month following surgery so I wouldn't have to worry about anything while I was recuperating. I took care of all my bills, arranged with my boss for the possibility of a month of leave, and had everything squared away for that month. As it turned out, I didn't need the entire month because I was back on my feet (or maybe I should say my legs) in a couple of weeks. But having taken care of everything ahead of time put me at ease and allowed me to concentrate on recovering from the operation.

—*Mark Biundo*

ONE THING THAT helped me cope was visualization. A lot of people think visualization is picturing Pacmen eating away at your cancer, but I needed a real emotional connection to make the visualization work and focus my immune system on healing. I just couldn't get an emotional connection to some Pacman eating my cancer. Instead I visualized things that meant something to me.

I had a brain tumor, and it really affected my balance. I couldn't play any sports. All I could do was walk—and even that I couldn't do very well. While I was walking, I would picture myself swimming in open water, which I associate with being very free and healthy and strong. I also went out and bought a brand-new pair of snow skis and a mountain bike and kept them in my room and visualized using them.

At first, when I tried to picture myself riding a bike or swimming or skiing, I would sort of choke or fall or wobble around. Even in my mind, I wasn't able to do it. I had to slowly build up from swimming one lap to two laps, three laps, and then on to open-water swimming. We have a house on a lake where I love to swim, and I'd picture myself there, going farther and farther out.

By the time I finally was able to swim after I finished my radiation, the doctors were amazed at how many laps I could do right off the bat.

—*Sheri Sobrato*

Moving from Fear to Peace

All emotions lie along the continuum of the two primary emotions that are themselves part of a continuum: fear and love. When we feel separated, we are operating in the realm of fear. When we feel connected, we move toward love. When we behave in self-destructive ways, it is from fear. When we gain self-knowledge and, as a result, are able to change for the better, it is through love. Love leads to inner peace. Fear goes in the opposite direction. Here are some healing lessons:

1. The essence of our being is love.
2. Health is inner peace. Healing is letting go of fear.
3. Forgiveness is the way to true health and happiness.
4. Since love is eternal, death need not be viewed as frightening.
5. We can let go of the past and of the future. Now is the only time there is.

6. We can become lovefinders rather than faultfinders.
7. We can learn to love ourselves and others by forgiving ourselves and others rather than by judging.
8. We are students and teachers to each other.
9. Giving and receiving are the same.
10. We can focus on the whole of life rather than the fragments.
11. We can perceive others or ourselves as either extending love or giving a call for help.
12. We can choose to direct ourselves to experience peace regardless of the events in our lives.
13. All minds can be joined.
14. Decisions can be made by listening for the preference for peace within us.

Blythe Ritchfield,
Executive Director, Life Center for Youth and Adults,
Santa Fe, New Mexico

I BECAME MORE religious during my illness. Many things happened that made me realize that someone was watching over me. For instance, the day my doctor told me that the disease would probably recur, my minister, whom I hadn't seen in many years, walked into my hospital room. I couldn't figure out how he knew I was there. Believing in God and in the fact that good always comes out of awful things made me feel a little easier about putting my life in His hands. And so much good came out of the experience. I awakened to how people come from out of the blue to help and thereby learned to do the same for others.

—Susan Laggner

I THINK A huge factor is attitude. At the time I was diagnosed, I had just been offered a teaching position at North Carolina State. My kids, Christopher and Megan, were only four and six years old, and my second book was a month away from being published. So being sick didn't work at that time for me. It was definitely not part of the plan. Part of what heightened my strength and resolve was my conviction that I was not going to die and leave my kids without a memory of me. I had very strong memories of my father, and I wanted them to have that too.

My experience with cancer prompted me to write *The Keeper of the Moon,* which is a novel reflecting my life. Eighty percent of the book is about my childhood, but threaded all through it is the myeloma and comparisons to my father's death from lung cancer. He was from a different generation in education and philosophy of life, and when he was diagnosed with lung cancer, he said, "That's it. I'm dead." And two months later, he was. He quit eating, and I think he starved to death as much as anything because there wasn't that much evidence of tumor in his body. But I had so much going for me; I took a totally different attitude, and it worked.

—*Tim McLaurin*

EVERYBODY IS GOING to have some bad and some good experiences. But the funniest things happen, and you have to try to have a sense of humor about them. My husband is a physician, and one day one of his patients, who is sort of the grande dame of our small town, came into his office—she is someone I've known since I was twenty years old—and she said to him, "Oh, I'm so sorry to hear that your wife is terminal."

My husband paused a minute and—I don't know how he did it—said, "Aren't we all?"

People would give me things like stuffed animals to cheer me up, and one day my son in high school came home with the cutest animal. But it was a stuffed buzzard. He didn't realize what he'd done. Of course, I laughed and didn't say anything to him. My husband nearly died laughing. I've still got that stuffed buzzard. If you can look at things in that way, you'll do very well. I think keeping an upbeat attitude—easier said than done sometimes—helps.

—*Elizabeth Martin*

Learning to Live in the Moment

Mindfulness meditation can be an important complement to traditional medical care in the treatment of cancer. When the diagnosis of cancer is given, fear is often our response. Mindfulness encourages us to be awake to this experience even if it is unpleasant. Learning to let the situation be as it is can change our relationship to it. Instead of clinging to expectations and agendas, we can learn to be present to the unfolding of the moment, to witness and observe what is happening.

Mindfulness is not magic. It is a practical approach to living in the moment—not in past regrets or future plans. It is not about fighting the disease process, but coming into relationship with it. It is about seeing and experiencing the truth.

The formal practice of mindfulness meditation consists of learning how to sit (or stand or walk) for periods of time while silently witnessing thoughts, feelings, and sensations moment by moment as they present themselves. It is a state of being rather than doing. There are no rigid rules for accomplishing it. Sitting on a cushion with the legs crossed or sitting on a chair are both acceptable. Some patients may have to lie in bed. What is important is the experience of the mind-body connection, the release of the body's tensions, and the noting and releasing of thoughts and feelings as they come and go. The focus is on the breath as it enters and leaves the body. Normally there is a tendency for the mind to leave the present moment, get lost in thought, and weave a story from the thoughts that come. When this happens, the patient observes where the mind went, watches the thoughts without identifying them, and then comes back to the breath. The breath becomes the anchor. Each time the mind wanders and we bring it back is the beginning of a new meditation. There is no failure, only increasing awareness.

The informal practice of mindfulness is a way of bringing the formal practice of meditation into daily life. It consists of being aware of the present moment in all of our daily activities, such as eating, bathing, walking, talking, and so forth. Often in the middle of these activities we find ourselves somewhere else. By noticing where we have "gone," we can bring ourselves back to the present moment.

By practicing mindfulness meditation for at least thirty, but preferably forty, minutes a day, patients can increase their sense of well-being and improve many physical and emotional symptoms of their illness. These improvements may include decreasing chronic pain through an awareness of its connection to fear, reducing the need for medications, and reducing anxiety, depression, and hostility.

Mindfulness recognizes the direct experience of being fully human. It is not about accomplishment, but about being.

—Eleanor McGehee, L.C.S.W.,
Stress Management Consultant, Sleep Disorders Center of Virginia,
Richmond, Virginia

BECAUSE MY IMMUNE system was suppressed by the chemo, I was put into isolation several times and had a lot of time to think. I started off thinking, "Why me?" I wondered what possible reason there could be for God to give me cancer at the age of twenty-five. But the more I contemplated, the more I came to believe that the question of why is useless. There is no answer to that question. I realized that I would have to be content with finding the answer to a different line of questioning: "Since this has happened to me, what good can I make of it? What can I learn? How can I turn this into something positive?" I think it was Nietzsche who said something to the effect that any hardship, so long as it doesn't kill you, will make you stronger.

—*Jonathan Pearlroth*

EVEN WITH A cancer diagnosis, there is always something to be grateful for. I was diagnosed with bone cancer in my left femur in 1978 and had to have my knee and thighbone replaced. I also underwent a year of chemotherapy. I have to wear a long leg brace, and I walk with a cane. Yet the way I look at it, I'm very lucky. If the diagnosis had come any earlier, I would have had my leg amputated. Everyone at the hospital called me "the miracle kid" because I was the first one to undergo the bone replacement surgery pioneered by my doctor, Michael Lewis. Perspective is everything! There is always a way to look at things in a positive light.

—*Donna Avacato*

CHAPTER FOUR

Getting the Most from Your Medical Team

According to the National Cancer Institute (NCI), in 1990 there were nineteen comprehensive cancer centers in the nation. Today there are nearly thirty comprehensive cancer centers, and more than fifty NCI-designated cancer centers in all. Local hospitals can also treat common cancers and help carry out more rarefied therapies. Clearly, the options for treatment are more numerous than ever and growing fast. (For a list of NCI cancer centers, call NCI at 800-4-CANCER; for more details on finding information, turn to Chapter Six, on page 117.)

Assembling your medical team and maintaining positive relationships with your doctors, nurses, and other medical staff is one of the most important aspects of cancer treatment. When you choose your primary oncologist, you are establishing a long-term relationship. Your treatment will last anywhere from several months to many years, and regular checkups extend at least five years beyond remission of the cancer.

Obviously, you need to feel comfortable with the physician on both a technical/professional level and a personal level. Of course, the correct analysis of the type and extent of cancer is the first essential. Next is the mode of treatment. How aggressive is the doctor? Are you comfortable with that level? Have the side and aftereffects of the proposed treatment been clearly discussed and considered? Have you been offered treatment choices based on what is important to you? These are important factors to consider when choosing a doctor.

One of the things that we cancer veterans almost unanimously agreed on is that no matter who your physician is, no matter what the credentials of the institution are, and no matter how much of a hurry you're in, you should have a second opinion. Any physician worth his salt should respect that and encourage it. If you are sensing otherwise, take it as a warning sign.

Among the many other aspects of the physician's care to carefully consider are his bedside manner and communication skills. Are you comfortable with the way he or she looks at you, touches you, talks to you? Does this doctor take time to explain treatments and answer your questions on a level you can understand? Does she really get to know you?

Right now these considerations might not be at the top of your list, but they become more important as you get deeper into the treatment. One woman found she had to instruct her husband to position himself in front of the door at the end of her examination so that she would have time to ask her questions before her doctor bolted. Needless to say, the relationship wasn't ideal.

Sometimes, it's hard for doctors, who spend every day dealing with cancer, to understand that you might never even have heard of an "oncologist" and don't know what "myeloma" is. There are plenty of doctors out there, however, who understand the need to explain and educate as they go. You have the right to ask questions and get answers that you don't need a medical degree to understand. If the explanation seems fuzzy, it's probably not registering. Ask again. No matter how ignorant you are about cancer and cancer-treatment terminology, you shouldn't be made to feel dumb. On the other hand, it's a good idea to read about your type of cancer so you can better comprehend and discuss your diagnosis and treatments with your doctors and nurses.

Don't underestimate your gut feeling and do consider the nuances. As Lou Ann Sabatier described her husband's decision-making process: "The second oncologist's course of therapy was only slightly different, but it was his manner and personality that caused Mike to choose him. Number one, he was older. The doctor who diagnosed Mike was Mike's age, and a little more abrasive. Mike didn't feel good about this guy, not that he was rejecting what he said, but with the second doctor, he walked in and just felt comfortable. That was as important to him as the credentials."

Finally, one thing most of us agreed on was that nurses are often a doctor's saving grace. They frequently provide the compassion that the doctors seem to hide, and they can slip into another examining room and ask the doctor the question you forgot to ask. Befriend the nursing staff, and your rewards will be ample.

The Bedside Manner Factor

WHEN IT CAME time to choose an oncologist, I consulted with several doctors. I'm not a person who likes to shop around for doctors—I've had the same internist since 1967—but since this was a person I was going to see for a long time, I wanted someone I could be really comfortable with. What convinced me instantly about the doctor I chose was that he, unlike the other three I saw, asked about me in a personal way, not just in a physical way. Did I work and did I want to continue to work? The fact that he indicated that I would be able to continue working meant a lot to me. He asked about my personal support system. Did I feel like I could get by with the help of my family, or did I need outside support? He delved into nutrition, which at that time was rather unusual. He asked if I was taking any vitamins and, unlike other doctors I've seen, didn't laugh when I told him my complicated vitamin regimen. When I saw him, he never failed to ask if anything new had transpired. He always wanted to know if I had questions. It was extremely personal treatment.

—*Toni Zavistovski*

WHEN I MET my surgeon, he barely looked at me. He never touched me or even smiled at me. I said to my husband, "He doesn't like me, and I don't want him to operate on me. We have to find somebody else." The doctor who recommended him said, "I can give you a list a mile long, but this is the man I think you should use." So I did, but I was angry that he never showed a human side. He put a wall between us.

When I went for my checkup after the surgery, I took him a copy of an article about a former surgeon that I had read in *The New York Times*. This surgeon had put up a shield between himself and his patients, and his coldness had caused him to lose so many patients that he had finally given up his practice. I gave the article to the doctor and said, "I think I understand now, but I have to tell you I'm very angry with you because I felt you never gave me any support. You're a wonderful surgeon, but you never gave me the feeling that you had any hope for me. You never touched me or smiled at me."

He said to me, "I have to tell you that when you came in, you reminded me of my wife. Because of that, I felt I couldn't help you, and that's why I was the way I was. I'm sorry. But I'm thrilled that I was able to help you." Then he gave me a hug.

Once he explained to me why he was so standoffish, I understood, but I wish he had told me from the beginning. I was glad, however, that I had said something to clear the air.

—*Bev Yaffe*

ONE DAY I was rushed to the emergency room because one of my lungs had collapsed. The physician on call decided that I should be admitted to the hospital. I found this out because I overheard her phone conversation with the floor nurse. During her conversation, she referred to me as "the lung." As weak and frightened as I was, I let her know that her behavior was inappropriate. She tried to ignore me, so I raised my voice and explained to her as clearly and loudly as possible that I was not merely a lung. She was not pleased, but I think she may have thought twice before referring to another patient as a body part.

—*Estelle Cooper*

I THINK THERE'S been a movement in the direction of better bedside manners, but with oncology, a lot of the doctors are pretty cerebral, and many are superstars in their fields and interested only in research. They can find patients to be something of an annoyance. We interfere with their research time.

I found that the nursing staff was the support system I came to rely on. They were always heroic and wonderful. And I found the same with the technicians. The support staffers in oncology tend to be really wonderful, special people and the doctors, a necessary evil.

—*Leslie Kaul*

A Good Doctor Needs to Be Compassionate

If I think they need it, I'll hug my patients. I don't care if they're fat or skinny, tall or short, old or young, black or white, or whatever. I'm a touchy-feely person. I think that's important. If you're afraid to touch patients, they'll pick up on that.

A good doctor needs to be compassionate. He needs to let the patient know he cares about them. You can be the smartest doctor in the world, but that patient is not going to get better if you upset them with your attitude. Some cancer doctors are burned out, and they get a little rude. Some protect themselves by putting up a wall, and their bedside manner is terrible. If you're not happy, there are other oncologists out there. You can switch.

If a doctor gets defensive about communication, there's something wrong. It's like a marriage. If you don't communicate, then you're just going to get more miserable. Express your concerns to the doctor right up front. Grab him by the white coat. Don't grab him by the arm. Don't grab him by the hand. Grab that white coat. That's the doctor.

I do the same thing with my patients if I think something's bothering them. I'll stop everything, put down my chart, put down my stethoscope, look them in the eye, and say, "What's wrong? Let's fix it." I think if you confront someone directly, you'll get it cleared up. It needs to be an adult-adult relationship.

—*Leland J. McElveen, M.D.,*
Hematologist/Oncologist, Baptist Medical Center,
Columbia, South Carolina

HAVING A DOCTOR who is understanding and cares for your emotional needs is as important as having a good technician. After my mastectomy, I was deathly afraid of seeing my breast, or lack thereof, so I told my doctor that under no circumstances did I want to look at my breast when he changed my bandage for the first time after surgery. He arranged to have a towel wrapped around my face, and I covered my eyes just to make sure all I saw was darkness. He changed the dressing, rebandaged me, and then buttoned up my pajamas with the loving care of a father preparing his daughter for bed. He told me I could open my eyes and that everything had turned out well—the operation was a success.

I will never forget my doctor for that small gesture of buttoning my pajamas. In that small act of kindness, he treated me like I was his family, not just his patient.

—*Rhoda Silverman*

Second Opinions

I WAS TOLD by two different pathologists that my lung cancer was the small-cell type—incurable and impossible to treat. My brother died of small-cell lung cancer just one week before I was diagnosed, and because of that, I believed that my fate was sealed. But I knew I had a fight in me.

I decided to get another opinion. I was examined by a different doctor who did a biopsy for his own pathology lab. The results came back inconclusive, which meant that I did not definitely have the small-cell type. I could be treated with drugs and surgery. I had hope. The fact that I went for a second opinion saved my life. Always get an independent second opinion—even with something that seems so black-and-white as a lab report—because sometimes cancer is not easily diagnosed the first time.

—*Maurice Chesney*

I WAS MISDIAGNOSED for the first four months of my illness. It was something I knew intuitively. I had a hell of a time trying to find a doctor to operate on me and remove the tumor, because the doctors thought my cancer was inoperable. Finally, I found a doctor who was willing to take a chance. He operated, only to discover that I did not have lung cancer after all, but an extremely rare bone/soft tissue cancer. Following your intuition and seeking a doctor who will work with you on your terms is a must

—*Kathleen Eldrid*

A FRIEND WHO had to get a bone marrow transplant later because he did not get the proper chemicals in the beginning insisted that I go to Houston to M. D. Anderson and get a second opinion about my chemotherapy. So I went there with my husband, and after looking at my records and asking many questions and learning that I had had kidney disease as a child, they decided they should change from cisplatin to carboplatin so that I wouldn't get kidney damage.

This was something that came out of an interview, a solid hour of questioning by one of the associates. They wanted to know everything I knew about myself and about my medical background, and I didn't get anything that thorough in Birmingham. At age three, I had had Bright's disease, which is an inability on the kidneys' part to filter poisons. It was caused by infected tonsils and adenoids, which were removed. But I had Bright's disease again when I was twelve. The adenoids had grown back, and they were infected, and the drainage from them caused the kidney problem again. Those things are a part of you—you don't forget when you lose three months of school in the seventh grade—but it hadn't been brought up until this interview.

I was really thankful that my friend insisted I get a second opinion. People should ask questions and not just accept the first thing they hear. Even if you hear the same thing twice, you have a better feeling for what you should do—two people have said this, so it must be right.

—*Ginnie Higginbotham*

RIGHT AFTER I was diagnosed, my doctor sent me to his plastic surgeon to talk about immediate reconstructive surgery. At that point, I didn't know anything about breast cancer or reconstruction or anything, and this guy explained what my options were—what kind of reconstruction my body could take because there are different kinds of reconstructive surgery—but he never once examined me. The only thing he asked me was, "What is your bra size?"

I said, "I don't know. We can look. I have one on."

He said, "No, that's all right. We don't need to."

I'm really small, but I could have said, "I'm a 38D," and he would have said, "Fine."

He never even looked at me, and at that point, I had no idea that that was wrong. But I went to see a surgical oncologist in New York at the urging of my sister, and he sent me to a plastic surgeon who he used. The difference between the two was like night and day. The second surgeon examined me. He took pictures. He showed my husband and me all the different things that they could do, like the various methods they use to reconstruct your breasts—which vary according to what kind of mastectomy you've had, the size of your breasts, and your skin and muscle tone—and the ways they can create a nipple once the breast has healed. He was so thorough I was shocked. The next time the other plastic surgeon was planning on seeing me was on the operating table. I was lucky that my sister convinced me to go beyond one doctor and one opinion.

—*Kristina Matsch*

A SECOND OPINION can be valid at any point in the treatment. I have a friend who went for one after her breast cancer recurred. Her first oncologist, who was in my doctor's practice, does a lot of research. Many of his patients fall into protocol guidelines, and he plugs them into the protocol, which gives them access to medicine they might not otherwise have. But that also has a tendency to make his patients feel like just a number. My friend felt like he looked at whether she fit the study or didn't fit the study, and that was the way he dealt with her, rather than as a young mother whose life was seriously threatened.

When the cancer recurred, his protocol was to give her pain medication and not to try to treat her. He thought that would be giving her false hope. She refused to accept that and switched to a new oncologist.

The difference in my friend's emotional state during these two episodes has been phenomenal to observe. She was very depressed and very negative initially even though her prognosis was not that bad. She was obsessed with having a recurrence, spent hours and hours researching things that were just minute details, and just couldn't focus on living and getting going again. Now, with the recurrence, she has had a horrible time, has been in the hospital two times on the critical list, but has remained amazingly positive throughout it all. She attributes that to having a physician who she feels cares whether she lives or dies. He hasn't given her a false sense of hope—he's been very realistic—but he is committed to healing and curing her.

She and I initially picked our doctors based on their credentials. As we got further and further into the process, we realized that the old bedside-manner factor really had a larger impact on our healing than the credentials did. Actually, you want both: access to the newest information and the best protocol and the most recently developed drug, but also a doctor who really cares.

—*Charlotte Wells*

I CONSTANTLY QUESTIONED my doctor and went for second opinions. I never put my doctors on a pedestal, and I asked for explanation upon explanation until I was satisfied that things were being done correctly. I read every book, pamphlet, and article I could get my hands on. I admit that I was a difficult patient. I am also here today.

—*Jerry Freundlich*

Communication

WHEN MY MOTHER was diagnosed, we were so overwhelmed that we didn't ask the doctor many questions. Then when we got home, we realized how much more we needed to know. I called the doctor the next day with a list of questions, and both he and the nurse were very helpful about making things clear to us. It made us feel a lot better.

You need to communicate with your doctors so you understand what is going on. The more you talk, the more comfortable you become, and the less scary the disease is. Communication takes cancer out of the realm of fear and taboo and brings it into the realm of hope and possibilities. Speak to your doctor as much as you need to in order to keep up on every detail of the treatment. Don't be afraid of your doctor—he is just human, after all.

I once had to raise my voice with the doctor and say, "Look, this is my mom who is sick, and you are going to have to give us all the time we need to understand what's going on." Always try to make a special connection with doctors and nurses so they remember you and don't just treat you like a case or a number.

—*Abby Drucker*

MY DOCTOR WAS wonderful from the very beginning. She explained everything clearly, and we enjoyed open communication. If I ever called her, she would call back immediately. I once asked her why she never asked me about what I ate and she said that she had never studied nutrition in medical school. They didn't understand the correlation back then. Yet, she was intrigued by my interest in diet and meditation. Years later, she began to study it more seriously. Open communication, not necessarily agreement or common perspective, is most important when dealing with your doctor.

—*Elsa Porter*

DURING THE COURSE of my treatment, I learned to speak up about what was important to me. For example, I felt strongly about being treated as a complete person, not just a diseased lung, but my oncologist wasn't of the same mind. When he first started to treat me, he never asked any questions about my emotional state.

I found out from his nurse, who was friendly and concerned, that he was a new father, so at the next session, I asked him about his daughter. We chatted for a few minutes about her, but he still did not ask about my family. After a few visits, I came out and told him that if he was interested in my recovery, as I was sure he was, he needed to inquire about all of me. He said that he didn't have time for chitchat and that his nurse would fill in those gaps. I did not give up. Each time I saw him, I told him how crucial my emotional well-being was to my recovery.

After a few months, he began to take my request seriously. When I came in, he'd relax for a few minutes and really talk to me. Our working relationship improved tremendously. In the end, he even asked me to meet some new residents and to explain to them how important the whole person is to healing.

—*Estelle Cooper*

I WAS TOLD by my doctor that my recovery from throat surgery would take two weeks. Luckily for me, a nurse told me it would take months. She said that the doctor was being optimistic and that the truth was that I was going to get my ass kicked. She scared me, but I appreciated her candor, and from then on, things became real. I knew that between the day of my first diagnosis and the day of full recovery, there would be a long darkness that I would have to deal with. But being prepared for the darkness made it easier to deal with, and I knew that eventually there would be light. I've learned that the truth, although painful, can be freeing. Ask your doctor to give you the plain, honest truth.

—*Tony Dalo*

WHEN YOU GO to the doctor, you want to communicate, but sometimes you simply can't. So in between, my wife and I would collect our questions in a book and then when we went to the doctor, we'd present all our questions. Then we'd have to write down his answer because a week after a visit I would say, "No, the doctor didn't say that," and my wife would say, "Yes, he did." And we'd go to the book, and the answer would be there. You just can't hear everything you want to hear at the time. Or you hear it through a warped listening process.

—*Frank Sheridan*

GOING THROUGH THIS process, one of the best things I did was keep my own medical file. Whenever you switch doctors or get referred to another type of doctor, it can be difficult to get all your records. You have to arrange to have copies released from every office you've been to. If you obtain copies at each visit, it's much easier, and you have a full history of your own. Each time I see a doctor, I ask for a copy of the doctor's report, or I leave a written note asking them to send it to me. I usually find the staff very helpful when I explain why I'm doing it. I tell them, "I'm keeping a copy because I've seen a lot of doctors, and I need to have a medical history so that I'm not writing to ten different places."

You have a right to your own records and results. But they can only release a report about the work they've done. So if a file has another doctor's stuff in it, they can't send that part. That's why I get a copy at each stop. Initially, a lot of my work was investigative. I was getting referrals and seeing many specialists. Having my own records certainly saved me tons of time. Later, I'd forget what happened six months or a year before, but I could go back and look at my history anytime.

—*Rachel Kaul*

ONE DAY AT the hospital I was almost given the wrong chemo. Incredibly, it was my doctor who made the mistake. The error was probably not critical, certainly not life-threatening, but it taught me an important lesson: If my doctor could screw up, then anyone and everyone could screw up. The hospital staff was made up of hardworking and caring professionals, but they were overworked and had too many patients to look after.

Up to that point, I had felt that my responsibility toward a cure was in the emotional realm—strengthening my will to live and finding the determination to fight and endure. But from then on, I also assumed control over the day-to-day management of my therapy. I could not allow myself to become passive. I told myself that this was my life, and I could not expect anyone else to care as much about preserving it as I did. So I kept a close watch over everything that was done to me, questioned every treatment that was planned for me, and noted every little detail of each medical procedure.

And I did have to intervene a number of times to protect myself against mistakes and omissions. For example, the evening before my stomach surgery, the hospital staff brought me a veal parmesan dinner. You don't have to be a genius to figure out that you shouldn't eat a heavy meal before stomach surgery, but what if I'd given in and allowed my zeal for Italian food to get the better of me? Can you imagine the surgeon's surprise when he opened me up and found a partially digested veal cutlet in my belly?

—*Jonathan Pearlroth*

Advice from a Doctor: How to Be a Good Patient

While you can debate endlessly about whether a healthy attitude has an impact on tumor growth, there is no doubt that patients who are optimistic and easy to deal with get more out of their doctors and nurses. Here are some suggestions for establishing a good relationship with your medical team:

Ask questions. The more you ask, the more informed you become. When you are better informed, you then ask better questions. It's a positive cycle.

Become a participant in your care. Even though doctors and nurses often seem rushed—and even brusque at times—it's because we have a lot to do, not because we don't want you to be involved.

If something is wrong, talk about it. If you have a complaint about your care, bring it up, but try to let some of the little things slide or you may put unnecessary strain on your relationship with your doctor. Try to understand how your medical team works in the modern-day hospital setting.

Express your fears to your doctor. Too many people feel they need to keep a lid on their feelings in front of their doctors. I want to know my patients' emotional status so that I can address their needs.

Michael Andreeff, M.D.,
Chief of Molecular Hematology and Therapy,
Stringer Professor for Cancer Treatment and Research,
M. D. Anderson Cancer Center,
Houston, Texas

My oncologist took a hard-line approach and was very strict and disciplined in his handling of patients. I liked his attitude, but it doesn't appeal to everyone. In one instance, when I was probably three months into my chemo and he was on vacation, one of his colleagues was overseeing my case. I was feeling bad and went back into the hospital two or three times because my blood counts were so low. I went home on a Sunday, and I was due to start chemo the following Monday. I asked this colleague whether I should come back for the chemo, and he said, "Oh, no, I'll let it go this time." Well, on Tuesday morning my telephone rang, and it was my regular oncologist. He said, "Where in the hell were you? I want your body here now." At the time, I was a little grumbly, but in the long run, his approach worked out best for me. That was why I had chosen a doctor who was going to be aggressive and hard on me and push me to undergo whatever he thought should be done.

—John Hall

I WENT ON a macrobiotic diet because it had been successful for others and would give me some control. While I was on the diet, I had mixed feelings—if I were to survive, I would have to eat that way for the rest of my life, and I wasn't sure I could take it!

As it turned out, I relapsed while I was on the diet. I went back to my oncologist, and when I told him about my diet, we wound up having an altercation. He was guilty of the worst kind of arrogance—he was completely contemptuous of my dietetic efforts. A doctor should never demean a person's attempts to care for himself, even if he doesn't think they work. I let him have it in front of a waiting room full of people. This was a very important event in my healing process because I realized I was capable of honoring my own perceptions and feelings, even if authority figures disagreed.

From then on, I went with my instincts, which made me an uncooperative patient. After my treatments, I refused to go only for quarterly checkups. That would have driven me nuts. I needed to be able to go in whenever I was concerned, not to wait for a predetermined time. So my doctor allowed me to come in three times a week or once a year, whenever I wanted. This gave me a sense of comfort and control.

—*Joe Kogel*

MY DOCTORS TOOK out my right ovary, and they wanted to take out the left one because they thought the disease would spread to it, but I wanted kids so I told them, "No way." I wasn't willing to accept their recommendation. The hospital said, "We can't release you because we think you should have a hysterectomy." I told them to jump in a lake and signed myself out, relieving them of responsibility.

My husband and I found a doctor who supported my desire for pregnancy. He watched me for a year until I got pregnant. Then he checked the left ovary to see if the disease had metastasized as predicted, but it hadn't. I got pregnant again a year and a half later.

I was in total denial of the disease, maybe because I was twenty-eight and too young to contemplate dying. My priority was to have a kid. The cancer was secondary. I was never afraid of the cancer. I don't know if that helped my health or not. But I focused on what was most important to me—having kids—and thankfully, I succeeded.

—*Madeleine LaPorte*

AFTER MY SURGERY, I was given a choice of protocols. I could go with the current standard or participate in a trial in which you were randomized either into the standard protocol or a newer, more aggressive one. The standard one had about a forty percent overall survival rate at the time. They thought the new one might be better, but they had no concrete evidence yet. It was much more intensive. You had to be in the hospital and be hydrated by IV beforehand. It was very invasive, and one of the potential side effects was deafness.

I think that was the most horrible time my family ever had—crying and screaming and everyone so upset. We were being forced to make a decision about a world we knew nothing about. Once I entered one protocol, I wouldn't be a candidate for the other, ever, and if that turned out to be the better one, I would have missed my chance. But possibly losing my hearing seemed like a high price to pay to test the new protocol.

Back then we were frustrated because we thought they all knew the right answer and were not telling us everything. Now I know that the doctors themselves really didn't know which was better. It was a test to find out. Brain tumors sound like such a highly scientific thing, but it's a very subjective world.

In the end, I decided to refuse the randomization and go with the standard. I knew that if I were in the newer protocol, it would mean a more debilitating day-to-day life. And I knew that if I was always sick, I would never have it in me to beat it. It turns out I made the right decision.

—*Katie Brant*

I HAD A very aggressive attitude that motivated me to beat my cancer and I did a tremendous amount of reading on melanoma.

In the beginning, I was the one who insisted that the doctor cut off the bump on my ear. Once the results of the biopsy came back, the doctor told me he had never known anyone to survive my kind of cancer and gave me six months to live. Well, cutting the bump off as I had demanded proved to be worthwhile. After one of my reconstructive surgeries failed, I suggested to my doctor how to redo it, based on information I had gathered from all around the country. He hadn't heard of that approach, but he tried it and it worked. Being aggressive—and informed—paid off.

As an aside, I think it's important to charm your doctors—charm them differently than others charm them so they see you as their special patient. If you can entertain them, they will want to help you. Their profession is practically devoid of laughter, so make them laugh and they won't forget you.

—*Bill Goss*

CHAPTER FIVE

Testing, Testing, 1-2-3

The Cancer Dictionary by Roberta Altman and Michael J. Sarg, M.D., describes over two hundred tests used for diagnosing cancer. Many of these will occur in the blood testing, so other than the finger prick to get your blood, they will be virtually unbeknownst to you. But a relentless battery of very obvious, and sometimes painful, tests is necessary with any cancer treatment. If ever you need a sense of Zen, in addition to a sense of humor, this is the time. Patience is a virtue in waiting to have the test done, in cheerfully allowing the test-takers the necessary time to achieve what they need to do, and in waiting for the results.

In most cases, you simply need to resolve to accept the waiting time and to try to make it productive. Instead of bashing your head against the wall in anger as you wait an hour to get in to do a ten-minute test, be sure to bring something to occupy your time—work to do, a letter to write, or a book to read. If you have a flexible schedule, tell the receptionist when you call to make an appointment that you'd like to come in early, late, just after lunch, or whenever the wait is usually the shortest. They'll almost always be glad to oblige you.

If it is a crucial test, and you need it as soon as possible, simply grab the first available appointment, and knowing how important the test is, consider the wait part of the test itself. Hey, at least the wait doesn't hurt.

Your veins will be poked and prodded and eventually you'll learn to quickly point out to new blood-takers the veins they shouldn't even bother with. If the nurse or intern is particularly inept at finding a vein, request someone else. Anesthesiologists are particularly handy at finding a good vein and inserting the needle; if you're in a hospital, and they're having trouble finding a vein, request that one be sent for. In any case, no matter what the test, demand professionalism and don't hesitate to ask for a doctor or supervisor if you think something is being done improperly.

Waiting-Room Blues

DOCTORS' WAITING-ROOM lines can be discouraging. They can make you mad—you're on time; why can't the doctor be? At first I was angry, and then I learned to use my waiting-room hours—yes, hours—constructively. All I had to do was get one fundamental thought set in my brain: No matter what else I wanted to do, no matter how sunny it was outside and how dark it was in the waiting room, the only truly important mission of my day was the one I had come to accomplish right there. Waiting was part of that mission.

Blood tests, X rays, CAT scans, MRIs—they're all part of the treatment and assessment process. So waiting to have those tests is part of working toward getting better. And I was glad for every opportunity to work toward getting better. Whether I was reading the newspaper or a novel, writing a letter, or doing a crossword puzzle, I learned to enjoy that time. It became bonus time because I was both *actively* working to get well and doing something else constructive.

—*Dean King*

IT'S FUNNY BECAUSE years after my treatment when I was doing volunteer work, I met a guy who had been in my doctor's waiting room during the same period I was, and I didn't recognize him. It was basically because I was completely and totally in my own space. I would read books about healing or meditations, or study the Bible for a class I was taking, or visualize—anything to use the waiting-room time effectively instead of sitting there getting frustrated.

—*Sheri Sobrato*

Blood Tests

IRONICALLY, ONE OF the most physically painful parts of my whole treatment was the finger prick I received at the beginning of each visit to my oncologist's office. It was administered by Nina, the sweetest ol' European lab technician to ever prick a finger. We'd talk about the weather as she wiped my fingertip with cool alcohol, and helplessly I would look off across the tiny lab space in anxious anticipation. It was one of those little gizmos with a prick on a pendulum that shoots down like a missile to your fingertip, ending in an ant-sized nuclear explosion of pain. Despite Nina's disarmingly sweet charms—You don't have to worry, she would lilt, I never hurt—it hurt like hell. And it kept hurting in the waiting room afterward as I pressed a cotton wad to my wound.

I dreaded that finger prick almost as much as anything. Several visits into my treatment, however, I noticed a strange sensation that overtook me as I squirmed in that cold, hard chair waiting for the missile to fall. The best way I can describe it is that my skin would start to hum all over, as if my nervous system was sending out a protective energy force. This force, or shield, somehow swallowed up the pain of the finger prick. Even today, when I return to the doctor for a checkup, I experience this. I am delighted by my body's ability to protect me.

—*Dean King*

I REMEMBER ONE intern—they are the ones who usually take the blood samples—who couldn't find the vein. This guy was just poking around. I said, "What are you doing?"

"Well, I'm trying to find a vein."

I said, "Could you get the resident and have him do it? I don't want you doing this." He was kind of in a huff, but he went and got the resident. You don't have to sit there and let somebody who's studying to be a doctor poke around in your arm to find a vein. If they can't find it on the second try, get them out of there.

—*Richard Brookhiser*

I HAVE ALWAYS been squeamish about needles. I dreaded blood tests and the daily ritual of the white coat coming into my hospital room with a needle and a vial. I asked my doctor if there was any way around this, and he suggested that I have my blood taken through my IV. That way I only had to be stuck once for each treatment. I also learned to ask for baby butterfly catheters, tiny little needles that hurt less with my small, rolling veins. These little things certainly made the trips to the lab less stressful.

—*Marcia Moosnick*

RIGHT BEFORE TRAINING camp, I went back to see the chemo-therapist who had diagnosed me. During my appointment, he found an elevation of an enzyme, alkaline phosphatase. It was a precursor to the cancer coming back. So he called to see if it had been elevated at my checkup three months before. It had been. Their response? "Oh, yeah, I guess it was. Gee, if we'd known who it was, we would have done something about it."

Basically, I think a doctor ordered a blood report, but nobody ever looked at it. One of the things I stress is that you have to be your own quality control. Another thing is that you have to tell the doctor, "Listen, I want you to be the coach here. Everything has got to come through one person, you. If you order a test, you look at the results. If you send me to another doctor, you see what that doctor says. You're the guy who has to coordinate everything because otherwise things like this can slip through the cracks."

I've heard that they now have nurses doing that at Sloan-Kettering. A nurse is in charge of gathering all the lab reports and making sure the doctor gets the information he needs. That's extremely important. If you're ordered to go have a test and nobody looks at it, what the hell good is it? Make darn sure someone looks at it.

—*Karl Nelson*

CAT Scans

MY FIRST CAT scan scared the living daylights out of me. Not only was I scared about the results, but the process itself freaked me out. I had to lie down on a narrow platform with an IV in my arm. The platform slid back and forth through a doughnut-shaped machine and I was told to alternately breathe and hold my breath as they took slides. You can't move, and the room is always cold. So ask for a blanket. . . . No, ask for several.

One morning I went for a CAT scan, and they told me to drink two enormous glasses of something they called "contrast," which highlights the scan for the radiologist. It had the thick consistency of a yogurt drink and a chalky bitter taste, coupled with the overly sweet lemonade flavor they used to try to make it more palatable. With each sip, I felt more nauseous. Later, I learned that you can request different flavors. In fact, eventually I took in my own favorite drink—diet black cherry soda—and mixed the contrast beverage myself. It was never more than barely palatable, but at least I got to choose the flavor.

—Karen Manheimer

IT HAD ALREADY been a long day when the computer linked to the CAT scan froze up while I was lying on the table. As I told the technician when he brought the hand-held urinal to the scan bed, "No problem. I've learned to live with a lot of things." We laughed. At that point I not only had an IV pumping dye into my bloodstream, I had four large cups of barium "bismal"—a murky, chalky pink drink—in my stomach, and just to round things out, an enema that had put who knows what into my colon. I lay there for a while praying the computer would come back up. It never did. Despite the inconvenience, I tried to take it all in stride. The same sophisticated high-tech machinery that can help save your life can also go on the blink.

I went back the next morning bright and early. With all the requisite goodies applied once again, I was back on the CAT scan's sliding bed, which moves in tiny increments through the middle of what looks like a giant, cored computer disk. The CAT scan made a noise like a rapid-fire View-Master as the forty-five shots of my neck were snapped. Once again, the computer bank jammed. So I just shut my eyes. The barium rumbled through my stomach like a go-cart in need of a tune-up. But the room was cool and the blankets on top of me were nice and warm, and I didn't actually have to do anything but lie there and relax. Sure enough, we finally did get the shots of my back taken too—just in time for me to sprint victoriously to the nearby bathroom.

—*Dean King*

I ALWAYS GOT my CAT scan results the day the scan was taken—before my oncologist even got them. I waited in the office until the doctor who read the scans gave me the results. He always prefaced it with, "I'm reading it while it's still wet, so what I can see is such and such, but don't hold me to it because the results may change once it's dry."

I'd say, "Okay. Just send me the report when it's dry." I did this because I wanted to have control over my case. After all, it's my body, and I wanted to know. But that's me. You could probably talk to fifty other patients who would say, "I don't want to know. Let the doctor tell me if he has anything to say." But I think that knowing first gave me power.

—*Bev Yaffe*

Magnetic Resonance Imaging (MRI)

NOW THEY HAVE modern machines, but when I was receiving treatment, the MRI was a tube you had to climb into. It was very small, and most people found it claustrophobic. They put you on a sled, and the sled slid into the tube.

They put me on the sled, and they tried to push me in, and the nurse said, "How ya doing?"

I said, "I'm stuck."

So they pulled me out, which caused me to burn my elbows on the walls of this thing. They turned me around and put me in feet first with my arms over my head, and then I fit into the tube.

When you get in there, you have to remain still for roughly half an hour, and that's a bitch. The top wall is about two inches from your face. To compensate for that, they have a microphone that picks up anything you say.

They said, "How ya doing?"

I said, "I'm here. I can deal with this."

So the nurse said, "What kind of music do you want to hear—classical or jazz?"

I chose classical. I'm lying there stuck in this tube, and they start playing, of all things, Mozart's *Requiem*!

She was a nice young thing, so afterward I suggested that when someone is stuck in a tube she not play hymns for the dead.

Anyhow, I found a use for my weird sense of humor. You need it at a time like that, when you're so vulnerable.

—*Frank Sheridan*

Bone Marrow Tests

I READ A lot of the literature on bone marrow tests, and all of it indicated that the test was really painful, even though you're given a local anesthetic. But when they did it, I was pleasantly surprised because it really wasn't that bad.

The aspiration is like having a tooth pulled. You can feel the pulling and the pressure, and sometimes just that feeling can make you kind of queasy. One time, I got very light-headed. They take the marrow from your lower back, those flat hipbones.

A bone marrow biopsy is a little different. With a biopsy, they take a little piece of the bone too, so it's a little more painful. Even though you are given a local, the pain shoots down the back of your leg. It's not so bad that you can't tolerate it. It's more uncomfortable than it is painful. They have to penetrate your bone, so the doctor's got all his weight down on the instrument—I can't tell you what instrument because I keep my eyes closed. I think mainly it's the idea of what the doctor's doing. The whole idea that he's penetrating my bone and taking something out makes me very uneasy. Each time he does it, my palms get clammy, and my heart races a little bit, but afterward I always say, "It's not that bad. I don't know why I get myself worked up over it."

—*Michele Fox*

THEY PUT THIS corkscrew device into your hipbone. You can actually hear the screw going in. This sounds stupid, but it's like opening a wine bottle—you can hear the squeak going through your bone. You can feel the pressure because they have to push hard. You know it's going in, but you can't feel the pain.

I was anesthetized. I was given a series of needles in the hip. They numbed my hip and then gave me another one deeper and then another even deeper and I think they actually anesthetized the bone. It hurt afterward like a bruise hurts, but that was nothing. It's not the pain—it's the squeak.

For me, the worst thing about the bone marrow biopsy was that there was a delay—it seemed to be interminable, a week or five working days—to get the results. I had learned enough about lymphoma to know that the most significant thing was the possibility that it had spread. So my feeling at the time was that the bone marrow test was a life-or-death diagnostic tool. Waiting for the results of the test was tough—sitting in the oncologist's office waiting for him to give me the report and knowing that in five minutes he might tell me I had six months to live.

—Jerry Dunne

I HAD A bone marrow test right at the beginning and, I think, three times in all. I'd meditate to get through each test, and it really helped me deal with the anxiety and the pain. You can take courses in transcendental meditation. They give you a mantra and you close your eyes and repeat the mantra, and it puts you into a semiconscious state—just brings you down real mellow— and really helps you deal with fear. It's like a prayerful state. You're lying on the table, and by the time they get to you and get all their stuff together, you easily have time to reach that calm and meditative state.

—Mamie Dixon

Rectal Exams

SOONER OR LATER—no matter what or where your cancer is— your internist, your oncologist, or your oncological surgeon, if not all three, is most likely going to want to give you a rectal exam. Better safe than sorry. But having been examined at different times by all three, I can tell you, it didn't have to be as painful as it usually was.

As they say in the movies, I'll never forget my first time. The surgeon, a small, ruthless Frenchman, told me to get on my hands and knees and push as if I were having a bowel movement. I don't know where he learned his technique—from a torture manual, I think. He shoved in his rubber-gloved finger fast and hard as I exhaled in agony. As he probed back and forth, I gasped in pain. I could barely sit down for the next two days. Only once did I have it done humanely, when the doctor actually took the time to smear on some gel and then slowly worked in his finger. Don't get me wrong—it wasn't a picnic in the park, but I didn't have to grunt in agony. And the recuperation time was shorter too.

Clearly, it's a difficult matter to talk about. This examination seems to both terrify and bring out the worst in physicians. It's as if they feel that if the act isn't wholly circumspect—i.e., painfully brutal—then it could impugn their integrity. I've never had it done by a female, so I can't draw any gender conclusions, but I do recommend having a frank word with your doctor before you proceed with the examination.

—Dean King

The Waiting Game

THE WHOLE PROCESS of reaching a diagnosis, of going through the initial testing, takes forever. One of the most difficult things to handle, with any disease, but particularly with cancer, is the sense of urgency you feel as a patient—"Oh, my God, I have cancer"—while the health-care machine takes it at a very different pace. On their terms, they're moving very quickly, but when you're talking about living in fear and ignorance about what is going on with you, it seems an eternity.

They did one biopsy on me and then another. Then I was admitted to the hospital, and I went through a week of tests—angiograms, gallium scans, I can't even remember—many, many tests. So I was in the hospital only for staging purposes.

It's not as if you go to the doctor, and you find out what you have and what you need to do about it. You go to the doctor, and you find out you have to call back in a week. And then they still don't have enough information, and it's a long, drawn-out process. The most difficult thing is to accept that you can't know stuff for quite a while because there's a lot that they don't know. And there's still a lot of guesswork, even when it comes to treatment. They can't guarantee anything. They can give you statistics. Everybody wants to know about their statistical chances, but all of that is pretty much theoretical information. It's not really practical.

—*Leslie Kaul*

I LEARNED TO never schedule a CAT scan, X ray, or other test on a Friday if at all possible. That's because when I had my bone marrow analyzed to see if there was any lymphoma in it, the test was done on a Friday morning, and I spent the whole weekend worrying about the results. Mercifully, when Monday arrived—it felt like a month—I was told that the test was negative, but I vowed never again to subject myself to a weekend's worth of torture. If possible, schedule your tests early in the week. It's much easier to reach your doctor or the lab on a Wednesday than it is on a Saturday.

—*Jonathan Pearlroth*

BEFORE I WAS diagnosed, I had a routinely scheduled mammogram. Usually they do two different views of each breast. This time they took third and fourth views of one breast. As soon as they took extra views, I knew. I got scared, right there. I found the lump myself the following Tuesday morning and called my nurse practitioner. She got me an appointment to see a surgeon that afternoon.

Later, after my first post-treatment mammogram, the radiology tech said to me, "You'll get a postcard with your results on such and such a day."

I said, "And if I don't want to wait that long, what do I have to do?"

She said, "Call back in a few days." That's what I did. I got the results in a few days but only because I persisted. Otherwise I would have had to wait an anxious week or two until they came in the mail.

I think people need to push their health-care practitioners to get results faster. At the hospital where I work, when somebody gets a mammogram after having had breast cancer, they can call back in a few hours and get the results. The HMO I use said there was no way they could do that, so I talked to the patient representative. I said, "I think you need to figure out a better way because people aren't sleeping, me being one of them." Now she's taken it to a higher level to see what they can do to get the results out faster.

—*Lorraine Anderson*

CHAPTER SIX

Taking the Information Search into Your Own Hands

Never before has so much information about cancer and cancer treatment been available to the public. You can start with the National Cancer Institute's hot line, 800-4-CANCER, from which you can order the free PDQ (Physician Data Query), which contains the latest therapies for your type of cancer, along with information on institutions and doctors conducting the most up-to-date research. Two different versions are available— one for physicians and one for patients. You may want to have them send you both. Start with the latter and proceed to the former, which is more technical.

Many people are also turning to the Internet, where various sites contain studies and discussion groups regarding cancer. For instance, on America Online, there is an ongoing BMT (bone marrow transplant) chat session, where patients and former patients can share their stories and ask and answer questions.

Because the cancer front is constantly changing—too fast even for doctors always to be completely up-to-date—the Internet and the PDQ are often excellent resources. There are also many books available on cancer, cancer treatment, and complementary activities and treatments that serve as an excellent basis for a general background. Among them, *The Cancer Dictionary* by Roberta Altman and Michael J. Sarg, M.D., is a solid resource for deciphering unfamiliar terms and understanding your illness. It presents factual information without overwhelming you with scary, dated statistics. The booklet "Cancer Information: Where to Find Help," which is published by the American Institute for Cancer Research (800-843-8114, or, in Washington, D.C., 202-328-7744), is another good resource.

For rarer or more challenging cancers, once you identify the medical centers that specialize in studying and treating your type of cancer, you may want to visit and meet with the doctors to hear their recommendations. What goes into finding the right treatment and the right team in these situations is a lot of digging for information, dogged pursuit of the doctors and programs with the most experience in treating your type of cancer, and, of course, a little luck. One recent favorite story is about a Dallas couple who traveled to Houston, Philadelphia, and Pittsburgh to talk to top melanoma experts. But while they were trying to make their decision on which treatment to choose, a chance meeting in a grocery store at home in Dallas led them to a local doctor who reported his patients were having success with a doctor doing a vaccine out in California. Ultimately, they headed west.

Good things happen to those who make the effort, whether high tech, low tech, or no tech.

WHILE BOOKS ON the specifics of cancer treatment can become dated fairly quickly, they are still an excellent resource for background information and for identifying the experts in the particular field with which you are concerned. My wife, who is very interested in why things happen, did most of our research on the why's and wherefore's of what was going on in the library of Southwestern Medical School—most university libraries are open to the public, at least for onsite research. She came across the writings of a doctor in Vancouver who was a specialist on Hodgkin's disease, and she didn't stop there. She picked up the phone and called him. He turned out to be very helpful, and throughout my illness, my wife carried on a series of long-distance conversations with him. He helped us make and reaffirm decisions concerning my lifestyle and my treatment. I wouldn't hesitate to pick up the phone and call anyone who you think might have an answer for you. If they don't, they might know someone who does.

—John Hall

I WAS TOLD that my chemotherapy protocol was called M-BACOD, the latest, most up-to-date treatment for lymphoma. The letters represented the names of five different drugs. I asked questions about each one, its side effects, and the subsequent steps of the protocol, and the chemo technician seemed pleased that I was interested. Most people, she told me, ask no questions whatsoever. For me, the more questions I asked and the more I learned, the more power and control I felt I had over my situation. And any amount of control I felt was an improvement over that sense of utter powerlessness I felt the day I was first diagnosed.

—Jonathan Pearlroth

AT FIRST, I read everything I could get my hands on. Every time a new study came out, I would grab the paper or carefully listen to whatever it was or call the doctor to see if he knew about this new study, and I found that inevitably, a few months later or maybe a year later, another study would come out contradicting the previous one. I would definitely caution against going overboard. I think it's important for every patient to be properly informed, but when it's done to excess, it's ill-advised. There are too many mixed messages out there, and reading everything in sight is part of dwelling on your illness.

While I was in the hospital, one negative thing happened that I'll always remember. An oncologist recommended by a physician friend came in to see me the day after my surgery. I didn't know anything about chemotherapy other than the horror stories that everybody hears. I had just been informed that morning that they had removed seven lymph nodes and five of them were malignant, meaning I had to have chemotherapy.

In walked this oncologist. He was a brazen man with an extremely strong personality. I was asking about the chemotherapy drugs, not only about the effect on me physically but about the effectiveness of the drugs, and he started talking about specific drugs and specific effects on cancer cells. Somehow our conversation went on and on and became more and more detailed in terms of the drugs. He gave me the names of all of them, which was fine, but then he said, "When you're dealing with cancer, and when you're dealing with metastases, you can't always be guaranteed that the chemotherapy drugs are going to effectively kill all the cells." That statement threw me for a loop.

I kept asking question after question, and I tried—quite successfully I think—not to freak out. The conversation deteriorated, and finally I wound up asking, "Then what is my prognosis?" And here I had this two-year-old and four-year-old at home, and I asked this really awful question, and he said, "Oh, I would say about fifty-fifty."

Then I broke down. I just found that answer so horrifying. And he said, "Well, just consider that the glass is half full instead of half empty." Now, whenever I hear a commercial on radio or TV about the glass being half full or half empty, I can't help but remember that. Maybe the lesson is to not ask too many questions from doctors you don't know because it might create more trouble than it's worth. There is a point at which a patient can ask too many questions, and I passed it with this doctor.

—*Toni Zavistovski*

WHEN DEAN WAS diagnosed, we kept hearing that Hodgkin's disease has something like a ninety-five percent cure rate, but one evening I was reading through a bunch of pamphlets from the American Cancer Society and found that for more advanced cases of Hodgkin's (like his), the numbers fell to seventy-odd percent. I got all upset. Then I thought, "These are just numbers. They have nothing to do with Dean. Each case is individual, and no statistic can tell you what is going to happen to that person." After that, I refused to focus on numbers—I'm still not exactly sure what his stage was—and never read any more literature. Instead, we got all of our information from those who knew his case best: his doctors.

—Jessica King

MY DOCTOR'S OFFICE was nice and had tons of magazines, and they were always pretty current, which helped. But I had a really bad experience in his waiting room one time. I made the mistake of picking up an article about cancer. It listed the ten or fifteen most deadly cancers, and, of course, leukemia was number seven. That put me in a hysterical state, and when I was called to get my blood test, I was a mess. So they removed that magazine, thank God.

My doctor talked to me about it and went over the statistics again and my prognosis. He said, "I'm not going to lie to you. People die every day of leukemia, but the remission rate is getting higher, and you're doing really well, and you're going to go for your transplant. Keep your chin up, and don't read those articles."

—Michele Fox

I KNOW A lot of people with cancer won't read a damn thing. I went to the opposite extreme. I went up to the doctors' library and got on the computer and found out the latest things that were going on. The first time I read about my cancer, the cure rate was fifty-three percent, and I was meditating on that, trying to deal with that.

My sister-in-law, who's a nurse, told the doctor, "You'd better check this guy out, because he's reading everything he can get his hands on." So when I went to the doctor, he said that he'd heard I was reading, and he started kidding me about it.

Then he asked, "What was the copyright date of the book you were reading?"

That book was the *Merck Manual*—a kind of comprehensive medical book that isn't too scientific. I told him that I didn't know, maybe the late eighties.

He said, "Don't read a damn word. Oncology is at such a stage that if you read anything from the eighties, it's automatically wrong."

So I went back and, of course, the book was from '87. I went out and bought a book published in '91, and the numbers for diffuse lymphoma were over ninety percent. Oncology is exploding. They come up with new things every day.

—*Frank Sheridan*

WE'VE USED THE Internet quite a bit. When Brian was diagnosed, we were out of state, and my sister called up articles on her laptop computer. The doctors were hanging around us in the hospital lounge in Florida, watching us bring stuff up, fascinated. Apparently they had never done it themselves.

It was a valuable research tool in directing us to who was doing the research, who was getting good results, who was doing experimental work. We used Oncolink and Medlink and looked under cancer and then multiple myeloma and found the University of Arkansas. There was a lot of information about the treatments that they were doing and the numbers. We were at Mayo Clinic, but they don't do experimentals for the most part. On the Internet, my sister found Arkansas was doing phenomenal research in the area of multiple myeloma and that they had written an incredible amount of data on having longer-term remissions.

I think I could have gone to a medical library and spent my life in there and not found the information I was looking for. I wouldn't have known where to look. The Internet cut to the quick.

—*Peggy Schmidt*

Surfing the Web for Cancer Info

In the past, if you were not a subscriber to America Online, Prodigy, or CompuServe, you did not have access to any of the cancer discussion databases or forums. The new technologies for the World Wide Web make it possible for anyone who has Internet access to post questions and receive answers. It really opens up the field for people who have questions that they're afraid to ask in person, or that they don't know whom to ask, or that their doctors are not answering. It can also be a way to sit back and view questions and answers without having to participate. I can't think of an easier way to find that kind of information—especially if you don't live near a library that has medical journals and books.

You can find all sorts of information about cancer, but you have to be sure you're looking at a reputable site. Avoid the ones that give you somebody's theory that because their brother ate peaches every day, he was cured of thyroid cancer. Use your common sense. Be wary if you don't recognize a site by name. And the bottom line is that no matter what you find on the Internet, you should check all advice with your doctor.

The American Cancer Society probably gets about forty to fifty e-mail questions or comments a day. Many are very specific, such as "My mother was diagnosed with stage-three breast cancer. The doctor is advising this treatment of drugs. What should we do?" We would pass the questioner on to either a physician or our breast-cancer expert to help her get the information she needed.

Some of the more helpful cancer sites on the Internet are:

CancerNet Information (National Cancer Institute Internet site)—gopher://gopher.nih.gov/11/clin/cancernet

Oncolink (University of Pennsylvania Internet site)—access CancerNet at the above address and then type in the following address: http://cancer.med.upenn.edu/

National Cancer Institute Web site—http://www.nci.nih.gov

Cancer Guide—http://cancerguide.org/mainmenu.html

Cansearch—http://www.access.digex.net/~mkragen/
cansearch.html

—Betsy Jubb,
Former Director of Multimedia Products, American Cancer Society,
Atlanta, Georgia

WHILE SEARCHING THE Internet for info, I happened upon the following site: URL: http://www.comed.com/IMF/imf_ocir.html (must be typed exactly as shown). It has links to dozens of fabulous sites. Here are some of the links you can access from this site:

American Cancer Society

Arizona Cancer Center

Arlington Cancer Center

Bone Marrow Donors Worldwide

Bone Marrow Transplant Internet Mailing List Archives

Bone Marrow Transplant Newsletter

Canadian Cancer Society

CancerGuide (patient resource)

Center Watch—Clinical Trials Information Center

Cedars-Sinai Comprehensive Cancer Center

Chanin Institute for Cancer Research—Albert Einstein College of Medicine

Cleveland Clinic Foundation

Columbia-Presbyterian Medical Center

Dana Farber Cancer Institute

Food and Drug Administration

Fred Hutchinson Cancer Research Center

German Cancer Research Center (Heidelberg)

Hebrew University—Hadassah Medical Center

Harvard Medical School

Kaplan Comprehensive Cancer Center (NYU)

Karolinska Institute, Sweden

Leukemia Research Fund (U.K.)

Mayo Clinic

Memorial Sloan-Kettering Cancer Center

University of Michigan Comprehensive Cancer Center
Home Page

National Cancer Center, Tokyo, Japan

National Cancer Institute's International Cancer
Information Center

CancerNet

Clinical Trial Search

Journal of the National Cancer Institute

National Institute for Cancer Research of Genoa (Italy)

National Institutes of Health (NIH)

National Organization for Rare Diseases

Myeloma

Bone Marrow Transplant Information

Chemotherapy

Medical Oncology

Radiation Oncology

Surgical Oncology

One Day at a Time—a patient's chronicle of his bone marrow transplant

Roswell Park Cancer Institute

Roxane Pain Institute

National University of Singapore Biomed Server

Stanford University Medical Center

University of Texas M. D. Anderson Cancer Center

U.S. Department of Health and Human Services

Waldenstrom's Macroglobulinemia Support Group

Oncology Research Cooperative Groups

National Coalition of Cancer Survivors (NCCS) guide to cancer resources

Good luck, and happy surfing!

—*Jody Levy*

WHEN THE CANCER recurred in my liver and I was told there was no hope, I started searching for other avenues. What I found out is that many different things are being done across the country. Each hospital seems to be taking a different course, and they're getting grants for certain tests and clinical trials or what have you. It's up to the individual patient or their family—whoever can do it—to scout out as best they can all the possibilities, to get a complete picture of what is being offered.

Bear in mind that there are also many rules and regulations for trials. Frequently you're ineligible because of your age or because you've already had another treatment. But because I was able to make all these phone calls and find out, at least I felt I was participating in my own treatment, taking care of myself. You just have to keep searching until you find your place.

—*Bev Yaffe*

CHAPTER SEVEN

It's a Man's Job: Visiting the Sperm Bank

All too often doctors forget about the issue of fertility until it is too late. But for any male about to undergo chemotherapy or radiation to the pelvic region who wants to conceive children in the future, it is crucial. Ask your oncologist whether the proposed therapy will have any effect on your fertility. If there is a chance that it will, then you'll probably want to visit a cryobank to store sperm as soon as possible.

Generally, by the time you are diagnosed, you want to start treatment as soon as possible too. So chances are you will only have the opportunity to store a small amount of sperm. Time is of the essence. Also, check with your insurance company. There is an initial cost as well as an annual storage fee.

Later, if in fact your therapy has caused infertility, which may or may not be long-term, you can have the sperm shipped from your cryobank to the fertility center you are using for the process of artificial insemination or in vitro fertilization. (For more information on infertility treatments, turn to "Making Babies," on page 373.)

MY DOCTOR TOLD me there was a fifty-fifty chance that chemo-therapy would leave me sterile and if I ever hoped to have children, the prudent thing to do was to store a supply of my sperm at a bank. Since this was a whole new world for me, I called the sperm bank to ask what I had to do in preparation for opening my "account." I was told that as long as I was eighteen years old, all I needed to do was show up at their office and everything would be taken care of.

As my girlfriend and I headed over to the bank, I felt the same vague expectation of adventure as on my first excursion to a topless bar. The place turned out to be a stylish combination of plush waiting room and high-tech lab with a white-jacketed technician who occasionally turned to check on something among the important-looking machinery surrounding her. I went over to the counter and waited for the technician to notice me. "Yes, may I help you?" she said pleasantly.

"Well . . ." I said, lowering my voice. "I'd like to . . . I've come to open an account, make a deposit."

"Of course. Just fill out this form and return your sample here." She handed me a small glass. "Here's the key to your room, down the hall, number three on the left."

It was all very professional, entirely discreet. My room was sim-ply, yet tastefully, decorated. A nice plant, a print of a famous paint-ing, a wooden table, a lamp, a big reclining lounge chair, and a few copies of *Playboy, Penthouse,* and *Hustler.* The magazines were the only tip-offs in the entire place as to the nature of the business, and even they were discreetly contained in plain leather binders. I asked my girlfriend to come in the room to help me do what I had to do, but since she was too embarrassed, I relied on Miss Novem-ber to help me out. I left the room with my sample and furtively carried it to the counter, feeling awkward about handing a perfect stranger—and a woman at that—a glass containing semen I had just produced behind a door not ten yards away.

The technician looked at my deposit matter-of-factly, as if she were a teller checking the currency I had just handed her, and told me that I could call in a few days to make sure that the motility of my sperm was satisfactory. If so, I would be billed an annual storage fee, and if I didn't pay after a few warnings, my sperm would legally become the property of the bank, to use or destroy as they saw fit.

"Aha," I thought, smiling. "So that's their game. They're going to hold my kids for a yearly ransom!" If I didn't pay, they would murder my children or sell them off to be raised by strangers. But then again, the four-hundred-dollar storage fee—compared to, say, the annual cost of orthodontics—didn't seem very much to pay for giving my kids a chance to be born.

I asked the technician how long the samples could be safely stored. She said that since they would be frozen in liquid nitrogen, and therefore couldn't be damaged by power failures or any other electrical mishaps, they could be stored indefinitely. I silently said goodbye to my babies and promised to return in a few days to produce a few million more potential brothers and sisters to keep them company.

—*Jonathan Pearlroth*

THE SPERM BANK said that I could "collect" my sperm samples at home as long as I could deliver them to the sperm bank within forty minutes. They gave me some clear plastic jars. I was living with my parents at the time, and the first day, my mother, who is a physician but who nonetheless euphemized my whole experience, said, "I'll wait in the car while you go get *ready*." So I went up to the bedroom and got my sample, but I didn't want to carry it in the clear plastic jar all the way to the sperm bank sitting next to my mother. I looked around in the kitchen and grabbed a little paper bag that was left over from my childhood. It was white with an orange pumpkin on one side and a black cat on the other, and it said, "Trick or treat!"

—*David Rakoff*

MY SPERM-BANK ODYSSEY began when they were plugging the chemotherapy into my arm and one of the nurses happened to say, "You've been to the sperm bank, right, Evan?" No one had ever mentioned a sperm bank to me. They unhooked the tubes from my arm as if they were defusing a bomb and sent me on my way to the sperm bank.

I was given a manila folder filled with I didn't know what and was sent to a little cubicle that was refrigerated down to about forty degrees. There was a metal folding chair, a little side table, and a box of tissues. I opened the folder and found a dozen or so pornographic magazines, which completely startled me, and I remember wondering if they subscribed to these magazines or if it was someone's job to go shopping periodically to keep the supply varied and up-to-date.

My girlfriend had come into the room with me because we had decided to make the sperm-bank expedition fun and to try not to lose touch with our sex life. But it became a very surreal thing in that I was about to enter a world of pain and torture, and here I was in this room for an activity supposedly associated with pleasure and had to give myself an orgasm in the midst of only humiliation. So I wound up coming into the little plastic cup while thinking about the story I would have to tell my children someday of how they came to be.

I made two trips into New York on two consecutive days, which is not the way you're supposed to do it. You're supposed to skip a day in between. Then before I went down to Baltimore for my bone marrow transplant, on a whim I had myself tested and found that there was still a viable sperm count. So I went to a sperm bank in Baltimore.

The Baltimore sperm bank had this elaborate system whereby you went into a room that had a reclining chair and magazines arranged in order of explicitness on a rack on the wall. If you wanted to pick one of the least explicit magazines, they were in front so you wouldn't have to glimpse the coarser material. You went to a little box on the wall that you opened. There was a plastic specimen jar with your name and patient ID number already on it. When you were through, you put the specimen back in the cabinet and left through another door. Your leaving through that other door alerted a technician on the other side of the wall to retrieve the specimen and let the next person into the room. So, in other words, after your doctor prescribed orgasm, you didn't have to face anyone.

In New York, I had wound up on a line of men each holding our little specimen jar waiting to hand it to a woman in a window who then weighed the specimen and announced the weight like at a boxing-match weigh-in and recorded it in a book.

So those were my two sperm-bank experiences. To top it off, the storage rates in New York have risen to $1,200 a year. In Baltimore, they've remained $100 a year.

—*Evan Handler*

Choosing and Using a Sperm Bank

Certain types of cancer surgery, chemotherapy, and radiation therapy can cause permanent sterility in men. If you want to have children after treatment, you need to consider freezing and storing sperm at a sperm bank. Here are ways to improve your chances of preserving fertility:

Talk fertility from the start. Don't wait for the doctor to bring it up. Discuss your case with the first doctor involved in your therapy. Many oncologists focus only on saving lives. They might not consider what will happen if they're successful.

Pick a good bank. You'll want one with proper freezing equipment and storage facilities, one that labels samples accurately and that you can trust to help you maximize your future fertility. Unfortunately, only California and New York license sperm banks, which makes it hard to weed out the less qualified operations in other states.

Your best bet is to talk to the experts and ask for recommendations. The American Society for Reproductive Medicine, or ASRM (1209 Montgomery Highway, Birmingham, AL 35216-2809; 205-978-5000), provides a list of more than one hundred recommended sperm banks in the United States and ten in Canada. The American Association of Tissue Banks, or AATB (1350 Beverly Road, Suite 220-A, McLean, VA 22101; 708-827-9582), will send you a list of their six accredited sperm banks. (Because accreditation is not required by law and the process is expensive and time-consuming, few volunteer to undergo it.) If you do not live near one of the banks on the list, ask the director of one of the accredited banks for a reputable bank in your area.

Contact an IVF center. Because doctors at in vitro fertilization centers rely on the samples stored in sperm banks, they are up-to-date on what to expect from a good bank. Ask for recommendations. There is at least one IVF center in every state. To find one in your area, contact the ASRM (see above).

Get a consultation. Once you have chosen a sperm bank, the ideal approach includes a preliminary semen analysis to determine the volume and quality of specimens and a test cycle of freezing and thawing to determine the survivability rate of your sperm. Because of limited time, however, collecting specimens in cancer patients often involves a series of compromises.

Store as many separate samples as possible. During intrauterine insemination, the standard number of postthaw sperm cells per stored sample used is fifteen to thirty million. Because pregnancy rates do not drop until you get below five million cells, separate the samples into as many frozen vials as possible. You can always combine them once they're thawed, but you can't thaw a sample, take a portion, and refreeze it because there is about a fifty-percent kill rate in the freezing-thawing cycle. The cost of freezing more vials should not be prohibitive.

Charles A. Sims, M.D.,
Cofounder and Medical Director, California Cryobank,
Los Angeles, California

DESPITE THE INTENSE anxieties of just having been diagnosed with Hodgkin's disease, I remember one recurring incident that did make me laugh. Before my first chemo session, visiting the sperm bank was my primary task. I worked in an editorial office, with several women my age and older, the kind of open-floor office where you overheard everything, and everyone knew what everyone else was doing. We were all friendly, but in a work situation, my trip to the sperm bank would have been an embarrassing topic of conversation. So when the hour of my appointment neared, I simply announced that I was going to the "bank." I always got a chuckle out of that as I walked down Third Avenue to the lab. The women at work never asked what took so long, and I never mentioned the nature of my deposit.

—*Dean King*

PART TWO

Going to War

CHAPTER EIGHT

Courage in the Face of Chemo

This is it. There are no conscientious objectors in this war. You've been through boot camp, and now you're about to enter the field of battle. You can do it. You *will* do it. We've been there and made it. And there have been some heartening improvements in the process since then.

One thing that most of us agreed on was that the anticipation of chemotherapy was tougher than the chemo itself. Sometimes things in life get blown out of proportion. Persevering takes strength and courage and fortitude, especially in the later rounds as the process wears thin on you. But the truth is you simply have to keep showing up. And you may have to grit your teeth a little bit.

Sometimes there is a burning sensation as the chemicals enter your veins. Sometimes you can feel cold or hot flashes. Some chemo you can taste. But these things are only nuisances compared to the benefits of the therapy. You'll have a nurse or doctor nearby to assure you that the reactions are normal and to check on anything that might be considered abnormal. Psychologically this is the important thing, to know that you are competently and compassionately attended. If something is bothering you too much, it can and should be changed.

After the initial fear of chemotherapy is long gone, the side effects—lethargy, nausea, ill humor—do tend to mount. The veins in your arms might feel like bamboo and you might have lost your hair. This, too, will pass. The best news is that the intense flulike nausea, which has long been associated with chemotherapy, has been greatly alleviated by a drug called Zofran. One patient who was treated in the pre-Zofran days told us he vomited all night after his first chemo treatment. "I felt numb, depleted, and disoriented," he said. "And the thought of having to endure six more months of chemotherapy came close to triggering a new round of nausea." Now many people who take Zofran never get sick at all.

That's not to say you'll rush right out and eat a feast of paella and sangria, but with the resources available today, including narcotics to calm nerves, much can be done to limit a chemotherapy patient's discomfort. The National Cancer Institute (800-4-CANCER) offers a free booklet called "Chemotherapy and You: A Guide to Self-Help During Treatment," which explains the basics of chemotherapy and how you can best work with it.

Preparing Yourself

I WILL NEVER forget what my nurse Carmen told me before my first chemotherapy treatment. She said, "Think of this as an army of workmen with sledgehammers going in to beat up the bad guys." For me it was the first effort at positive visualization, and it really worked. Looking at it like that made me feel like I was getting stronger with each session. It gave me a slight mental edge, a reason to look forward to those otherwise unpleasant treatment days. Instead of an enemy that made me feel bad, the chemo became my ally.

—Dean King

I HAD A relaxation tape of ocean music that I took along to chemo sessions. I'd play the tape in my Walkman, and that helped me wind down before the sessions. I'd listen to it for about the first half hour. It relaxed me and helped me to focus on visualizing the cancer cells being killed. After that, I would chat with the nurses in the clinic or the friend who had brought me (a group of my friends, who were all nurses, got together and juggled their schedules to make sure someone could drive me to each chemo session).

Also, very early on, after I was diagnosed, a friend at work gave me a videotape of scenery—four different sections—with music that was a useful visual stimulus. I used it the first two weeks after I was diagnosed, while I was recovering from the surgery, and into the first couple rounds of chemo. It helped me unwind in the evening.

—*Lorraine Anderson*

WHEN IT CAME to chemotherapy, I put my favorite groups on my Walkman, turned up the volume, and just rocked, jazzed, and funked right through it. The positive vibes helped me to deal with the side effects of treatment and project a healthier attitude.

—*Blythe Ritchfield*

ANYBODY GETTING CHEMO needs to plan on extra rest. Sometimes the oncologist will tell you, "Oh, you can continue to work." With many of the regimens you can, but you're going to have a reduced level of energy after work. You shouldn't be discouraged by that. It's normal. It's hard to explain how chemo makes you feel. It's just a total body involvement. But when you feel painful results—whether it's being tired, feeling nausea, or losing your hair—you have to remember that those are signs that the chemotherapy is being effective, that it's doing something. Think of it as eating up little cancer cells. At one point, they began to tell children at the National Institutes of Health to think of the cancer cells as being eaten up by Pacmen, which are the chemo cells. It's a good visualization for adults as well.

—*Elizabeth Martin*

AS I WAS going into my first chemo treatment, I decided I wasn't going to make up my mind that it would make me sick or not make me sick. I was just going to go with the flow and see what happened. I forced myself to think, "No matter how bad I might feel afterward—even if it makes me absolutely, completely green with nausea for three days—I can handle it. I am somehow going to do this, and I will be okay when it's done. I just need to get rid of these bad cells. That's my job—to get rid of these bad cells."

—*Jodi Levy*

AT MY FIRST treatment, I sat in the room for over half an hour asking the nurses a million questions even though I knew the answers. I dreaded starting the treatment. Finally one of the nurses told me my not-too-favorable odds of surviving without the treatment. I guess that did it. It was cold, hard, and irrefutable. I told them to start the IV.

—*Marcia Moosnick*

I GOT THROUGH chemotherapy by connecting with other patients. At each treatment session, I talked to the other people at the doctor's office. I asked plenty of questions and shared my quota of fear and anger. I was able to express my feelings, and I learned from others that the side effects I was experiencing were normal.

—*Frank Narcisco*

TO MAKE IT easier on me when the nurse was poking my veins ten times to look for a decent one to put the chemo in, I sat in my Jacuzzi beforehand and wrapped my arms up in hot towels and then asked for fresh hot towels when I got there. I also took in little hand pumps and pumped up my veins.

—*Sheri Sobrato*

TO MAKE MY chemo easier, I opted to have a port inserted under the skin in my left arm. This small metal device worked like an electrical outlet. A catheter was threaded from the port to a major vein. The nurse would just puncture my skin each time and plug the IV directly into the port. This allowed me to have chemo without an IV hookup each time, and it saved my peripheral veins from corrosion.

—*Karen Manheimer*

Train in Vein

I have patients who don't have good veins. Sometimes they get hard from the chemotherapy, and some people just have small veins. I usually tell them, "I will attempt to go in, but after a couple of treatments, you might not have any usable veins left." They can see a surgeon and have a port-a-cath or Broviac catheter put in, which makes both our lives so much easier. After that, I only have to prick the skin on the surface. We have a mainline right there, and it's ready for use. No more picking and poking to find a usable vein. Patients having a stem-cell transplant, which involves taking a lot of blood, almost always have these put in.

The port-a-cath is a tubular device that's inserted under the skin in the chest wall, and it goes into the aorta. The patient doesn't take care of it. The nurse does. The patient only sees a bump on the skin. The Broviac is a double-lumen apparatus that sticks out of your chest from a hole that's made surgically and that goes into the aorta. The two lumens stick out, and the patient pins them to his clothes. The patient learns how to flush it and take care of it. A nurse helps until the patient is comfortable enough to do it alone.

Both kinds of catheters are usually removed right after chemo is finished.

—*Carmen Lopez,*
Oncology Nurse,
New York, New York

Controlling Nausea and Other Side Effects

I, LIKE EVERYONE else, was terrified—aside from the large, looming terror of losing one's life—mostly of the nausea. At the first treatment, my doctor gave me an injection of Compazine to combat the nausea, and I remember going home and waiting around to see what would happen. And nothing happened. Of course, I was greatly relieved. So from that time on, I would schedule my treatments in the morning and then I would go straight to rehearsal—I'm a violinist with the Metropolitan Opera—and then continue with my day as usual.

After several months of treatment, some friends of ours invited us to use their house in the Hamptons for a weekend. So I had my treatment on Friday morning, went to the rehearsal, and then my husband and kids and I all got in the car and drove out to the Hamptons. There was an incredible rainstorm that day, so we were on the road forever, and by the time we got there, it was dark and we were starving. We got in the house, and we were trying to figure out what to do about dinner, and suddenly it dawned on me that the nurse had forgotten to give me the Compazine that morning. And there I was, stuck out in the Hamptons, and I thought, "Oh, my God." But then I realized that I had gone the whole day without any nausea at all. I was stunned. After that, I never took any more Compazine injections.

—Toni Zavistovski

I HAD A difficult time with the side effects of chemo because it took a while for me to find an antinausea drug that worked. One drug made me jumpy. Another made me sleepy. And a third did absolutely nothing. Finally I found Ativan, an antianxiety drug, which reduced the stress I felt at the beginning of treatments and lessened the severity of the vomiting.

Even with the Ativan, I still had some nausea and vomiting, and the way I dealt with it was to count off the hours after each chemo treatment. I knew that the side effects would end at around two or three in the morning. Sometimes I would doze off between fits of nausea, and then an hour or two would elapse without my even being aware. No matter how bad I felt, it was comforting to know that at a certain magical hour in the middle of the night, I would begin to feel better again. Even the worst experience can be handled when you know there's an end to it.

—Jeanne Clair

THE ANTICIPATION OF chemo was almost worse than the chemo itself. While it made me feel horrible, I never actually vomited after treatments. But I was so nervous the day before that I became extremely nauseous. I couldn't even eat dinner that night. Finally, halfway through my year-long chemotherapy, my doctor gave me a narcotic to take before chemo sessions. It was basically like having amnesia. After the treatments, my girlfriend and I would rent a video, and the next day I'd have to ask her what we watched. It was a weird sensation, but it helped me get through the last six months of chemo.

—*Scott Cox*

I WAS ON CMF chemotherapy. It was a pretty low dosage, and I didn't lose my hair, but I definitely got sick. The first time they gave me Compazine, but it didn't work. I was really sick. Months two through six—I went every three weeks for eight periods— they gave me Zofran, which helped. Eating helped. I ate afterward, when I felt sick. I would eat something to settle my stomach. Crackers. It's almost like when you're pregnant.

I would go on a Thursday afternoon. I would take Friday off and go back to work on Monday. The periods of feeling bad got progressively longer, but I was still able to keep that schedule. There was only one period, at the four- or five-month level, when I couldn't go back to work for a couple of days because my cell count was off. I had to prolong my chemo one more cycle because I had to skip that treatment.

—*Claire Noonan*

OVER TEN MONTHS I took two protocols. The first one was called CHOP, a combination of four drugs. The second one was called ASAP, otherwise known in medical books, unfortunately, as "salvage therapy," which gets the point across.

My doctor treated me very aggressively. With the first regimen, I got my "juice" once a month as an outpatient. One of the drugs was a steroid, so I was on an up for five or six days. Then I'd crash when they stopped the steroids and become a wet rag. They gave me another drug called Zofran, which was magnificent because it kept me from vomiting. In ten months, I think I vomited less than seven times, which is almost a miracle. And when I did, most of the time it was because I goofed and didn't take my Zofran in time. It was first given to me by IV, and then I would take vials of it home to drink every six hours. Now it's in pill form. Zofran is more efficient and more effective than marijuana.

After six months, the doctor put me through a number of tests, and they all came out very positive. He explained that there are billions and billions of cells in your body, and there are billions and billions of cells that are cancerous, and statistically even when they have a successful regimen, there are still some cells that are resistant. His point was that it was going to come back. He was so certain that he strongly suggested a second regimen—three sessions with heavier juice.

Each month I went into the hospital for five days. There were four drugs, but the heaviest was platinum, or cisplatin. It's a drug that gets to your kidneys unless you take constant fluids. You get fluids for five days, and basically you pee for five days to wash out your kidneys. Other side effects that I had were neuropathy, or lack of sensation on the bottom of my feet, and tremendous problems with my digestive tract, both upper and lower. Gas pains, cramping, waking up in the middle of the night farting.

One thing that is very important—and I was stupid about this, especially in the beginning—is not to say, "I have to tough this out; after all, I want to live." Don't be macho or stoic or heroic and say, "Well, I can put up with this and with that." Pain and discomfort are now a field for nurses and doctors. There are people in the hospital who walk around with buttons with the word "pain" surrounded by a red circle with a dagger through it. Even if you're most seriously affected by your cancer and you're in tremendous pain, they can help. Nobody is supposed to put up with pain. I was supposed to be a little bit more connected with medical people than the general public because I work in the medical field, and even I didn't know or believe it. We live in a culture that says you have to put up with it, but you don't.

Whatever it is, they can counteract it ninety-nine percent of the time. If you have intestinal distress, you go and say, "I'm up in the middle of the night with gas pains and diarrhea." They give you something. I'd say, "I can't sleep at night," and they gave me sleeping pills. You're supposed to tell them what's going on. Be honest and tell the medical people what your problems are. If they can respond to them, they will. And if they can't, they'll tell you.

—Frank Sheridan

THE DOCTORS STRONGLY recommended I get a catheter put in, so I did, and that was another minor surgery. Then I started my chemo treatments at the doctor's office—a combination of MOPP and ABV, as in ABVD. I didn't have the D because my doctor thought with everything else the D would just make me sick and wouldn't give me a whole lot of benefit. That's the one that makes people sick. I had my first treatment on a Tuesday, and my wife gave birth to our second daughter two days later. Luckily, I felt well enough to be there for the delivery. That was important to me.

The MOPP I handled well. It didn't make me feel too bad, although the one time I got sick was after a MOPP treatment. I think I just talked myself into it, but another time after a MOPP treatment, we went to Rusty's Ribs. I ate a whole rack of ribs right after treatment.

One weird thing that the MOPP did was as soon as the doctor started putting it into my body and I got the mustard taste in my mouth, my sinuses would open up and my nose would run incredibly.

I took Compazine before I got the ABV, but it really knocked me on my ass. Afterward, I'd go home and sleep for a couple of hours and be worthless for a day and a half. I never got sick, but I lost my hair. It was falling out, so finally I just shaved it all off.

I had had a mustache since I was a sophomore in college, and it was falling off as well. I got tired of it falling into my food, so one morning I shaved it off. At the time, I was also taking prednisone, and my face was all puffy and my skin was gray. When I walked downstairs that morning my wife looked at me and ran out the door. She came back a couple of minutes later and said, "Don't you ever do that to me again." She didn't recognize me and thought I was a strange guy walking in the house.

Because of the prednisone, I was so wound up, I couldn't sleep. I had to go on sleeping pills for six months. The steroids made all my joint aches and pain and arthritis and tendinitis and all that stuff go away, but at the beginning, I had a side effect my doctor had never seen before—it felt like somebody kicked me right square in the nuts. They ached. That's the only time I broke down and cried. I was lying on my bed thinking, "If this is what it's going to be like, I don't know if I can make it." I had to ice them to get some of the pain to go away.

I went and saw a urologist, and he thought maybe I had an infection in there, but it turned out to be just a side effect that I had for some reason. It affects everybody differently. With each cycle I went through—and I went through seven—the pain was less severe, but even on the seventh, it was still there.

—*Karl Nelson*

I'D HEARD SO many horror stories about the side effects of chemo—the nausea and the vomiting and the bowel problems. I did have those problems, but the medications made them very tolerable.

My first treatment took away my appetite completely, so they had to feed me intravenously. I couldn't fathom eating any-thing—even my favorite things, like ice cream. Just the thought of food turned my stomach. There was a span of about twelve to fifteen days in which I had nothing to eat at all. Just water, barely.

Once they stopped feeding me intravenously, I started with soups and crackers and stuff like that, and even that was really hard to get down. It took everything I had. I didn't want to eat and had no appetite. When I swallowed the food I felt like it was going to come right back up. But I closed my eyes and tried to do the mind-over-body thing and forced it to stay down. It slowly got better.

One of the reasons I had no appetite might have been because the hospital food was just horrible. My mom would cook food at home and bring it in for me. It was great because not only was I used to her food, but she's a good cook. She could only do it when I didn't have neutropenia, which is a blood condition where you don't have any neutrophils, a type of white blood cell that is crucial to fighting infection. She knew not to bring in fresh fruit or vegetables. She cooked everything really well and made sure that the meat was well done and things like that. It was a big help.

Sometimes I did vomit no matter what they gave me, and it didn't matter what I had eaten. It just comes, and there's nothing you can do about it. But I really expected it to be a lot worse.

On top of the nausea and the loss of appetite, the metallic taste in my mouth was hard to deal with. I always wanted gum or something to suck on. Fruit-flavored Life Savers worked best for me. I had bowel problems too. I think that's pretty common—cramping and diarrhea. Unfortunately, on top of all that, I developed hemorrhoids.

I think the hardest part for me was having insomnia. They gave me a mild sleeping pill called Restoril, which helped. I think rest is important when you're dealing with something like this. It wouldn't let me sleep the way I would at home—a good eight hours—but I was at least able to get five or six hours' sleep a night.

—*Michele Fox*

ONE OF THE medicines made me very constipated, and I didn't realize it at the time. It sounds ridiculous, but one summer it got to the point where every single time I ate, I would immediately feel nauseous and throw up. My boyfriend and I would go to dinner, and by the time we'd get outside, I'd be throwing it up. We laughed because the dinners were often really expensive. The doctors told me, "You are so constipated, your system will literally not take anything else." Then they put me on medicine so that every time I ate something, I had about a few seconds before I had to get to a bathroom. It gave me tremendous diarrhea.

I was in West Philly at the time and knew the layout of every single restaurant in the area because when it came, I had about three seconds to get to the bathroom. I'd drop everything I owned and take off. It was always funny but always terrifying too. I was scared I wouldn't make it to the bathroom. I'd be crying and running and banging down doors at McDonald's and stores. I lost a lot of weight that summer.

—*Katie Brant*

THE PHYSICIAN I consulted at M. D. Anderson said that my first doctor had given up on me and, therefore, undertreated me. He suggested a stronger chemo. This dose of chemo was so strong that I had to be put in a sterile environment to prevent infection, which left me behind a plastic wall that had an opening through which they stuck their gloved hands when they needed to touch me. They even had to sterilize my get-well cards before passing them through the slot.

Time in these situations loses its meaning. I read the cards I

received, did some crafts, watched TV, and did visualizations. My
kids came to visit from Florida, which was very helpful for both
my husband and me. The time passes because when you don't feel
well, you become somewhat removed from the normal rhythms
of life. This is a coping mechanism.

Later on in my treatment I was able to get chemotherapy as an
outpatient. At M. D. Anderson, they have developed a delivery
system for chemotherapy that the patient can administer at
home. It fits into a fanny pack and enters through a port-a-cath.
This enabled me to continue with my life and lifted my spirits by
letting me stay in my own environment. I recommend it!

—*Judy Weiner*

DURING THREE OUT of the seven cycles, my white blood cell
count—this was before they began using the drug that keeps
your white blood cell count up—dropped so low that I ended up
in the hospital. The first time it happened, I was in the doctor's
office. I was running a fever of a hundred and one or a hundred
and two degrees and had no infection, so he wanted to put me in
the hospital. The doctor told my wife on the phone that he had
once seen a guy going through chemo who seemed perfectly
healthy and then started running a fever. Three hours later he was
dead. There were no white blood cells in his body to stop
infection. Well, that's not the thing you should tell my wife. I
wanted to stop at home to get my stuff, and she said, "No. Get
the hell to the hospital."

I ended up in the hospital for five or six days every time that
happened. I'd have to wait until I stopped running the fever, and
then I'd get out, but I'd have to go on oral antibiotics for a couple
of days. It happened again on the last cycle, and then I developed
an infection in the catheter. So they had to take it out. It actually
saved me a week or a week and a half of having the catheter in
there, which I thought was wonderful.

—*Karl Nelson*

IN MY MIND, half of oncology nursing is actually education. They
are supposed to tell you—and they often don't—the symptoms

that you should be expecting. If you knew what was coming, it would be much easier.

When I got sick, a friend on Long Beach, Long Island, offered to let me use his home, a block from the ocean, for the week after I had the juice. So my wife and I went out there the day that I stopped the steroids. They hadn't warned me—or maybe they had, and I didn't hear it—but we got out there, and I crashed. My legs were heavy. My body was heavy. I was tired all the time.

It was pleasant out, but I decided that before we took a walk, I was going to take a nap. I slept all afternoon. My wife woke me up for supper, and afterward I went for another nap and slept all night. The next morning I got up and ate breakfast and said, "I gotta take a nap." I couldn't believe it. I couldn't move.

That's what happens when you're on the month cycle. You go for five, six days on the steroids, and then you collapse. Over the next three weeks, you work yourself out of this crash until you almost feel normal, and then they take a blood test and say, "Oh, back to normal," and hit you with another dose. That's the whole plan, but I didn't know that the first time.

—*Frank Sheridan*

THERE WERE A couple of weeks on my first chemo round when all I could eat was watermelon. Everything else tasted horrible. But that changed. For about two months, I hardly slept at all, and I ate cereal at night and read *The Wall Street Journal* and other newspapers. I didn't really watch TV, but a lot of people I've talked to stayed up and watched it all night long. I tried to eat good food, but I was constantly hungry. On the way to work downtown, I'd have to stop at a McDonald's. I usually had about six meals a day.

—*Brian Schmidt*

I HAD A bad reaction to the vincristine, with numbness in my hands and my feet. My hands got so weak that I couldn't button my shirts up all the way. My hands would cramp constantly, so bad that I had to take the other hand and straighten out the fingers. The thumb was especially weak. I could shoot a basketball, but I'd miss by three feet to the left. I had no strength in my thumb to control the ball with.

My feet were the worst. I developed drop foot. I could walk fifty yards, but after that I didn't have any strength to pick up my foot, so I just kind of threw my foot out in front of me and let it flop down. I had no feeling in the bottom of my feet, so I couldn't tell if my foot was landing flat or not, and I twisted my ankle a number of times.

My hands came back pretty good, I'd say about ninety-five percent, but the bottoms of my feet even to this day—and it's been seven years now—still feel like they're asleep, that sandy kind of feeling. It's worse if I don't get enough sleep. For a long time I didn't work out because my feet bothered me so bad. I couldn't run or anything like that. But eventually I started some light jogging to get the confidence back in my feet and legs. Now I run on a treadmill for a couple of miles two to four days a week.

—*Karl Nelson*

I THINK THE doctors underestimate the power of the stuff they give you. They just tell you to go home and be tough. They had me on steroids for four days and off four days. They artificially keep you going, and then when you come off the steroids, your system crashes. I was basically shaking and anxious, so anxious that I didn't want to wait at stoplights. My mind and heart would race, and I would walk around the neighborhood several times to try to calm down. Sometimes it just didn't work. The heat and the mugginess were a factor. It was hard to adjust to normal outside stimuli.

Initially, I also struggled with depression and got no help from the doctors. But a counselor at the hospital at the University of Arkansas told me, "Seventy-five percent of people who have chemo get medically induced depression, and I believe you have that." She referred me to another doctor who gave me Zoloft. It made a big difference. They say that stuff usually takes a couple of weeks, but my wife thought I was demonstrably better in three days.

—*Brian Schmidt*

I HAD ABVD every two weeks for six months. After the first treatment, my oncologist told me I'd probably notice some changes right away, and sure enough, my night sweats went away, and the fevers weren't coming around. So I had confidence that everything was fine.

The day I had chemo, I would not feel good at all, but I never threw up. They gave me one of the antinausea drugs. I'd still get nauseous, but I'd be okay as long as I stayed pretty low-key afterward. My skin would be burning and tingling and kind of flushed. I didn't get too sick or fatigued until after the first couple of treatments. It accumulates with each dose. After my third treatment, when the chemo was making me feel lousy, I smoked pot, and that really helped. It helped with my appetite too. Some people have an aversion to marijuana use for medicinal purposes, but I don't, and I don't have a problem telling people that it can help them out. I'd usually go in to get chemo on Mondays. I'd get my run in, and then my appointment would be at two o'clock. I'd be there until about four. By five, I'd be lighting up. It helped more than the nausea drugs.

—*Mark Conover*

ONE SUNNY DAY after a chemo session, I arrived at the doorway to my apartment and decided I wasn't going inside—to hell with being embarrassed about getting sick in public. Instead, my wife and I walked over to a nearby park. We stretched out in the outfield of a softball field under the warm rays of the sun. After that I never spent another post-chemo afternoon inside on the couch, dozing in and out of consciousness, waking every half hour to throw up. Outside, I remained much more alert. I was still nauseous, but I was able to maintain a sense of control. I read the box scores in the sports section of the paper and enjoyed the times when I didn't feel too bad.

—*Dean King*

A FRIEND WHO went through cancer treatment before me told me about a prescription lozenge for chemo mouth sores called Mycelex Troche, which I would not have thought to ask my doctor about. I took them before my sister's wedding, and they helped alleviate some of the pain so I could eat and enjoy myself.

—*Tali Havazelet*

ONE THING THAT I found to be helpful was frozen fruit bars. They helped relieve the pain of my chemo mouth sores.

—*Monica Ko*

CHEMO DOES CRAZY stuff to you. It made me uninterested in reading or even watching TV. It made me grouchy (I told my dad to stop hovering over me). And it made me extremely sensitive to odor. I asked all my visitors to wash off their perfume, and I had my family distribute the many flower arrangements I received to other patients on the floor.

—*Karen Manheimer*

YOU REALLY DO have big mood swings. The chemo makes it worse. One minute you're fine, and then someone says something, and you're crying your head off. You have to try not to be upset by this. It's very normal. This is true about depression, denial, the whole gamut of emotions. One person may feel all of them. One person may feel none of them or anything in between. Most people are unprepared for anger, but anger is very common, and anger is constructive. Studies have shown that people who are angry and determined actually do better than people who are very accepting.

—*Elizabeth Martin*

THE GIANTS WERE great during my whole battle with cancer. They provided a limo to take me to and from my treatments—I just had them at my doctor's office and then went right home afterward. Well, when the limo companies clean a car, they use baking soda, and I started to associate the smell of baking soda with the chemo treatments. Every time I got into a limo and smelled that baking soda, my stomach turned. Then one day my wife cleaned our bedroom carpet with a baking-soda solution, and I about killed her. I walked in and turned right out. I couldn't handle it.

—*Karl Nelson*

THE DOCTOR TOLD me there was a high likelihood I would lose my hair, and I remember one afternoon I was taking a shower, and I looked at the bottom of the tub. There were these gigantic mats of hair, so I called Carol, my wife, in and said, "Well, it's here." It was not just the hair on my head; it was also my body hair. A number of weeks passed, and I realized that my nose tended to run a lot. I discussed it with my doctor, and he said, "Well, John, it's because the hairs in your nose likewise have thinned out." It had never occurred to me, but that is precisely what happened. I've talked about that with a number of other patients, and it's always the same: "Oh, I never thought of that."

—John Hall

WHEN I WAS undergoing chemo, I'd blank out in the middle of a conversation and forget stuff that I'd never forgotten before. People kept saying that it was stress-related or because I had so much on my mind, but a friend of mine who also had cancer talked to her oncologist about it at length. She said that there is a short-term memory loss related to chemo, and it depends on the chemo you're taking and how long as to whether it permanently affects you. It's something that I've heard over and over again from people who are going through chemo. They get so frustrated by this blip in mental efficiency. It's just little things, but now I can blame it on the chemo—or else on the fact that I'm getting close to forty.

—Charlotte Wells

WHEN MY IMMUNITY was down with the chemo, I was very susceptible to bladder infections. I would get a bladder infection, like clockwork, and then they'd put me on amoxicillin to take care of it, which would inevitably give me a yeast infection. I went back and forth from a bladder infection to a yeast infection for a solid year. I felt so gross. It took about three years. I can't pinpoint a moment when all of a sudden it was better, and I can't say that it ever got one hundred percent perfect, but it did get much better.

—Katie Brant

Maintaining Your Appetite

CHEMOTHERAPY KILLED MY appetite, even for foods I had always loved. After each blast, I felt sick for twelve to twenty-four hours, during which time I couldn't even think of eating. Then, for the next two or three days, there was a lingering queasiness that continued to suppress my appetite. I had to force myself to eat something simply for the sake of getting some food into my system. This "forced feeding" taught me a lesson: Never force yourself to eat any of the foods you love during chemo periods. If you do, you might always associate them with how you felt during chemo, and you won't be able to eat them again. It happened to me with peanut butter and jelly, something I had always been crazy about. I had some during one of my first chemo periods, and even years later, I can't hear the words "peanut butter and jelly sandwich" without wanting to throw up. It's the same with lasagna, which I ate on the day I was given my first chemo. And there used to be nothing in this world that I liked better than lasagna.

I learned to eat strategically in order to avoid bad chemo associations. The hospital gave me some vitamin-packed chocolate shakes that supposedly provided a full day's nutritional requirements. They tasted exactly like what they were—a chemist's version of a chocolate shake—but I chugged one down every morning, gagging with every gulp, because it allowed me to get my vitamins for the day without screwing up any favorite food associations for the future. Another thing I ate was oatmeal, which I deliberately made plain and barely palatable. I added just a drop of milk and no sugar. After I finished my chemo, I went back to the foods I love.

—*Jonathan Pearlroth*

I SCHEDULED MY chemo sessions after my last class of the week on Thursday afternoon. My mother picked me up from class and drove me to the hospital. I would eat a sandwich on the way. I would spend the afternoon hooked up to the IV bag. Afterward, I was always very tired. I slept all day Friday and most of Saturday. On Sunday, I did homework, and by Monday morning, I was ready for class.

My mother cooked up a storm on those chemo weekends and stocked the fridge with matzo ball soup and pot roast with kasha varnishkes. She thought that Jewish soul food would help me get through chemo. It did.

—*Karen Manheimer*

GOING THROUGH CHEMO was like having morning sickness twenty-four hours a day for two years. Usually I had the chemo on Friday, and by Wednesday, I would start feeling better, to the point where I could actually eat something, but then I'd start thinking about having chemo in two days and I would get anticipatory nausea. My nutritionist gave me some really good recipes for protein shakes so that I wouldn't lose too much weight.

—*Lisa Hollingsworth*

Life Goes On

THE ZOFRAN KEPT me from getting sick. They gave me a small bag intravenously before and after my treatment and two tablets to take the next day. A couple hours after my treatment, I would go to work. Once I forgot the tablets, thought I was fine, didn't go back, and I woke up at about three o'clock in the morning terribly nauseated. I've thought about it since, and maybe I'm glad I got sick that one time because it helped me to understand what other people have gone through with chemotherapy and how good it was that I had the Zofran to keep me from getting sick.

My second treatment was on opening night of *Love Letters,* a play I was in. There were only two people on the stage, and I was concerned about carrying this thing off, for two solid hours, with just one other person. I'd been in plays over the years but never with something like this hanging over me. I thought that because this was opening night, the doctors might change my treatment, but they already had them all set up, an exact schedule every four weeks at a certain time, and they didn't want to make any changes. It's a very crowded place. So they said, "We'll make sure you don't get sick." They gave me an extra booster shot that morning, and both doctors who were treating me came to the performance. They were ready in case I did feel nauseous. *Love Letters* tells a beautiful love story, the trials and tribulations of a couple. I got through it just fine, and people loved it.

—*Ginnie Higginbotham*

AFTER CHEMO, I would be out of it for two days. When I'd come around, I'd drag my shoes on, drag on whatever I needed to get out, and I'd walk to the corner. That was my goal, even if it took me three hours to get out of bed, out of my room, and down the stairs. Sometimes I could barely put one foot in front of the other, but I thought, "Boy, I'm going to make it to the corner." If it was freezing cold, I'd put on my long johns. I was just determined—even if someone had to hold my arm and help to get me there. I felt better if I could do that. I felt like that exercise injected me with something good and lifted my spirits.

The next day, I'd try to make it a little farther, and sometimes a car would pass by and they would have to take me back home because I would get there and couldn't get back. But I thought, "Walking releases endorphins, and that has to be good." Physically I felt better. That was my main thing. I was just not going to be defeated by it.

—*Mamie Dixon*

WHEN I COULD, I usually tried to swim two times a week—maybe a thousand yards. Not the distances I do now, but I did swim. My chemo was once a month, three times in a week, and then I'd have a miserable week. The week that I was recovering from the chemo, I normally would not swim. Then the next couple of weeks, I'd get to feeling pretty good. So I'd swim maybe two and a half out of four weeks.

It was important because it was a psychological lift. Although my internal body was being destroyed to some extent, I was still able to move physically. Other patients were often surprised—I think even my wife was surprised—that I was able to do that, but I don't think it was so much physical strength as mental.

—*John Hall*

ON THE DAYS that I went for chemo, I did something for myself, as a gift. I would sit down and watch *All My Children* in its entirety before making my way to the hospital. I took my own sheets and clothes for an at-home feeling. My husband would spray the bed with Chanel No. 5 perfume, and I'd set up an Eskimo statue, which a friend had given me as something to watch over me and keep me well. Only after I had completed this little routine did I go through the treatment.

—Ivy! Gunter

I GOT THROUGH chemo by holding a carrot out for myself. I knew that my chemo would last from October to April and that it would take me at least through May before I felt like doing anything fun. So I planned a big night out in the big city in June. I bought tickets to the Broadway play *Amadeus* and made reservations at a nice restaurant. I asked one of my nurses to join me. Planning the big night out was helpful to me because it gave me something to look forward to. It was a goal, a reward for making it through all those difficult days of treatment. I always tell people to plan a vacation or some sort of celebration for when it's over. Give yourself something to shoot for.

—Kevin Shulman

LAUGHTER HELPS YOU get through something like chemo. I had a very weird sense of humor about losing my hair. I went back to LSU for a couple of visits, and sometimes I'd yank my wig off and try to laugh and make a joke about it. One girl said, "Put that back on. I don't want to see you like that. That's gross." I laughed about it, but it really hurt my feelings. I had another friend who laughed with me until three o'clock in the morning watching my shadow on the wall from the light behind me. The way we formed the thin hair on my head made it look like a giant Hershey's Kiss. Another time, I walked into a Häagen-Dazs store with my wig on. Then I yanked it off and asked them if they would fill it up with two scoops.

—Lisa Hollingsworth

THERE ARE SOME advantages to chemo. I got the hair back on my head, but never in my armpits or on my legs, so no more shaving. Not bad!

—Clara Trusty

CHAPTER NINE

Radiation: Taking the Heat

Half of all cancer patients are treated with some form of radiation. Receiving the radiation itself is not actually painful, although for most of us it seemed somewhat sinister. You know you're being treated with something very powerful and hazardous if mishandled, and the fact that you feel no pain during its application is slightly freaky.

What the radiation is doing is penetrating cancer cells to destroy their DNA and thereby killing the cells or preventing them from growing. The doctors determine the amount of radiation it will take to kill a patient's cancer and then calculate the number and strength of treatments needed. The effects and side effects of radiation are cumulative. In general, nausea and lethargy increase, although for many people who receive radiation as a secondary treatment, neither may be a factor.

Constant application to a single area brings about other side effects that must be dealt with. Topically, skin can become irritated and inflamed. Radiation to the head and neck can cause various glands to cease functioning. Among other things, special dental care must be considered if saliva flow, which acts as a natural tooth cleanser, is decreased. Nausea and loss of appetite are also problems for people receiving radiation to any part of the digestive tract. For patients being treated around the sexual organs, the potential for infertility must be considered.

Radiation can now be given either externally or internally. For more information about radiation treatment and its side effects, request a copy of the booklet "Radiation Therapy and You: A Guide to Self-Help During Treatment" from the National Cancer Institute (800-4-CANCER).

MY FIRST RADIATION session was scary. I was put in a room alone, behind a closed door that looked like something out of a vault. The door made a low thud when it closed, and my claustrophobia was intense. I started to hyperventilate. I felt like I was going to faint. A voice came through the speakers and startled me. "Is everything okay?" the voice said.

"I'm scared, and I feel panicked," I said.

"Don't worry, we are watching you, and we can stop the radiation at any time."

I asked them to continue talking to me, and I began to calm down. The following sessions were much easier because I had the friendly voice over the loudspeaker to reassure me that everything was going to be just fine.

—*Susan Fischer*

THE FIRST TIME I went in for radiation, nobody told me that I'd be naked from the waist up in a cold, sterile examining room with several strangers. I felt a complete loss of dignity. They put a chin strap on me so I couldn't move as they tattooed me, and they gave me instructions as if by rote. I felt like one more slab of meat at the butcher that day. I wanted to scream, but instead I tried to remove myself from my own body. I closed my eyes and thought about the times I'd gone to a topless beach, transporting myself to the sea and imagining that it was my choice to be half-naked in front of a bunch of strangers.

—*Jeanne Clair*

AFTER DEAN FINISHED his chemotherapy, our oncologist recommended that he have some radiation to the chest, where the majority of the cancer had been. He said he wouldn't need much, but he wanted to take that precaution. We went to see the radiologist he recommended, and her staff explained that radiation would probably make him tired and might make his throat dry and that he should avoid exposing the radiated area to the sun. Then they told us to come back a few days later.

When we went back, they took us down to the radiation area and told Dean to undress for his tattoos. "His what?" I asked.

"He has to have tattoos so they know where to radiate him," the nurse said.

"Are they permanent?" I asked.

"Yes."

While he was being tattooed, I sat in the waiting room and wondered why I was bothered about something as minor—in the scheme of things—as a bunch of tattoos. I realized that it wasn't the tattoos themselves that upset me, but the cavalier manner in which we were told about them. The nurse's manner implied, "You're lucky he's alive. What difference do a few tattoos make?" The point of view I was coming from was more along the lines of "We've been through all this, and now we find out he has to live the rest of his life with tattoos?"

I also took time while I was sitting there to review the radiation plan, and it occurred to me that the radiologist was not only intending to radiate much more of his body—his neck, chest, and pelvis—than his oncologist had suggested, but she was also planning on giving him a much higher dosage of radiation than the oncologist had led us to believe was necessary.

When the doctor came through the waiting room, I told her that I would like to ask her a few questions. "What do you want to know?" she said. I hesitated in front of the waiting room full of patients, but I sensed I was not going to get a lot more time out of her, so I said, "I don't understand why you're planning on giving Dean so much more radiation than Dr. Waxman recommended."

"Your husband had a lot of cancer," she said. "This is what is necessary to make him better."

Luckily our insurance company made us go for a second opinion, and even though Dean had to get another set of tattoos, it was well worth it. The doctor we ended up with not only recommended a radiation plan more in line with what our oncologist had suggested, but he and his staff treated us like human beings.

—*Jessica King*

Tattoos Explained

Patients having radiation therapy are often tattooed beforehand. We map out the area that we're going to treat using tiny tattoos. In each radiation room, we have lasers, and we align the lasers up to the tattoos. That way we know that we are radiating the same spot during each session.

When people first hear the word "tattoo," they worry. Their first image is of a butterfly or naked lady, but it's just a tiny black or blue dot of ink at three different points. If you take a pen and mark it on your finger, it's probably smaller than that. Once they see that it's a small mark, they relax. It's like a birthmark—so small you can barely tell it's there.

As with decorative tattoos, the technique involves putting ink under the skin, where it remains indefinitely. There are several ways you can do it. Some people put the ink into the needle, and then poke that into the patient. I put a drop right on the patient's skin and pick at the skin a little bit with the needle. As far as pain goes, it depends on who does it. It's like drawing blood—some people are a little rougher than others. It should feel like a mosquito bite.

—*José M. Dieppa,*
Senior Radiation Therapist, Cabrini Medical Center,
New York, New York

INITIALLY, I WAS upset at the thought of my body being tattooed for radiation, and I was afraid that my breast would look like a ticktacktoe board. In the end, the tattoos were really nothing to make a fuss over. They looked like tiny birthmarks and were barely noticeable.

—*Susan Fischer*

I WASN'T TATTOOED. Instead, they used stickers—they were kind of corner markers—and told me, "When you shower, just shower around them; don't rub them." They stayed on for about a week, and then every week they replaced them. They wanted me to have the tattoos in case I ever needed more radiation, but I decided that I had enough scars on my body. I was convinced I was not going to have a recurrence. You have a limited amount of radiation you can withstand in one lifetime. My level of radiation was relatively low. Maybe they would have insisted on tattoos if it had been higher, which would have left less room for error in the future.

—*Jodi Levy*

I WENT IN to do my lead blocks and had purple *x*'s and *o*'s and arrows painted all over my body. Not really purple—more of a hot pink, sort of a radioactive color. They drew a box around the actual tumor that they were going to shrink with the radiation, and they tattooed me on my abdomen, at the sternum, and right below the navel. That was all pretty interesting. It was in the summer, and I had worn a sleeveless blouse, so the technician lent me his lab jacket so that I could go home on the subway.

—*Leslie Kaul*

ABOUT THREE OR four days after my laparotomy/splenectomy, I went in and they laid me on the table to do the dots—the tattoos—for the radiation. Because of my size and my muscle density at the time—I was two hundred and eighty-five pounds, six feet six, and in pretty good shape—I caused them a lot of problems. Normally they keep the source of the radiation a certain distance from the body. They had to raise it up in order to have the beam spread wide enough, and also with the muscle mass, I was thicker and denser than most people. So they had all sorts of physicists in there trying to calculate things.

I went through twenty radiations of the mantle area, both front and back, and then three conedowns, right on the mass. Then they decided I should have the abdominal area done as well—another twenty treatments. I wasn't thrilled about that because they'd originally told me twenty and that should have been it. Basically my wife said, "Shut up, and let's make sure we get it." So I did the extra twenty in the abdomen.

On the floor where I had the radiation treatments, nobody else could smell anything, but it smelled like radiation to me. As soon as the elevator doors opened, I could smell it. That odor was nowhere else in the hospital. It bothered me as soon as I walked out of the elevator. But only once did I get sick from the radiation, and that's because I let myself get worn down. I hadn't slept well for a couple of nights in a row, and I was outside moving some heavy wet dirt and rocks and just got overtired. I came inside and got sick and said, "Boy, that was stupid." You have to listen to your body. If it says you feel up to doing something, do it. If it says don't, then don't do it.

—Karl Nelson

AFTER MY SURGERY, I received the maximum amount of radiation possible. The mouth sores caused by the radiation became so bad that I could only swallow liquids, so friends would bring me everything they could run through their Cuisinarts. The food wasn't delicious, but at least it was homemade, and it meant that I had lots of visitors.

—Laura Eastman

Keeping the Mouth Healthy after Radiation

Radiation therapy focused on the head, neck, and face causes a variety of side effects on the salivary glands, facial muscles, jawbones, teeth, and tiny blood vessels of the mouth. Here are three of the most common dental side effects caused by radiation treatment, followed by tips for prevention:

Postradiation tooth decay: A rotting of the teeth caused by xerostomia, or dry mouth, which occurs when radiation knocks out your parotid salivary glands, located below each ear on the corner of your lower jaw. Saliva bathes the teeth and helps prevent cavities. When these glands shut down, decay can set in within a few months.

Postradiation decay can be prevented almost one hundred percent by good oral hygiene and the use of custom mouth applicators to give yourself a fluoride treatment. Each night put one-percent neutral pH fluoride gel, which is available by prescription, in the applicator and leave it in your mouth for five minutes.

You should also avoid mouthwashes containing alcohol because alcohol is very irritating. There are specific products, such as Biotene, that are made for people with dry mouth.

Trismus: A type of lockjaw caused when radiation stiffens the jaw muscles.

With trismus, you can't open your mouth very wide. If you let trismus occur, it's almost impossible to get rid of it. Before you begin radiation therapy, measure your mouth's maximum opening. To make sure you can always open your mouth to that width, do the following simple stretching exercise five or six times a day, throughout the therapy: Cross your thumb and middle finger, as if you had just snapped them. Then put the middle finger on the edge of the bottom teeth and the thumb on the edge of the top teeth, and force the teeth open. It's like stretching before running. You want to keep the jaw limber.

Osteoradionecrosis: Bone death that occurs when radiation closes small blood vessels that feed the mouth.

The same thing can happen to soft tissue in the mouth.

You need blood in order to heal. If you have radiation therapy to the jaw, and then you have a tooth removed, the hole in the bone where the tooth was removed may not get enough blood, and you'll get bone death, which is very painful and difficult to deal with. The key is prevention. Get a thorough checkup—and have any dental work done—*before* the radiation therapy. You don't want to remove a tooth from an area that has been radiated. If you have bad teeth, and you are about to start radiation therapy to the head and neck, it may be best to remove them first. It is also important to maintain good follow-up care with your dentist.

—*Alan Sheiner, D.D.S.,*
Assistant Clinical Professor, Mount Sinai School of Medicine,
New York, New York

THEY WANTED TO stop the radiation because my skin was breaking down and getting ulcerated, so I went to a skin-care specialist at the hospital and got various products that would help my skin heal so I could continue. Actually, I started using skin-care products before my first treatment. Over the entire area that was being radiated, I put high-concentration aloe vera gel—something you can buy over the counter. It protects the skin so that there isn't as much breakdown. The hospital said they had not seen it written up in the literature yet, but they had done it with enough patients to feel that it makes a positive difference.

But even so, the radiated skin started to break down. It was like a really bad sunburn, and then it became ulcerated, blistered. After dealing with this for nine months almost on a daily basis, I said, "There's no way we're stopping with only a week or ten days left. What do you have?"

We placed gel pads—called Vigilon—on the skin and then wrapped my chest with Kerlix, like an Ace wrap. The pads come in a couple of different sizes; I think the one I used was six by six inches. They're water-based, and they maintain moisture in the area for you. I slept with them on all night long—a concentrated time when my skin was exposed to the gel pad and nothing else. I had hydrocortisone cream and other creams that they had given me to use before that, but when my skin was really ulcerated, the gel pads worked best. We turned my skin around in two days, so we could keep going with the treatment.

—*Lorraine Anderson*

THEY RADIATED MY stomach, and almost up to my chest and down to the mid-thighs. For the first couple of days, I felt like crap. The first day, I just lay there in bed all day and threw up a little bit. The second and third days, I didn't feel too well. I didn't feel like getting up and doing anything.

I had about twenty treatments. With the last three, I was taking treatments in the morning and then playing for the Phillies in the afternoon. I played the first three or four games fine, but then after that, it hit me all at once. I went in to play one day, and I was just yellow. They said, "There's no way you're playing. Go home and get in bed." I was real weak. The first three days I was so excited to be playing again, and then, boom, that wore off, and I slept for two or three days.

That whole year—1994—I never did regain full strength. I think I pushed it too fast. I started working out—light running, batting practice, and stuff—while I still had stitches in my feet from the lymphangiogram, which was kind of stupid. I just wanted to get back to playing and forget the word "cancer." I wanted to get back to doing the only thing I knew how to do, but I should have taken more time.

—*John Kruk*

THE RADIATION GAVE me a hypothyroid condition, so I've been taking medicine for the last three or four years. Sometimes it makes me lethargic, and it can cause weight gain and hair that gets wiry. I use Synthroid, a prescription drug that I take once a day, to regulate the situation, and it works pretty well.

—*Bill Thomas*

A COUPLE OF things happened with radiation. I had transferred to a new school, and I'd meet people and couldn't remember them. It was so frustrating. I mentioned it to my doctors, and they said, "Oh, you've been through so much. You're at a new school. We're sure it's that."

I kept saying, "No, that's not what it is." One thing I've always been extraordinary at is knowing people and names. I could go into a party and know everyone's name and phone number by the end of the night. Now I couldn't remember anybody. The change was so dramatic for me that I knew something was going on, but every doctor kept saying, "No, no."

I was having other short-term memory difficulties too. My friends and I would study, and I'd tutor them. I knew the material cold. Then I'd get into class and not remember a thing. Everyone I tutored through the class got an A, and I failed. I had never had to study before and always did well, but all of a sudden I was studying and not performing.

What was so frustrating for me, though, was that I was having these symptoms that I knew were real. They weren't just psychological, and everyone was second-guessing me to death. Several years later, on a train ride home from New York City, where I had been interviewing for a job, I sat next to a guy who turned out to be a neurologist. I said, "Oh, boy, you've got a case next to you." We started talking about brains and brain surgery. He asked me if I had any deficits. I said, "To be honest, I can't remember a face to save my life."

He said, "Prosopagnosia."

I said, "Excuse me?"

He said, "Prosopagnosia—'prosop' means 'face' and 'nosia,' 'memory.' That's not uncommon. And what's amazing is that I studied under the world's leading researcher." I nearly fell over.

This doctor validated everything. It was wonderful. I'd known it was not just psychological. I think that for so many people going through cancer or through any kind of sickness, to have a doctor validate what you know is true, when everyone else is blowing you off, is so empowering.

—*Katie Brant*

IN THE CROWDED waiting room of the radiotherapy department, we decided that the dastardly prankster who designed the hospital gowns needed to be treated him- or herself. The remarkable thing about them was that no two were exactly alike. Each one had a unique way of fitting or tying in an inconvenient way— sometimes strangling, frequently with ties that didn't mesh, and even more often hiding all too little. At the time, however, the possible exposure of our bodies was not all that important to any of us, and we were a pretty randy lot. Sitting around half-naked and chattering about the Gulf War, the weather, and our evil gowns, our thighs and boobs inadvertently popped out when we moved, only to be nonchalantly tucked back in again.

But one instance of incorrigible body parts had us all in stitches. The waiting room, with its two curtained dressing closets that faced our chairs as if on a stage, was packed that day. I was relatively new to this, and as I emerged with my striped boxers hanging below my gown, a woman suggested that I put another on and pointed to a very trim older man who had improvised. He had carefully tied a second gown sideways around his waist. Looking down at my boxers, I said, "I'm okay as long as I'm not offending anyone." She said, "No, honey, you're decent." And I sat down among my fellow cancer patients.

Soon, the old guy with the two gowns was called by Fabian, the technician. He stood and took a step away from us, revealing that his efforts at modesty had been in vain. The gown tied around his waist reached only about halfway on his backside. As he walked past me and the ladies, a prize set of family jewels trailed behind him, dancing back and forth. Shoulders heaving, we tried to smother our laughs, to little avail. When he returned to his seat—he had been called out of turn—he had fastidiously recinched the gown.

Finally, the old guy's turn did arrive. And needless to say, all eyes were peeled on his backside as he repeated the trek to the radiation room. This time his gown covered everything—that is, except for one little open triangle. Sure enough, as he passed us, his privates pendulumed—to our uncontrolled howls of delight—through that little opening.

—*Dean King*

CHAPTER TEN

Hospital Strategies

Moving into a hospital is both comforting and disconcerting. On the one hand, there is a great sense of relief that now you are in expert hands, that now your symptoms will be closely watched and administered to, and that now in some major way you are about to directly address your illness. On the other hand, you are moving from the comfort of your own home and the company of your family into a big, cold institution—quite possibly into a room decorated with mint-green wallpaper, chairs that look like they were created for a dentist's office, and a roommate you've never met before and who probably has a snoring disorder among other gory afflictions. That's not to mention the food, which generally does live up to its reputation for being a notch below airline fare.

It's a lot to take in all at once. But while you don't ease into a hospital room like a warm bath, you can mitigate its impact on your psyche. From insisting on a different room to redecorating, we've done it all, as you will see in this chapter. And more than one of us has picked up the phone and ordered in egg foo yung. Heck, if

the delivery boy can penetrate the lobby of your apartment building to leave menus, he can certainly find your hospital room, where
he'll be received and tipped—no doubt—like a savior angel.

Beyond that, we also found it was important mentally to claim
the space we were temporarily occupying. Hospitals have many
rules and regulations for the safety of their patients and staff. But
there are ways to tailor the experience to your own personal
needs. The advice below should help make your stay bearable—
even pleasant—and more healing.

MY HOSPITAL—AT the University of Nebraska—assigned us our
own coordinator who handled all the doctors and nurses in the
different departments. The social workers asked me questions
that helped me get to know myself better—questions about life
and death, about who I wanted around me, and who I needed for
my support. The hospital never allowed us to do anything without the coordinator or another support person guiding us
through it. It was wonderful.

—*Elsie Stone*

I WANTED A single room, even though I would have to pay extra
for it, but at first they said one wasn't available. They put me in a
double room, and it was a lousy one, configured oddly, so that I
was stuck in a corner by the bathroom. I just said, "To hell with
this. Where is there a single room?" I appealed to my doctor and
got a new room.

Usually if you're a cancer patient, you're in the care of a doctor
who has some clout, especially if you've had an operation. Surgeons are like lords of the earth. And oncologists, too, because
cancer is a big deal. Use your doctor's clout. Tell your doctor,
"Look, have them get me the better room or get me a time when
it's convenient for me." Don't be afraid to insist on these things.

—*Richard Brookhiser*

YOU WOULDN'T BELIEVE what my room looked like. I made it as
homey as a hospital room could be. We even brought in furniture. I had one of our bedroom tables with a CD player on it. I

had pictures of everybody along the window ledge. People brought me all sorts of things, and I placed them around the room. I had an afghan thrown over the chair. When I was being admitted for the second time, I went in to decorate my room before my stay. I had to make it me, or I wouldn't have been comfortable there.

On the bone marrow transplant floor, there was a guy who asked, "Is Karla going home today?" When they said I wasn't, he said, "Well, I just saw her husband with a big load of stuff."

The nurse told him that it was just the first round: "She's going home tomorrow, but she's got two loads. They can't get it all in one."

—*Karla McConnell*

Room Sweet Room

In my ten years visiting patients as a social worker, I've found that the more familiar and homelike patients can make their hospital room, the easier their stay will be. Some of the following items can help you feel connected to the life you have temporarily left behind:

- framed photos of family and friends
- poster or small piece of artwork from home
- stereo
- VCR and several videos
- computer and computer games
- electronic organ
- dictaphone for taking notes or keeping a journal (if you don't feel like writing)
- telephone answering machine for when you have visitors, you're sleeping, or you just don't feel like talking on the phone
- hot plate and equipment to make tea or soup
- daily newspaper or weekly magazine delivery

—*Jill Kaplan,*
Social Worker, Memorial Sloan-Kettering,
New York, New York

I USED TO think that staying in the hospital allowed you to rest. Not so. Your vital signs are checked around the clock. They wake you up early in the morning to weigh you. They wake you up several times each night to draw blood. I was even taken for X rays several times in the middle of the night. But I learned that you can say no. If you don't want to get weighed early in the morning, then just tell them to come back later. Same for X rays.

—*Karen Manheimer*

I HADN'T BEEN in a hospital since I was born, and, honestly, I had a much higher expectation of what my doctor's care was going to be. It's the nurses, the interns, the volunteers who are actually there on a day-to-day basis. The doctor comes in, looks at your chart, spends four minutes with you. To most doctors, you are a chart—even in the best of hospitals. It's not that they don't want to answer your questions, but they are not going to think them up for you. So, as you think of them, write them down, and the next time they're on rounds, you ask another three questions, and the next time, and so on.

—*Claire Noonan*

CHEMOTHERAPY FOR LEUKEMIA is given in the hospital for a month at a time or longer, so I brought all kinds of things into the hospital room with me. But my experience there was pretty harsh for a long time. The night of my diagnosis, I had watched *Broadway Danny Rose,* the Woody Allen movie, at home with my girlfriend and my parents and laughed. So I took my VCR to the hospital but was told I wasn't allowed to plug it in because all the electrical outlets were reserved for emergency equipment. So I just put the VCR under the bed and plugged it in. I realized that first day that the way to get through was to disobey.

I also brought in music. I would put on headphones with a fifteen-foot-long cord, and I would dance every morning or stretch, at least as much as I was able to. I would be dancing, and I'd turn around, and there would be four nurses peeking in the room giggling at me and wondering what I was doing and why I was dressed in street clothes. The rules were not geared for me to bring my life into the hospital. Because of the dancing and the psychic healers who came to see me, I had quite a few looks and laughs directed my way.

Another issue was the hospital food. I was told to eat it because it was nutritionally balanced, even though they were giving me cereal packed with BHA and BHT. But I discovered that I could have food delivered to the hospital. I could call any Chinese takeout place I wanted to. That was quality-of-life information that no one offered me.

I became fueled by my anger and outrage, and I found a great deal of motivation and inspiration. I also got a lot of use out of refusing to participate in the community. I avoided getting to know any of the other patients. I didn't want to consider myself one of them because I saw them succumbing in larger numbers than I thought necessary. I saw them participating in the destructive systems of the hospital that weren't working to their benefit, and I became kind of a loner.

I grew to believe that anything I did that sent a message to my body and soul, that reminded me of the pleasure available in life, was a chit on my side. I made sure to get up every day and put on clothing I liked and that made me feel good and to move my body in ways that felt good, to music that sounded good to me. Exercise is important. I don't think anybody should lie in bed all day if they are well enough to get out of bed. After being diagnosed with a terrible illness and thinking I was going to lose my life, dance and exercise felt like a privilege. I made sure to exercise those privileges as much as possible to continually remind myself of what I wanted to get back to. I think that was invaluable.

I became outraged at all the ways the hospital system interfered with that. I don't understand the concept in our society of illness as a taboo. People are sent to special places to be ill. If you're too ill, you're even hidden away somewhere within those places. And in those institutions, there are all kinds of rules about how your suffering is allowed to proceed. I think it puts one into the position of having to become an incredible nonconformist in order to go about it in a way that makes more sense. And I encourage people to do that.

—*Evan Handler*

ONE THING YOU can do in the hospital is talk to strangers. Sometimes a little conversation with someone you don't know has a big effect—whether you talk, cry, or just smile and listen. Sister Rosemary Moynihan came to see me almost daily, and even though I'm not Catholic, I think I became one of her favorites. She never failed to give me a boost, and I never let her leave without giving her a kiss on the cheek. Peter Borbon, a social worker, would go on for twenty minutes about the Mets' prospects for the season. Dr. Posner, a psychiatrist, didn't talk a lot but always left me with the feeling she'd said a good deal. And then there was Nilton Bonder, a cool Brazilian rabbi. He gave me the Psalms of David to read, and we schmoozed about the day I'd visit him in Rio and we'd lie on the beach, watching the girls and discussing the Talmud. Sister Rosemary, Peter, Nilton, and all the other heart, brain, and soul people who came to see me provided spice, serendipity, and a spiritual boost merely from the fact that they were there when I needed an ear.

—*Jonathan Pearlroth*

I READ MY chart every day, and I found it to be very interesting. I knew exactly when the doctors were coming on rounds. I had done a lot of reading—not in an obnoxious way but in an involved way.

I looked mostly for things like the drainage, which had to be at a certain level before I could go home. During surgery, they had taken the breast away and put in what I called the Reebok pump to expand the muscle over the next six months so that they could then put in the saline implants. So there was a pouch, and there was fluid, and it had to get down to a certain level before they would allow me to go home.

I would also monitor the different painkillers that they were giving me and under what kind of time frame. Right before I was leaving, they almost gave me the wrong medicine—I'm allergic to penicillin, and it was right on my chart. They started to give me something that's sort of a subset of penicillin. I told the intern that I couldn't take it.

—*Claire Noonan*

TO KEEP MYSELF busy, I would check on the cleaning staff by putting a Life Saver under my bed, write down what day I put it there, and watch to see when it was finally swept up and who did it.

One day I listened to my horoscope, which told me I should be critical of everyone that day. So I took a pen and paper and sat in the hall all day writing down criticisms. At the end of the day, I realized how fast it had passed and how unimportant the faults on the paper were in the big picture.

I hated the food in my hospital, which was actually rated as having the worst hospital food in Indiana. So I used to send reviews back down to the kitchen every so often with the leftovers on my tray.

I read somewhere that people who relapsed all had one thing in common—stress. So, while I don't think I approached it the way most people do, I approached it *my* way. My lawyer sent me a singing rabbi. One of my friends sent me a dancing nun. You can only cry so long, but you can laugh a lot longer. I didn't worry about what other people thought of me. I did what I needed to do in order to live.

—*Clara Trusty*

I DIDN'T LIKE sitting in bed. It made me feel like a sick person. So I would get up and pace my room. A lot of times, when no one was there, I'd turn my Walkman on, put my headphones on, and walk around the room, singing or dancing. I've always enjoyed dancing, and it made me feel better, like I was exercising a little bit. I was using my muscles, and I was passing the time. It helped me think I was still normal: "I can still dance. I can still get up and walk around. I'm not confined to the bed."

The pacing got my muscles going, even though it wasn't very far to pace. At first, I would pace for about twenty minutes and my legs would get tired. Then I noticed that I'd go through a whole tape, so I knew that I was pacing longer.

—*Michele Fox*

I WAS IN the hospital during Thanksgiving, Christmas, New Year's, and my birthday, and to cheer me up, my coworkers sent

Care packages and special gifts like pajamas, slippers, a robe, magazines, and books. Best of all, they made videos of staff parties and sent them to me.

—*Monica Ko*

ONE THING THAT made me feel better in the hospital was to put my makeup on every day. Unless I was just deathly ill, it made me feel better not to look so sick. I always tried to coordinate my jammies with my turbans. When I first was there, I was in isolation, and I couldn't go to the sink—it was on the other side of the glass—so I put my makeup on in the bed. I had my own mirror. But when I was on the bone marrow transplant ward, they had just started allowing patients to go to the sink as long as the door was shut and nobody was in the room.

—*Karla McConnell*

THEY KEPT ME in the hospital forever—ten days after surgery. I felt fine, and that was the hard part, that I had to stay even though I felt fine. Everyone thought that I was a patient's daughter. Most of the people who were in there were my mother's or grandmother's age, and here I was, thirty years old, bopping around, not in a hospital gown, but in shorts and a sweatshirt. I had a positive attitude through everything. I think the burden of the illness was taken away by my confidence in the doctors.

I escaped from the hospital once just to have dinner with my friends at a diner. I walked out the front door, and we went across the street for three hours.

—*Claire Noonan*

THE NURSES AND doctors at my hospital were great. My boyfriend actually stayed the night and slept with me in my bed a couple of times. They used to say, "If he wants to stay, we'll bring a cot in." A couple of times he would start to fall asleep in his cot, and I'd say, "Why don't you lie in bed with me?" He would climb in bed, and we would lie there together. The nurse would come in, and she'd say, "I just need to check your temperature, and then I'll leave you guys alone." And she said, "I won't be back for another five or six hours." She was really good about giving us our private time. The doctor too—the next morning he knocked on the door before he came in and introduced himself to my boyfriend. It was nice to know that we could have privacy in a place like a hospital.

—*Michele Fox*

WHEN I WAS admitted to the hospital, they took me to my room, and a nurse came in and said, "I'm Jane, and I won't be here tomorrow for your surgery but I want you to know that we're thinking about you, and you're going to be okay. I'll be here to take care of you next week." And when I woke up in ICU at four o'clock in the morning, this beautiful blonde in white was standing over me. I thought she was an angel and I hadn't made it. It was Jane. She'd come there on her day off because she wanted me to know that I was loved and that everyone was pulling for me and that she would be there to take care of me.

—*Melanie McElhinney*

I DON'T THINK hospitals necessarily have to be places set aside for suffering and horror. I think that life can be integrated a great deal more. I visited a children's hospital outside San Diego, which is just an incredible playground of a place. Everything is done in colorful ways; the floor designs, tiles, and carpets all have clues to help you find your way to other places. The kids' rooms circle around the nurses' station, and there's a dinosaur section, for example, and instead of room numbers, one room has a picture at kids' eye level of a dinosaur and a snowflake, another a dinosaur and a flower, another a dinosaur and an ant.

The charts are kept at their eye level, everything to impress upon them that they are part of the process and to make them feel at home and comfortable. At night, little pinpoint lights in the ceiling look like stars. They have created a wonderful atmosphere. Why couldn't a hospital like that be created for adults as well? Any setting that brought a sense of passion for life into it would be great. Everyone has their own aesthetic, but it's certainly not orange plastic institutional furniture.

Personally, I think a sense of humor would be the best way to go when designing a hospital. An eye toward packing as much enjoyment as possible into an atmosphere where a certain amount of suffering is unavoidable makes sense to me. In the hallways of this San Diego children's hospital, the artwork on the wall was interactive. It was all puzzles that you could put your hands into and move parts around. There was this incredible mobile sculpture with moving parts and ball bearings that moved and spun around on wheels. Why couldn't there be puzzles on the wall of an adult hospital and little mindbenders and teasers all over the place? The CAT scan area of this hospital had a giant picture of cartoon cats all over the place. Personally, I would have enjoyed that as the way to find the CAT scan area in my hospital better than little green signs that said "CAT scan."

—*Evan Handler*

CHAPTER ELEVEN

Coping with Surgery

Among us, we've had myriad biopsies, cancers reduced or removed, as well as organs removed and limbs amputated. Our dealings with surgeons have been among the most and least satisfying. We've found them incredibly skilled, creative, able to make important decisions at the operating table, even sensitive to our concerns about superficial scars. In other cases, we've found them taciturn, arrogant, and callous.

Because surgery requires a high level of skill, physical stamina, dexterity, and the ability, literally, to think on one's feet—not just to think, but to make life-and-death decisions—there seems to be a high degree of bravado among surgeons. They have been called the prima donnas of the medical world. Which can lead to problems with patient relations. Keep this in mind when you're meeting with prospective surgeons. Ask the extra question, so you can better gauge the tenor of the relationship you're likely to have. You must feel able to constructively discuss your fears, concerns, and preferences with this person.

It not only helps to have some insight into the way surgeons tend to think, but it also helps to physically and mentally prepare yourself for surgery and the important recovery period following surgery.

If your surgery involves amputation, there are special concerns: See "Making the Best of Amputation" on page 188, where we talk about what it's like to lose a limb, how we bounced back, and some of the ongoing concerns.

I STARTED HURTING on a Saturday, a week after I had felt a strange foreign something in my right side. It was one of those things that sometimes was there and sometimes wasn't. It was a busy time at work, so I had just made an appointment to go in the next week. After reading a medical book, I decided that it was my ovary and that it might be swollen and could be a tumor. My book explained how they sometimes burst, and I had a friend who did have an ovarian tumor burst in the middle of the night. She was in a lot of pain, had to have an emergency operation, and then had to go back for more surgery later. That kind of frightened me.

So I went to the emergency room. They did an ultrasound, and it was a tumor on the ovary the size of an orange. My doctor sent me to Birmingham, where they do these operations every day. I went on Tuesday, and on Wednesday morning I went in for surgery.

I take good care of myself and didn't want a big scar unless absolutely necessary. I'd heard about the bikini incision for hysterectomies. I asked about it, but the doctor thought the tumor was too large to come through a bikini incision. He said it was too important an operation to be thinking of vanity at that time. He was going to pass right over it: "No, I don't think we can do that."

Here I was in an emergency situation, so I was at a disadvantage in my argument. But it bothered me that he was going to make a big incision right up the middle of my tummy. So I let him know in a nice way that I was serious about him getting by with a bikini incision if at all possible.

My husband also pitched in. He explained that he could see I was determined about this and that because I exercised regularly, he could see why I didn't want my abdomen scarred any more than necessary. The doctor said, "Yes, Ginnie has taken care of herself, and being thin is the reason she was able to find the tumor in the first place." He said, "Most people go around for years with this tumor, which gives it time to break out into the colon and other areas."

I said, "Well, maybe we could start with the bikini incision, and then if you need to, make the other one." He felt that was fair enough. If he found he needed to make another incision, fine, he had permission, but at least he'd try to get by with a smaller one. I stood up for how I felt but not in a way that made it hard for him to work with me. I think he appreciated that and understood how I felt.

It's more comfortable for the surgical team to have a bigger incision. But they had a young female associate who took her tiny hands and lifted out the tumor, and it worked. They did take out the other ovary and found that it had cysts but no sign of any cancer. But because of this doctor with very small hands they didn't have to do the other incision.

The fact that they could understand my desire as a patient meant so much to me. So many times I've heard the story: "If I'd had time, I would have gotten a second opinion or found out exactly what they were going to do." I'm glad I persevered and got what I wanted.

—Ginnie Higginbotham

I WENT BACK for another cone biopsy of my cervix not two months after the first one, and it was so different. This time the surgeon walked with me into the operating room, talking to me the whole time. The first time, the doctor had sort of said hello and disappeared, and I hadn't known what was going on.

The first time, the anesthesiologists discussed how they were going to put me out without looking at or talking to me. This time, Dr. Cash introduced me to the whole team and told me who they were and what they were doing in there. When he went to wash up, they continued that process, asking me questions and telling me what they were going to do and what various things were for. I found that comforting.

The first time, they wheeled me to the operating room and made me scoop myself from my bed over onto the table. The operating table, because it's a female surgery, has a hole in it where your vagina is—it's kind of strange to have to do this. This time, they put me to sleep while I was in my bed. I didn't have to do anything. It was very dignified. I didn't feel awkward or exposed or anything. The intern asked me if I minded if he was in there observing. That was really cool.

Then—here's my favorite part—the first time I had this surgery, I remember waking up confused and in a lot of pain. I was in a room with twenty other people, nurses running around, and I asked for painkillers. The nurse came over and said, "Let me see what we can do." She called my doctor, and he said, "Just give her Advil." Then they wheeled me out. The second time, I woke up from my surgery, and Dr. Cash was standing there holding my hand. I looked at him and said, "It hurts a lot more than it did the first time."

He said, "I'm going to get you some drugs." He got me drugs and told the nurse that he wanted to see me before I went home. He went and got my mother and brought her in to sit with me. He came back before I was released and sat down for a few minutes. He always does this—sits down and looks very comfortable, like he has nothing else to do. He has a hundred people waiting for him at any given moment but always acts like he's only talking to you. He told me how the surgery went and how I'd be feeling and gave me his home phone number and his pager number.

It was so different. The funny thing was that it was the same hospital. So the OR staff were the same people, but the experience was one hundred percent different. I think the key is finding a doctor whose style you like because the nurses and other staff members take their cue from the doctor.

—*Rachel Kaul*

I HAD A good local doctor who knew when to turn it over to somebody else. He told me what options there were. We discussed whether to take the whole esophagus out or to go for bits and pieces of it. What I was told is that this particular cancer hops; it does not stay in one place. The doctor who was doing the operation thought we should remove as much as possible because otherwise I was taking a chance that it would come back.

When I asked if there was anything I could do to get ready for the operation, they said, "Get into as good a physical condition as you can. You want to be as strong as you can." I've always been a very active person. I'm not a traditional jock, but I like to walk and play sports. They said it helped a lot to be strong. So I started running again. This was about three months before the operation.

The operation lasted nine hours, and it was pretty rough on them. The doctors would bring me back to consciousness once in a while so they could tell me how things were going. I thought that was cool. They said, "Obviously we won't turn the pain stuff off, but we will let you know how things are going." They would sort of bring me back and say, "Okay, open your eyes. You can't do anything, but we want to let you know that everything is okay so far."

My friends who knew about my Peace Corps service gave me a life preserver that they had written messages on. I took it with me to the hospital and hung it on my bed, and all the doctors and nurses on the team came in and wrote messages on it.

—*Rick Asselta*

What You Can Do to Prepare for Surgery

Walk a couple miles a day to improve your strength, and make sure you keep eating well; good nutrition and physical endurance will help you better tolerate the surgery. A well-balanced diet helps the immune system and the body's ability to heal. Patients who are in good physical shape can usually get out of bed much sooner and do their respiratory therapy much more easily, which helps them avoid complications like pneumonia.

Cancer-surgery patients tend to have a high incidence of clotting. They often produce more platelets, and their blood has a tendency to be stickier, particularly in the pelvis and legs. Patients who have well-conditioned lower extremities have much less risk of developing thrombosis, or internal blood clotting.

—Jeffrey J. Smith, M.D.,
Senior Gynecologic Surgeon, Clinical Associate Professor,
University of Oklahoma Health Science Center,
Oklahoma City, Oklahoma

WHEN YOU FIRST feel yourself waking up out of the anesthesia, somebody told me, just keep your eyes shut for a little bit longer and breathe really deeply for a while until you feel your own equilibrium. Then, open your eyes slowly. Just as you slowly count backward when you go down, allow yourself to wake up the same way. It eases you back into a state of consciousness. I did it, and it really helped. I think I would have been frightened initially otherwise—waking up in that big room with all those people who had just come out of surgery. One of the things they don't tell you is exactly what this process is going to be. You're sitting on a gurney with fifty other people all at the same time— it's not *General Hospital.*

—*Claire Noonan*

AFTER THE OPERATION, I was in a lot of pain. In fact, the first few months after the operation were worse than having the cancer. The pain was almost unbearable. It's kind of hard to describe. It was my whole body—my nerves were on fire. The doctors couldn't tell me why. I couldn't stand. I couldn't sit. I couldn't stay still. So what I did was keep moving, keep busy. The only thing that seemed to stop it was cold, so even during the winter, sometimes I'd go onto the back porch and just let the cold numb it. After about three months, it just disappeared. It was like somebody threw a switch and it stopped.

There was some problem with my spine related to the anesthesia. I still have a lump there, and part of my back remains numb. In addition, I was adjusting to the fact that I didn't have an esophagus anymore. My stomach was rebelling, and it was easy to choke. Swallowing was difficult. I had to adjust, and it took a while.

To try to overcome it, I started walking and then running again. When I first started running, I'd have to stop a lot. I had a route I ran near my house. There's a cemetery near it, and I liked to read the names on the stones. When I started, it was February, it was March, it was April, and then spring came. One very cold morning—so cold I hadn't even wanted to run—I passed that site and saw the trees and buds breaking through the winter, and that particular point was very poignant. The sun began to break through and warm my back. I stopped and looked at the flowers and started to cry. I realized I had made it.

—Rick Asselta

I HAD BRAIN surgery and was treated with radiation afterward. And to this day—I reached the ten-year mark in August of '96—I don't have any repercussions from it at all. It's pretty amazing, actually. The doctor gave me a list about as long as my arm of things that could happen as a result of the surgery, such as blindness, aphasia, not being able to speak, paralysis, and even death. My son was ten months old, and I just sort of laughed at the doctor and said, "I'm not going to die." But I never thought I'd be as normal as I am today.

I was up and about in no time, begging them to let me out of ICU so I could get out of bed. I was making my bed in the hospital, and the nurses just couldn't believe it. I figured I felt great because they had gotten that thing out of my head, but it was euphoria from the prednisone, a steroid they had given me. After I stopped taking it, I didn't have the kind of superenergy I had had on the drug, but I was still amazed at how good I felt.

Now the only aftereffect I have is a very slight equilibrium confusion sometimes when I reach over. I might lose my balance a little, but never to the point where I fall. I'm able to catch myself. That's it. I've worked ever since.

—Cathy Owen

I DIDN'T EXPECT to get sick so much after surgery. I've always been a very healthy person, but every three weeks I'd come down with something—an earache, a sore throat, a this or that. Apparently that's not abnormal when your immune system is being attacked.

—Rachel Kaul

TO TREAT MY melanoma, the surgeon removed the mole and cut away tissue until he reached an area competely free of carcinoma. This meant cutting through muscle and tendons, lifting the shoulder blade to gather tissue beneath, cutting from the back of the neck across the shoulder, and making a thorough examination of the shoulder-bone area and the lymph nodes in the armpit and neck. All of this for a mole the size of a half-dollar.

Thankfully, the doctors determined that no lymph nodes were cancerous, and the surgeon believed all of the melanoma had been removed. The surgeon took a graft of skin from my lower back and buttock and placed it over the abyss. I was tightly bound with my hands across my chest to keep the graft in position while it healed.

After the surgery, I was heavily sedated. My mind was like mush. People came and went, moved me, asked questions, and checked my vital signs. My chart gave orders not to disturb my wound's dressing, but someone failed to read the instructions and mistakenly uncovered it, which moved the graft. Infection and gangrene set in. I developed a high fever and grew very ill. Antibiotics helped, but the doctors had to cauterize a great deal of the graft, which left me with a large scar with ridges and bumps throughout. The skin graft is very thin, and there are no nerve endings on the scar itself. The area on the lower back, where the graft came from, was extremely tender and took quite some time to heal. It also left its mark.

Then came the process of recovery. Because there had been so much trauma to the right arm, the shoulder, and the neck area, I had very limited use of my right arm. There was also the psychological side of the recovery. I had such a horrible scar. Though I never thought of myself as vain, I couldn't look at my back. In my mind I was disfigured and disabled. Everyone helped me. My husband, God love him, treated the scar with antibiotics for three months to hasten the healing. When I cried at how horrid I was, he assured me it didn't matter and encouraged me to exercise my arm so we could play tennis together.

A lady from the American Cancer Society visited me and showed me her double mastectomy. She was years younger, absolutely beautiful, and didn't care a flip about her breasts. She was alive, well, and looking forward to a long life. That helped open my eyes. My children also encouraged me. They helped at home, took care of me, and, though I know they were frightened at the possibility of losing their mother, they never showed their fear or talked about it until much later.

I began to think I could use my arm again and started exercising. Breast surgery patients will tell you about the "climb the wall with your arm" exercise. You draw a line on the wall and climb it with your fingers. Each time you raise the line it's another step ahead. When you finally draw a line taller than you are and manage to raise your arm above your head, it's time to celebrate.

Rehabilitation was not easy for me. I've never been a very disciplined person and sometimes reading a good book seemed more enticing. The trauma to the muscles and tendons around my shoulders, the shoulder blade, and the ball-and-socket joint had left me in considerable pain. To avoid this pain, which increased during the exercises, I simply wanted to stay in my room. But I came to realize that I would heal faster and get back to my life more easily if I improved my attitude. I worked at it every day. Fearful sometimes that stretching would rip my graft (although the doctor assured me this wouldn't happen), I began swimming. I went to the fitness center at six-thirty every morning and swam laps, always with a shirt covering my scar. After six months, I was up to sixty laps and felt I could do anything. I played tennis after eight months, which surprised even the therapists and the doctor.

—*Ruth St. John*

THERE ARE TWO nerves in the esophagus that are vocal-cord nerves, and in the course of the operation, they can be cut. The surgeon told me the odds were that I'd lose my voice, but he was going to do everything he could to save it.

After the operation, the nerves were okay for one vocal cord, but the other one looked gone. Talking was laborious and sounded pretty crummy. I sounded like Marlon Brando in *The Godfather*. I made the mistake of going back to work too soon. I got out of the hospital in February, and by May I went back to work for the end of school. I was using a portable mike attached to my throat to talk to the kids. The kids were real nice about it, but I think going back to work so soon made my recovery take longer.

One vocal cord was so badly damaged that it looked like they'd have to operate again and move the one that worked closer to the one that didn't so it might vibrate off the other. About three or four days before that operation was to take place, I was driving with my daughter to the hospital, and I was kind of joking around, and all of a sudden it was like, *pow*. It just came back. The nerve recovered. I started singing and said, "God, I can sing!" My daughter looked at me and said, "No you can't, Dad." Thanks a lot, kid.

She said, "I guess we can put this operation off."

The funny part was that we wound up getting a bill for the operation. I called the hospital and said it never took place. They said, "Oh, yes it did."

I said, "You tend to notice when someone puts a knife to your throat."

—Rick Asselta

Making the Best of Amputation

WHEN I WAS fifteen years old, I was diagnosed with osteogenic sarcoma, which is a rare form of bone cancer. At the time, I was a cheerleader at my high school, I had horses that I loved to ride, but the most important thing to me was my dancing. I was training for an audition for the New York City Ballet Company. The way that works is you have to audition for an audition, and I'd gone through the first audition and was preparing for the second one when I started feeling a lot of pain in my left hip and down my left leg.

I attributed it to all of the exercise that I was getting as a cheerleader coupled with all of the training that I was doing for the upcoming audition. I was dancing seven days a week and was either in class or teaching classes to children. The pain was getting significantly worse, but I thought that if I kept training, it would eventually work itself out. Finally, it got so bad that I went to a chiropractor. This was about three months into it—in January of 1980.

Unbeknownst to me or the chiropractor, a tumor was growing on the sacroiliac crest in my hip. The chiropractor would crack me and manipulate everything and I'd feel great when I came out of his office. But I'd go on to dance class, and in a couple of hours be in extraordinary pain again. It got to the point where I was losing weight rapidly, my hair was falling out, I was losing color, and I was obviously sick. But nobody knew why.

The chiropractor referred me to a neurologist in Richmond. At first we thought it was a slipped disc that was pinching the sciatic nerve or a ruptured disc or something like that, and then through a series of tests, the neurologist discovered that there was a large tumor about the size of a grapefruit growing in my pelvis. After a biopsy, it was determined that it was sarcoma. It turns out that my chiropractor had been manipulating my sciatic nerve away from the tumor—which was why, for a time following my sessions with him, I'd be free from pain.

While it took about six months to diagnose, after diagnosis everything moved really rapidly. Three days later, my left leg and hip were amputated. They considered doing a hip replacement of sorts but were unable to do that for a variety of reasons. One of the characteristics of osteogenic sarcoma, the way it was explained to me, is that it quickly breaks off and travels to other parts of the body, and so to make sure that they got all of the tumor, they needed to remove the hip and the leg. I then had six months of chemotherapy. I was on the drug Adriamycin, which was actually in clinical trials at that time but is now the protocol for osteosarcoma.

I had my surgery in May of 1980, took the chemotherapy through November of 1980, and then in January of 1981, actually on my sixteenth birthday, I received my artificial limb and went into rehabilitation with that. I did rehab for about two weeks, came home, and went back to school. I had been doing homebound school the whole time, but then I went back to classes in February of 1981. I also went back to dance class.

It sounds trite, but part of my will to keep going was my desire to dance again. When I was told that I had osteogenic sarcoma and what the prognosis was, which wasn't good, and what the protocol would be, the first question that came out of my mouth was, "Will I be able to dance again?" There were about twenty white coats surrounding my bed, and they all just looked at each other. Nobody wanted to be the bad guy and say, "Probably, no."

My surgeon had the misfortune of explaining that it was very difficult to sit with this type of amputation—even with a prosthesis. There are very few people in the entire world who even have true hemipelvectomies, like the one I was to receive. He never said "Never" because he is wonderful, but he made sure that I understood that it was going to be difficult. A year later, when I did dance in a recital, he wasn't able to be there, but he called me to wish me luck, as did all of the other physicians involved.

—*Melanie McElhinney*

I WENT FROM having a little bit of pain in my chest to where you could see the tumor growing every day. By the time they did the surgery, you could tell where the tumor was because my chest was sticking out. It was the size of a baseball and, being underneath my pectoral muscle and pushing out, it caused excruciating pain.

When they sedated me to do the biopsy, it was the best day I'd had in months—the first time I'd been out of pain in a long while. It had gotten so bad several weeks before the surgery that my wife was going to the pharmacist in the middle of the night to get all kinds of things.

I had a four-quarter amputation—my shoulder blade and all my arm. They took out the majority of the ribs on the right side of my chest where the tumor was. They rebuilt my chest wall with a piece of muscle from my leg. It was radical and aggressive, but that's how you had to treat it. Surgery, at that point, was a relief. By the time I came to afterward, there was pain—don't get me wrong—but it was a different kind of pain.

—*Dale Totty*

EVEN THOUGH I was in my twenties, I was in the pediatric ward after my amputation because osteogenic sarcoma is normally a childhood cancer. Before I got the prosthesis for my leg, I painted my crutches and put rhinestones on them, used them to practice moving all about, and kept a positive attitude. During my time in the ward, I noticed that the little girls in the room began to shed the blankets from their laps, show their amputations, and get up to walk around on crutches. I realized that I was inspiring them to have fun with their crutches and get active. Knowing that I was helping others helped me even more.

—*Ivy! Gunter*

AFTER MY AMPUTATION, they wanted me to go through therapy, to write the alphabet for hours on end. I just couldn't do it. They wanted me to fit the scenario of someone who has lost an arm. I got real frustrated. I just refused to do their therapy. Instead, I went home and restored an antique car. It was one of those things I'd always wanted to do. A friend of mine had one when I was in college, and we used to tinker with his. That was my therapy, and that was how I learned to use hand tools. I just did it.

Cancer made me stop and think, "What's important?" I had been all set to go work in the corporate world, and I said, "I can't do that. We've got to change something here." I had been doing everything for the future, for my career. There's nothing wrong with that, but at the same time, if you're not really aware of what's going on, you're missing a lot. I didn't even know if I was going to be alive in six months. People get so bogged down in what they're doing, how important they are. They have to have this and that—the money, the car, the house. I think people lose awareness of what's really important. They don't spend time with their kids. It's terrible. I feel fortunate because I was woken up at an early age.

I'd always wanted to be a full-time wildlife artist, and I decided this was the time. So I painted while I finished college and got myself back together physically.

I love the outdoors. Nature is a good place to figure out what's going on. You can see where you stand in the whole realm of life. You can reflect. You're kind of small in the whole picture. It helped put me into perspective. At the time it seemed like I was barraged—school, hospitals, doctors, people—always something to deal with, so I turned to hunting, and hunting became therapeutic. Now I duck- and bird-hunt a lot. I grouse-hunt. I hunt with one hand. I'm a big person—six feet eight and two hundred pounds after losing my arm—so I'm blessed with a big hand. That helps me do these things one-handed. It wasn't easy because I had to change hands too. At first, I missed a lot. It took many a year to change from right- to left-handed.

I don't use an artificial arm or anything. I wear a shoulder-cap prosthetic, which pretty much just puts the shoulder shape back, so at least my clothes will hang. I won't use the arm; it just gets in the way. It's actually limiting and even a crutch, in my opinion. They gave me all kinds of living aids, and I have hardly used any of them. I said, "How am I going to fit in if I've got to have something special for everything I do?" The only thing I use that's specialized is a knife they gave me to cut food with.

I've adapted some equipment. To fish, I wear a fiberglass harness I developed that fits around my waist. It's got a tube where I put the fishing rod, different sizes for different rods. It has interchangeable pipes that you can fit different diameter rods into. After you catch a fish, you put the rod in, and then you can reel.

I do some tough stuff, but that's my mentality. If anything is a real challenge, that's what I like to do. I really started the hunting because I needed to walk. They took out a large section of muscle covering from my leg, and I had all this swelling and blood retention. I was also working on just one lung, so I felt I had to get going, or I'd never be able to make it.

I guess everybody gets their therapy in a different way. I just keep on getting it. I do the things people say you can't do—paint, fish, hunt, restore cars, build boats. I just do it. I kind of have an attitude that way. There are things that I have to overcome that most people don't even think about. I'm in a frame of mind now where I just find a way to do it.

—*Dale Totty*

WHEN I WENT back to the hospital for my rehab, unfortunately I was placed with stroke victims. They were all fifty or sixty years older than I was, and I thought, "I'm going to do what I need to do and get the heck out of here." It was incredibly depressing.

For hemipelvectomies, you kind of sit in your prosthesis, and it wraps around your stomach real tight, and that's what holds it on. To walk, you take your first step with your sound leg, and the forward motion will bend the artificial knee, and then you learn to use your back muscles and the momentum of going forward to swing the artifical limb through. Acquiring a natural gait takes a lot of work and a lot of practice. I think my being a dancer helped me because learning how to use my new leg was really rigorous— nine hours a day of just walking and being really uncomfortable and really sore. The dancing and discipline helped at that point.

They put a mirror in front of me and a mirror behind me, and I walked on parallel bars all day. Back and forth and back and forth. For a break, I'd take a cane and go out in the middle of the floor and walk in a circle. They had to teach me how to fall again and get back up gracefully. I wanted to walk really well because if I walked really well, then that would help me to dance again.

After two weeks, I came home and went to dance class that night. I was so excited, and I wanted to show off my new leg. I was proud of it. I have a dimple in my right knee, and the prosthetist carved a dimple in my new left knee, to match exactly.

My dance teacher said, "Absolutely, you're going to be back on that stage again." I'd never thought about being in an actual recital. I had talked about going back to dance class and seeing my classmates, but it had never occurred to me I could be in a real performance. I was holding on to the bar with both hands, trying to get my balance again, and she came up to me that very first night and said, "Okay, we're going to figure out what you're going to do and how we're going to work this. You need a partner." She was incredibly supportive and really worked with me to figure out what I could do and what I couldn't—different ways to do turns and how to use my arms to my best advantage and use facial expression to make up for the lack of movement.

Well, I did dance again about a year later. I was not, by any stretch of the imagination, gracefully pirouetting across the floor like I once had, but I was there, and I did accomplish the goal of dancing again. It was in our local dance company's annual recital.

I was very nervous. All along throughout the diagnosis and the hospital stays, the Fredericksburg newspaper—I grew up in Stafford County, which is very close to Fredericksburg, Virginia—did an update article on me about once a month. They first wrote about me before my diagnosis—about my audition with the New York City Ballet, about the dance troupe, all that kind of stuff—and then a month later, they did an article about my getting sick. They took an interest in it and continued to follow it, so the day before the recital, I did an interview. I was nervous about people not understanding why I wasn't leaping around the stage—I was afraid that people wouldn't know what had happened and that they would not understand why this girl was out there just kind of moving around, moving her arms. I didn't realize that the entire audience would be an incredible support system.

So I was very nervous. I had to dance with a partner because I'd only had my limb for about two months, and the hardest thing about learning how to walk again was trusting something that I couldn't feel. Stepping off a curb was just terrifying because I didn't know that the knee wasn't going to buckle. That was the most difficult part to overcome when trying to learn how to do some simple moves in the middle of the floor again.

I walked out with my partner, who was one of my parents' best friends. He was a Fairfax County policeman. He took a lot of ribbing for it but ended up being named Policeman of the Year that year. He's really wonderful. It's difficult to put all of those emotions into words, but when I got out there, the smell of the rosin and the bumps of the toe shoes on the stage—all of it—was exhilarating.

The stage started black, and the music began, and the spotlight hit us, and we came out from the wings. We walked out, and he had his arm around me, and I had one arm up and the other one out, as in first position. We bent and swayed at the appropriate times, and I could do what is called a balance, which is step with your right foot, put your left foot behind, step with the left, and step with the right, so that you're making a back-and-forth motion. I could turn on my artificial limb if I rocked it the right way, and Tim, my partner, was standing there to catch my hand and make sure that I kept my balance. I could do pirouettes or piqués, and I could do chaînés, which are little tiny turns. I did a couple of those. But no leaping. There was no muscle control. My left leg had to remain straight. It was just combinations of simple moves. All I had ever wanted to do was to be on the stage dancing, and being back on the stage was exhilarating, even though I wasn't leaping. It was wonderful.

At the end of the performance, there was a rousing standing ovation, which was really incredible. I'll never forget it. It was truly overwhelming.

—*Melanie McElhinney*

AMPUTATION DOESN'T HAVE to slow you down. There's an explosion going on in technology and resources and new devices. Golf clinics, water-skiing clinics, snow-skiing clinics, bowling. Even though I lost a leg, I play golf and swim. They taught me to run, but I've never really kept up with that. It's very physically intensive. The main thing that I was really active in all through college was swimming. I'd do laps and laps without any problem. I do it now for pleasure. I used to snow ski too, but then I ruptured a disc in my neck, which scared me off skiing for a while. I've learned how to ride a stationary bike, and I've ridden a two-seater bicycle with my wife. I'm still working with a physical therapist who wants to teach me to ride a regular bike.

—*Frederick Duckworth, Jr.*

After Amputation: Phantom Pains

THEY USED TO take me down to talk with folks who were in the electrical-burn unit. A lot of these guys—many power-line workers—had lost arms or lost the use of their arms from electrical accidents. Most people have these things called phantom pains. I probably talk to more people about that than the cancer. The arm actually feels like it's there, and it drives you nuts at the beginning. It feels like someone is bending your fingers backward and you can't stop it. It feels like you're breaking your arm or your wrist. It's terrible.

My doctor prescribed some kind of narcotic, but I felt like I was drugged up all the time. I said, "It's still not helping."

He said, "Listen, it's not going to go away. You're going to have to tough it out." And I did. I came to believe that the phantom pain provides you the balance you need to survive. I still feel like I have everything on that side. As I told a guy in the electrical-burn unit who was going nuts, "Believe it or not, the phantom pain is serving a purpose. It's going to make you feel whole down the road. It'll still bug you at times, but you'll get used to it."

I still have episodes of phantom pain from time to time. I get all kinds of feeling down in that arm. I think it's from stress. Now they have all kinds of pain therapy and electrode therapy, but at the time that wasn't a real popular thing.

—*Dale Totty*

MY FATHER HAD a friend who was a psychiatrist, and he helped teach me relaxation techniques, which were very important because I had a lot of phantom pain from my amputation. Sometimes it's just a sensation where you feel like your leg is still there, but sometimes it's actually pain. They've come a long way now with different kinds of treatment, but a lot of people are still bothered by it. Pain medicine helped some, but it made me a zombie. I was trying to go back to school, so it was hard to take narcotic pain medicine and come home sleepy and not be able to study.

My psychiatrist taught me relaxation techniques to overcome the phantom pains, and I used them to help me with the chemo too. The main one that he taught me was to start at the tip of my toes and visualize both sides of my body, even though my whole left leg wasn't there. Imagine your toes going to sleep, then the front part of your foot, then the middle of your foot, and then the back part of your foot. Continue up your ankle and calf, knee and thigh, and on up until you're totally relaxed. It really worked. I would lie on the sofa or floor or bed and would just feel this warmth come over me as I got my whole body to relax that way. It would make the pain go away. It was amazing.

I still get some phantom pains every three or four months, in the middle of the night. But when I get them now, they're different—more like fleeting electric shocks.

—*Frederick Duckworth, Jr.*

CHAPTER TWELVE

The Big Guns:
Bone Marrow Transplant

In the past ten years, the improvement of bone marrow transplant techniques and procedures has brought cancer treatment a long way. In fact, bone marrow transplants have been a major breakthrough in the treatment of certain cancers. These days they are not only used for people who have had a cancer relapse, but more and more as a front-line procedure. Women with breast cancer having ten or more positive nodes are frequently advised to have an autologous (using the patient's own bone marrow) transplant. They can then be given much stronger doses of chemotherapy, killing many more cancer cells.

Most transplants nowadays are done with stem cells—the most immature blood cells, which re-engraft more quickly. Restrictions for isolation are less severe, and drugs to combat graft-versus-host disease are now available. The technology has evolved, but the premise remains the same. They bombard you with chemo and radiation in order to kill the cancer, which at the same time destroy your immune system. Afterwards, they have to give you back your previously harvested marrow, or that of a donor, in order to rescue your immune system and get you back on your feet.

This is some heavy duty stuff, but the results make it worthwhile. Volunteers at the Bone Marrow Transplant Family Support Network (800-826-9376) will discuss all aspects of the process with patients or family members. They have an extensive list of advisers who have been through the treatment for many different kinds of cancer.

SINCE MY DOCTORS didn't give bone marrow harvesting much priority, I had to push them to do it just in case conventional chemotherapy didn't work, and I needed a transplant.

The bone marrow harvest was a piece of cake compared to the major surgery I had already had to remove part of my stomach. The morning of the harvest, I was wheeled down to the operating room and was knocked out with general anesthesia. I woke up an hour or two later in the recovery room. I had very little pain, just soreness in my hips and sternum, but nothing that a couple of Tylenols couldn't take care of.

I was sent home the next morning. The doctor told me that he had inserted a large needle into my hip and sternum area and sucked out enough marrow to do the transplant and have plenty for backup. He said that bone marrow regenerates quickly so that removing a couple liters had no effect on my immune system. The marrow was treated with chemo and then frozen in liquid nitrogen to be held indefinitely in case I needed it at some point thereafter. Nowadays, they are doing more and more stem-cell transplants, which don't even require general anesthesia. Blood is taken from the donor's vein, the stem cells are separated, and the rest of the blood is then returned to the donor. The procedure is like giving a blood donation—you're out of there in a couple of hours.

Harvesting my marrow turned out to be a smart move because I relapsed soon after my first remission, and the tumor had grown back to the size of a football. Since conventional chemo had failed, my best—and possibly only—hope was a bone marrow transplant.

—*Jonathan Pearlroth*

WITH THE VERY first chemotherapy treatment, I immediately started getting better. Six months later, I was in total remission. I had very few problems with the chemo. I'd be in the hospital for four straight days per month and would get out and feel kind of bad for a day. I always rebounded. I never lost my hair or anything like that.

At the end of six months, I was disease-free, and then the doctor popped something on me that I didn't expect. He said, "What do you think about going for a bone marrow transplant? The reality of myeloma is that it will probably come back, and it comes back a little worse each time. Right now you're healthy and young, and maybe we can just knock this out totally." The bone marrow transplant was a big step. Here I was, totally healthy with the possibility that the disease would never come back, and now I would be taking a chance of dying, with a certainty that I was going to be very physically altered at least temporarily.

I thought about it and talked with my wife. I thought the transplant was the course to take because if I waited five years and it came back, I would be five years older and not as strong. There was a sixty-percent chance that I'd make it through the transplant and a forty-percent chance that I wouldn't, and I was pretty resigned to that. Fortunately, my brother turned out to be a perfect match, so we took off for Seattle in late April of 1990 and had it done. It was four months of pretty intense stuff, but I walked out of there disease-free, and I still am today.

—*Tim McLaurin*

I HAD MY bone marrow transplant in 1986. I'll never forget the details. On my first day, at 8:30 A.M., I was taken down to Nuclear Medicine for my first blast of total-body radiation. The radiation technician strapped me onto a support pole, which—I apologize for the lack of a better description—looked like a crucifix.

I was strapped in tightly, because the radiation, they said, might make me feel faint and possibly even lose consciousness. I received forty-seven rads over a period of twelve minutes to the front of my body, and then I was flipped over like a pancake to have the same amount applied to my back side. The lead lung protectors, which had been custom-made for me, were precisely positioned on my chest according to an X ray of my lungs.

The radiation was invisible, odorless, and painless; the buzz of the radiation machine was the only thing that let me know that something was happening. Afterward, I felt very nauseous, but as in chemotherapy, each patient has a different reaction and to a different degree. The process was repeated at twelve-thirty and four-thirty in the afternoon, and then again, three times a day, over the course of the next three days—Tuesday, Wednesday, and Thursday. On Friday, I received only the morning and noon treatments, which brought to an end the radiation portion of the transplant.

Saturday was a day for rest and recovery, and on Sunday, the chemotherapy protocol began. On Sunday, Monday, and Tuesday, I received VP 16, a mysterious-sounding chemotherapeutic agent, and on Wednesday and Thursday, I was given massive doses of Cytoxan, another chemotherapy drug. The Cytoxan wound up the chemo phase of the transplant.

Afterward, I was under constant observation by the doctors as they waited for my blood counts to fall. Once my counts reached zero—how odd it was to have zero as a goal—my marrow, which had been harvested from my hips previously, was brought from the lab's liquid nitrogen freezers and injected into my system through my catheter, very much as if I were receiving a blood transfusion. The rest of the transplant procedure involved waiting and coping: waiting for the marrow to engraft and for my immune system to restore itself, and coping with the unpredictable side effects of radiation sickness. I had no immune system for at least two weeks, which meant I had to deal with infections, diarrhea, mouth and gastrointestinal-tract sores, and fevers. I had to take plenty of painkillers, and I felt thoroughly weakened throughout the period.

Since I was vulnerable to any and all infections, it was necessary to place me in "reverse isolation" during the critical period when I had no immune system. Reverse isolation is protection against infections that come from the outside world. It's the opposite of the common form of isolation where people in the outside world are protected against being infected by patients with contagious diseases, like chicken pox or tuberculosis. But while the reasons for the two kinds of isolation are different, the practical effect of both is the same: I wasn't able to leave my room. It meant that everyone entering my room had to wear a cap, gown, mask, booties, and gloves. No one was permitted to get too close to me, and if any visitors weren't feeling one hundred percent well—if they had so much as a sniffle or sneeze—they were barred from my room. Once my immune system returned to an acceptable level—my white cell count had to reach 1.0—I was taken out of reverse isolation. The process took a total of five weeks.

I coped with the weeks of isolation in my small room by trying to assert as much control over my daily life as possible. I asked as many questions as I could. If someone came with a needle to draw blood, I asked them why and what for. If the nurse's aide wanted to weigh me at some ungodly hour of the morning, I'd tell her to come back later, at a more civilized time. I also learned how to ask for help and how to communicate with the staff. There is nothing wrong with making a friend or two. Talk to your nurse or doctor. Ask them about their personal lives. It's important to get beyond the formal medical relationship. It helps pass the time because you have someone to talk to, and it makes you, the patient, more than just another "case" for the staff.

But I didn't let friendship get in the way of what I needed. When I was in pain, I rang for my pain med until I got it. When I felt nauseous, I asked for something to help me get over it. If something, anything, was not right, I let the staff know where I was and what I was feeling. As competent as the doctors and nurses were, they were overworked and had plenty of other patients to take care of. I had to be the wheel that squeaked if I wanted to get the grease.

Many things about bone marrow transplants have changed since then. The reverse isolation isn't as strict; the doctors now use a growth factor to help speed your immune system's recovery; the pain-and-nausea management has improved; and they now perform stem-cell transplants, a milder alternative, as a first option. But the basic procedure remains the same. They blast you with medicine intended to kill the cancer, and at the same time they kill your immune system. That's why you need the transplant. It gives you back your immune system and your life.

My nurse at the time told me something I've never forgotten:

"The transplant will probably be the roughest thing you'll ever go through, but I know you're going to make it. Then the rest of your life," she said, her big brown eyes glowing at me, "will be a piece of cake!"

—*Jonathan Pearlroth*

I KEPT A journal of my bone marrow transplant. It helped me keep my perspective.

What I choose to forget:

1. Anxiety and fear
2. Visitors with masks
3. Severe vomiting
4. A ten-by-ten-foot room with a closed door
5. No hugs
6. Coming in
7. Going home
8. Coming back
9. Round-the-clock painkillers
10. No privacy
11. Fevers
12. Bone marrow biopsies
13. Infections
14. One bad nurse
15. Mouth sores
16. Swollen glands
17. Feeling ugly
18. Being bald

What I choose to remember:

1. The big picture window with a bright open view
2. Hanging fabric in my room with two friends
3. Monique to make up my room and bring fresh water
4. Long mornings in bed with a book and telephone

5. The warm, wonderful staff
6. Colored macaroni drawings of undersea life sent by my niece
7. Lots of time to get ready for the day
8. Afternoons of reflection on life: past, present, and future
9. Meeting with friends
10. A soothing environment
11. A peaceful and quiet sense of self
12. Perfectly controlled temperate air
13. Snuggling with a stuffed white bear that perfectly fit all my hurt places
14. Deep, detailed, and fulfilling conversations with my husband
15. Staying up as late as I wanted to
16. People always happy to talk to me when I called
17. Music of my choosing
18. Letters and gifts from friends and strangers
19. People who gave their lifeblood
20. Good advice from people who cared

—Jeanne Clair

MY EXPERIENCE AT the hospital in Baltimore, where I went for my bone marrow transplant, was much more human than at the New York hospital. They sent me a package of materials to let me know what was in store for me. It reminded me of going to summer camp: Don't forget to bring insect repellent and extra batteries for your flashlight. When I got there, the room numbers had been covered by each person's name cut from colorful construction paper, and all the patients were given giant calendars to put on the wall to record their blood counts and to cross off each day leading up to their release date.

They even had something called the evening of elegance. Everyone who made it through the transplant was entitled to an evening of elegance of their own design the night before they were released from the hospital. Usually it consisted of a waiter arriving in a tuxedo with an elaborate dinner—like filet mignon and wine and parfait desserts—from some local restaurant that would be served to the patient and their guest. It was included in the price of the stay. I thought that was a brilliant psychological tactic.

—*Evan Handler*

A Perspective on Bone Marrow Transplants

I worked as a nurse in the bone marrow transplant department from 1978 to 1985. I was doing direct patient care, and I also have a friend who had a bone marrow transplant a couple years ago. So I have experienced bone marrow transplants from a lot of different angles.

We are using much better diagnostic procedures and tools than we had before, and Zofran and better IV access for patients have greatly improved the process. Respiratory problems for bone marrow patients are much better understood than they were in the past. Now there are preventive measures and more aggressive treatments for these problems.

For certain diseases, transplants can even be done on an outpatient basis now, without the long isolation period. That's quite a leap. It's possible for some breast cancer patients, for example, to go in to get their chemotherapy and transplant and leave the next day. They go back to the clinic for frequent checks, but they're only hospitalized if they have complications. It's also possible sometimes to leave the day after the bone marrow or stem-cell infusion for other diseases as well. For most transplants, though, you still want the patient in the hospital and isolated. Even the breast cancer patients who leave the hospital are essentially isolated wherever they are, whether it's a hotel room or an apartment or whatever. They're not out walking around shopping or going to a ball game. They're confined, but not to the extent that you might be as an inpatient. The whole process is a lot easier on patients with the advances that have been made in the last few years.

—*Lorraine Anderson,*
Oncology Nurse Educator, University of Minnesota Hospital and Clinic
(and breast cancer survivor),
Minneapolis, Minnesota

IT'S NOT UNCOMMON for a couple or a whole family to relocate temporarily to the city where the medical treatment is being given. My son Evan went to Johns Hopkins for his bone marrow transplant. I had never been to Baltimore, and now all of a sudden I was going to be living there for anywhere from three to six months.

My husband and I looked into renting an apartment there, but we had no clue about which part of town to look in or which apartment complexes might be in a bad section or hard to reach from the hospital. We had no idea how the rents compared. So I made some phone calls. I knew somebody who travels all over the country for dog shows. Sure enough, she had a good friend in Baltimore, and they knew somebody who was the manager of a hotel downtown.

I thought this was going to be a good resource for me to find out the part of town to look in and a realtor to contact, but when I called, he said, "Look, I manage this hotel, and I'd be delighted to rent you a small apartment at a residential rate. You don't need to go to an apartment complex."

I told him, "I don't need daily housekeeping service. Just have them come in once a week to clean and change the linens." The big expense of a hotel room is housekeeping, so he could give me a rate that compared competitively to renting an apartment.

It turned out to be wonderful. The room was nicely furnished, and the hotel had a barber shop, restaurants, excellent security, and all the activities a hotel offers. We could get taxis if Evan needed us in the middle of the night. It was much easier than staying in an apartment.

Once you're in a new town, go to the public library and read the bulletin board and find out everything that is going on around town. The Yellow Pages are important, too, if you're looking for support groups through religious affiliations or through ancillary medical services or if you're trying to find things to do to fill the time. The patient is in the hospital, but the family has an awful lot of empty hours.

I found out that Baltimore has coffeehouses and bookstores. When my husband had to return to New York, it was a wonderful place for me to be alone because I was surrounded by things that gave me good vibes. When he was in Baltimore, we got to explore the city. We'd go to the library and to meetings and events. We managed to get to the symphony and to art shows, and we began to feel more at home. It's so easy to let your whole life revolve only around the hospital. You begin to shut out the rest of the world. But it's essential to have the perspective of life going on, that it's not all illness-related.

By not being totally enveloped in the medical aspect, we also made it more appealing for Evan's friends to visit him. They mostly came from New York, so they usually stayed in the hotel overnight. We were able to be better hosts. We'd have brunch for them in the morning in our apartment. It was a way of lightening things up. It's hard enough for young people to visit a friend who is so deathly ill. It helps to create a sense that life is going on.

—Enid Handler

CHAPTER THIRTEEN

Battling Breast Cancer

Breast cancer is the most common cancer among women. While annual incidences of new cases of breast cancer have been increasing by about three percent annually since 1980 and have now risen to around 200,000 a year, more breast cancer is being caught at earlier stages because of better screening techniques and greater awareness. This has led to increasingly successful treatment using surgery, radiation, or chemotherapy, or some combination of the three. In recent years, the use of autologous bone marrow transplants and high doses of chemotherapy have made strides in the battle against more advanced primary breast cancer and metastatic breast cancer.

With mastectomy, breast reconstruction often begins before you leave the operating table. That makes forethought doubly important. The Y-ME National Organization for Breast Cancer Information and Support (800-221-2141) provides hot-line counseling, educational programs, and self-help meetings. The American Cancer Society's Reach to Recovery program (800-ACS-2345) can often arrange a personal visit from a breast cancer survivor.

Encore, a YWCA-sponsored program for breast cancer patients, offers a forum for discussion and exercise classes for patients who have had breast cancer surgery. For more information, contact your local YWCA or the Encore National Board (212-614-2827).

Dealing with Mastectomy

SELF-ESTEEM IS awfully important in the case of breast cancer. My husband was so supportive that there was never a question that I would be less attractive with one breast than with two. I didn't suffer because of that.

Also, because there are so many of us out there who have had breast cancer, and it is so out in the open now, it's not as hard to accept—at least as opposed to the stigma that was attached to it twenty-five years ago, when my mother had breast cancer. I remember when she told me, it was so shocking, and it seemed at the time that it was something that had to be kept quiet—kept quiet because the patient herself wouldn't want people looking at her to see if one side looked different from the other side. I imagine it was harder in those days because there was so little written about it, and there was no Betty Rollin (author of *First, You Cry,* about her experience with breast cancer).

I just can't help thinking that it is easier to deal with now than it was then. Not easy, but easier, because there are places where you can go for advice and because you can read about the experiences of others.

—*Toni Zavistovski*

I ASKED EVERY question I could think of, but I never asked what the scars would look like. I just trusted them to deal with it cosmetically. I had a fabulous plastic surgeon, but the guy who makes the initial scar is the breast surgeon, and we never talked about the scars. Mine go all the way across my chest and almost meet in the middle. They didn't need to.

I compared chests with a good friend of mine who had breast cancer the year before me. Her scars are minimal compared to mine. So I confronted my surgeon about it. I said, "I can't wear V-neck T-shirts or bathing suits, and my friend's scars only go from the nipple to the outside."

The surgeon was honest with me. He said, "The bigger the incision, the easier it is for me. When we have a young woman, we really want to do an incredible job, particularly in cleaning out the breast tissue and making sure we get it all. But, no, it didn't have to be that big."

I would explore options. There is a new procedure at Johns Hopkins where they just make a circular cut around the nipple and do the entire mastectomy through that circular cut. When they reconstruct the nipple, there is virtually no scar. You can't tell. Ask about the scar. It's important.

—*Charlotte Wells*

WHEN I WAS diagnosed, my surgeon recommended lumpectomy, chemotherapy, and radiation, so that's what I chose. I had medullary cancer, and we didn't think it was going to be that bad, but then we found out that it was a very aggressive tumor. It was over two centimeters, poorly differentiated, and grade three.

They checked seventeen lymph nodes, and all of them were negative. However, I had a very strong family history of breast cancer, so I had to have chemotherapy. I did four cycles of CAF, which is Cytoxan, Adriamycin, and 5-FU, and then I did four cycles of Taxol. That's a new experimental thing for people like me, who although they have negative nodes, are at a high risk for recurrence.

Then my oncologist suggested that I have my breasts removed. He's promastectomy in younger women with aggressive tumors like mine. For some reason when he told me that, I felt relieved. I hadn't been ready when I was first diagnosed, but at that point, I knew it was the right thing to do. I didn't want to have to spend the rest of my life worrying about a recurrence. With the aggressiveness of my tumor and all the breast cancer in my family, removing my breasts just made sense to me.

When it came time for the surgery, I was ready. I don't think I ever shed a tear. That's the type of person I am. I wanted the harshest chemo. I wasn't afraid of that. I've met women who are really scared to have chemo, but I felt like it might save my life. Of course there are no guarantees, but I do feel good about the decisions that I've made. If I had a recurrence, I would never look back and question my treatment.

—*Leigh Abruscato*

I GOT SEVERAL opinions on my surgery, and I was given real options. One doctor discouraged me from having a double mastectomy. I don't remember the exact numbers now, but I had maybe a twenty-five percent chance of it recurring on the other side. He said, "You've got a seventy-five percent chance that it won't." But I was young and had young children, and I didn't want to risk a recurrence in the remaining breast. So I opted for aggressive surgery. I made that choice, and I don't have any regrets. The statistics are not good with recurrence. That's why I opted for the big-gun treatment. I knew the full range of my options and took responsibility for the choice.

—*Charlotte Wells*

I WOULD NEVER say that I'm happy that I had to have a breast removed—I certainly wish it hadn't been necessary as far as appearance goes—but it's not something that I really pine about. I was just thankful I found out early enough so that it didn't involve anything else. I didn't have to have chemotherapy. It wasn't something that would handicap me or change the way I was living. I can still do the same things I did before. Because of that and the support and encouragement of the people who loved me and the conviction that this was something that God had planned for my benefit in the long run, I never got depressed about it.

I felt that it was a chance for me to know God in a way that I wouldn't otherwise have had. I felt that it was going to make me more effective in helping other people, and that has certainly been the case.

—*Katherine Arthur*

IN LIFE THERE are different ways of looking at yourself. You can look down at your body; you can close your eyes and imagine what your body looks like; you can compare yourself to someone else; or you can choose to look straight at yourself in the mirror. I chose to look straight at myself in the mirror because I knew that if I was going to learn to accept myself and love myself again—for what I was and not what I wanted to be—then I would have to face myself front and center in the mirror.

The only way for me to get past the pain was to go through it. It took me four and a half years to completely accept myself for who I was: a woman with one breast. But having come to a full acceptance of who I was, I realized that I was so much more than I ever was before. My self-love became so strong that when reconstructive surgery came into vogue, and my doctor suggested it, I told him that I didn't want anything to do with it. I was comfortable with myself as I was.

—*Rhoda Silverman*

FOR A WHILE I thought that I would live with an impaired left arm. I had numbness in my left hand because of all the lymph nodes that had been removed. Then, a year later, I was doing exercises designed by Moshe Feldenkrais. (They are written up in a book called *Listening to the Body,* by Jean Houston and Robert Masters.) During the exercises, I suddenly had a severe pain in my left side, and then all the original feeling returned to that hand. It was explained to me that these exercises, most often used for stroke victims, reprogram the nerves. Feldenkrais's work has astounded me. His exercises allow the body to do things it didn't know how to do before.

—*Elsa Porter*

ONE THING THAT nobody told me was that my arm movement would be restricted at first. My mom, who'd had breast cancer before I did, mentioned that I would have to do exercises after the surgery, but she intentionally didn't overwhelm me with the recovery part.

I had a double mastectomy, and they had to cut the muscles under my armpits to take out the lymph nodes. So both my arms were out of commission after the surgery. I couldn't raise my arms even to shoulder height. I couldn't get out of bed by myself. There were days when my five-year-old had to come and prop me up, because I'd get stuck. I'd get stiff from sleeping, and fall off the pillows and be lying flat with no strength in my arms. I literally couldn't get up. That part was really tough, but with a lot of physical therapy, I was able to get that mobility back.

—*Charlotte Wells*

I ENCOURAGE WOMEN who have had a mastectomy to be very frank with their husbands. The patient is dealing with losing a part of her body that is closely associated with who she is as a woman, with physical limitations after the surgery, with fears about being unloved or even dying, and she needs to be able to share all of these feelings with her husband. He may have trouble dealing in the emotional realm. Here he is, worried sick about the woman he's shared his life with, yet he's holding on to his stiff-upper-lip upbringing. Some men may need help learning how to listen to their wives' feelings—and how to express their own.

—*Elizabeth Martin*

THE BIGGEST ISSUE for me after my mastectomy and implant was dating. When do you tell someone? Somebody who is forty or fifty might have heard of this before, but my peers don't know. At first explaining that I had had a mastectomy was my biggest fear. You're no longer going to have the perfect body in someone's mind. But finally you realize that if you're seriously involved with somebody, it really doesn't matter.

I met the person I'm with now after the surgery, and we've been together for two and a half years. It was a cross-country relationship, so the first time we actually were sitting down together having dinner—we had only known each other for about a month—is when I told him. He reacted wonderfully. He said, "Okay, that adds an interesting element but not a negative one." It wasn't a big deal for him, and I think that's one reason why I'm with him still.

After that, I remember watching *My Breast*—a TV movie made from the book by Joyce Wadler—with him. The author happened to have the same doctors I did. He asked me so many questions throughout the movie that I finally had to shut him up, but it opened up a frank discussion between us, and that's how we worked through it.

—*Claire Noonan*

I WOULD TELL someone whose wife has had a mastectomy to focus on her needs, rather than on your own. She is already worried that love isn't there and that she can't perform. Be very careful, even though you're missing sex right now. It's a very difficult situation. A wife needs to know that she is still desirable but without feeling pressure from her husband to perform. Do whatever you can do to reinforce her sexiness. It might be buying a pretty camisole so that she's comfortable and feels good about the rest of her body. It's a common thing for women who have had mastectomies to feel uncomfortable being totally nude. Talk about it; be very open. While making love she may always have been on the bottom, and now the weight on her chest is extremely uncomfortable. Ask her what she is comfortable with.

The positive side of this is an opportunity to be creative. If you look at it as a chance to overcome inhibitions, to say, "Okay, now we're going to try different positions," then it can be fun. I'm more comfortable being on the top because I'm petite anyway and the pressure on my chest was uncomfortable. The problem with that was that it made my chest more visible too. That's why for a long time I wore a camisole. Also, sex from behind—I think that's a position people feel is kind of taboo, but for me early on, it was the most comfortable because my husband wasn't staring at my chest while we were making love.

The most important thing is to make her feel loved and desired, yet allow her the space she needs to deal with the disfigurement. That's the hardest part—even with reconstruction, you still feel disfigured.

—*Anonymous*

To Reconstruct or Not

I HAD IMMEDIATE reconstructive surgery. At first, they gave me a temporary implant, which sort of looked like a square breast, but at least I never had to wake up and not have a breast. I didn't have a nipple, of course, but I had a breast. I was able to wear low-cut things or a bathing suit without any problem. It looked a little weird, but I really didn't care. When I went to Cape Cod that summer, everyone was saying, "I want one of those too," because it's bigger. We just laughed about it.

—Kristina Matsch

I'M A LITTLE bit uneven, but not terribly. Depending on what I'm wearing, I might have to put a small pad into my bra or something like that, but for the most part, it hasn't been an issue. Obviously, you're never going to look the same as you did before, but nobody knows. I've moved to California from New York, and my new oncologist, when he looked, said you just don't get work like that out here. So I guess my plastic surgeon did a great job.

—Claire Noonan

THE DOCTOR REMOVED my breasts and put tissue expanders in. Then over a period of about a month and a half, he gradually filled them by adding saline through a port under my skin. Now I'm waiting for my implants. I decided to go with the silicone implants, which are very hard to get because of all the legal problems. I've read a lot about it, and I don't feel there's enough evidence to prove that the silicone implants are unsafe. My doctor recommended them because my skin is very thin and transparent. He said that the silicone would ripple less than the saline and look more natural. I still have breasts, but they're not the same. In some ways, they are better—they don't sag, which they had started to do after I had my baby. My husband's been very supportive about the way I look, but it's taking me a while to get used to my new body.

—Leigh Abruscato

THE LOSS TO me was not the breasts themselves but the nipples. I was flat-chested, so it was kind of ironically exciting to me that I was finally going to get a figure—not the way I'd want to get it, but still it was almost a positive side of the cancer. But I wasn't prepared for the loss of the nipple, its appearance, its sensitivity, and its involvement in my sex life.

They reconstruct the nipple. I had friends who lifted up their shirts and showed me their reconstructions. That was really helpful, because you have this fear of what you're going to look like after surgery. They show you photographs, but it's not the same. One friend of a friend, whom I'd met but didn't know well, came over one day and said, "You know, you don't know what the surgery is going to look like, and if you're comfortable, I'll show you what I look like." It was very helpful and a wonderful gift.

My reconstruction was not as successful as hers. Sitting across the room when she showed me her chest, I couldn't tell which breast was which. With mine, you can tell. They don't look real. They took the skin that was on the breast, and they kind of puckered it up and twisted it and made it the part of the nipple that protrudes, and they tattooed the areola, the round circle, to simulate the color and the shape. It usually works really well. My problem was that because I was so small, the skin stretched by the tissue expander was very thin. There was not that much to pucker up. They couldn't tattoo very deeply, and they didn't get it dark enough because they were afraid of puncturing the implant. Saline implants wear out, on average, in five to ten years, so if I have them replaced, then I'll get them to try and redo the nipple.

There are other small things. It's a little painful to lie on my chest because the implants feel like water balloons, and I'm afraid that if I get too much pressure on them, they might pop, although the doctor assured me they won't. In a bathing suit, you can kind of notice the ripples in the implants, but generally, I'm really pleased with the way I look in clothes.

Nipple sensitivity played a big part in my sex life, so losing that was hard for me. On the other hand, my sex life is better than it ever has been, because we've found other ways of doing things. My husband, having dealt with the possibility of losing me, is more appreciative of me. He's a more sensitive lover. And because my chest was sore for so long, that was out of the picture, so we had to look for other ways to stimulate and nurture. That part has been great.

—Anonymous

BEING AN ATHLETE, I've had a lot of trouble with my breast implants: They've deflated. I've had fifteen surgeries between the reconstruction and these deflating implants. My surgeon throws his hands up and says he doesn't know why I'm having problems. He says he has some bodybuilders who have had breast augmentation surgery, and they do very heavy weight training without any problem. But I have discovered an FDA article that advises against doing strenuous exercise. I swim thousands of yards—heavy-duty swimming with a coach and time trials—and I weight-lift hundreds of pounds. So it has to be that. But whatever the reason, reconstruction has been an absolute nightmare for me.

Many women going through breast cancer call me and say, "I'm going to wake up with a breast."

I say, "Forget about it. You're not." I tell them the truth. You don't have a breast as soon as you wake up. You just have this little sack in there. I think that emotionally you need to go through a mourning period—whether you lose a breast or a finger or any other part of your body. I think you should go through that mourning period first and then augment your breast if you want to.

But when you're diagnosed, the first thing the surgeons do is to soften the blow by telling you not to worry, because you're going to have breasts. You don't deal with the issue that you're losing your breasts. In my case, it's been nearly a year and a half since the last surgery, and I'm still not done with these things. I'm considering getting rid of them. Now I'm faced with dealing with the loss of my breasts and how it will really be without them. I got over cancer, but I guess my next goal is to get over the loss of my breasts.

—*Charlene Sloane*

I DECIDED NOT to have reconstructive surgery. This was long before the controversy about silicone implants—in 1985 it wasn't thought to be a dangerous thing or even a questionable thing—but I felt that the surgery was difficult enough without risking complications from elective surgery. I also didn't like the idea of putting a foreign object in my body for the long term.

—*Katherine Arthur*

I DIDN'T MAKE a big deal out of my mastectomies. My husband wasn't hung up on women with breasts. In fact, it didn't even occur to me to have reconstructive surgery because of both his attitude and mine. I wouldn't think of taking on another risk by putting in silicone implants. I did wear a prosthesis for many years, but ultimately I just wound up using puffy scarves to minimize the apparent flatness, which has worked very well throughout the years.

One of the most difficult things in terms of public exposure is swimming—how you look in a bathing suit. I found tank-top leotards to be most practical for hiding scars. Luckily, flatness did not upset me—to the point that I even went to a nude bath once. I figured if others were uncomfortable with it, that was their problem. I wasn't going to allow a lack of breasts to interfere with my taking advantage of life. If your concern about your breasts does interfere with your life experiences, I recommend that you think about your life, put everything into perspective, and determine whether or not breasts are all that important in the scheme of things.

Mastectomies cause difficulties, yet it is important to remember that there are advantages to having a double mastectomy—you can no longer get breast cancer, and running doesn't hurt anymore.

—*Elsa Porter*

WOMEN WHO HAVE just had breast surgery should wait until all swelling is gone before they buy a prosthesis. Reach to Recovery, an American Cancer Society program for breast cancer patients, can provide a temporary prosthesis, which is important for some people's self-image. Or you can make one yourself with cotton and an old bra, but when you've got staples and swelling and so forth, you can't do a whole lot.

When you're ready to get a prosthesis, the first thing to do is to check your insurance coverage because prostheses are quite expensive, starting at about $150 at a place like Sears and going up from there. There are organizations that will help you pay for it.

You should take someone with you. If you've got a daughter, take her. If not, take a friend who will be very honest. Make an appointment because you want to make sure the person who is trained in fitting is there. It's good to go to a place that carries more than one kind because then you can compare. Wear the tightest thing you would ordinarily wear. Turtlenecks or knit dresses or T-shirts. And try several. Don't buy the first one you try unless you really think it's perfect.

You're looking for a normal appearance and comfort and, when you poke yourself, a normal feel. The prostheses are mostly made out of silicone with various kinds of liners. For the most expensive kind I know of, they take a mold of your other breast and create one that's a good match. You use an adherent to make it stick, which you have to replace from time to time. Another kind uses a piece of Velcro that sticks to your chest. That's good for two to three weeks, and that is very satisfactory. With that, you don't have to wear a bra if you don't want to.

They need to be replaced from time to time when you're lucky enough to have been a survivor for as long as I have. I'm having to fight my insurance company right now to get a new one. But most of the time the insurance companies are pretty cooperative. Sometimes they provide special bras as well. Anybody who has breast cancer, whether they've had a Reach to Recovery visit or not, can call the American Cancer Society and get a list of stores in their area that carry prostheses.

They are being improved all the time and are very natural-looking now. Even so, I tell women who have had breast cancer surgery to look around and realize that nobody is shaped the same on both sides. Some women get very, very self-conscious about it, but even normal people don't necessarily match.

—*Elizabeth Martin*

When Breast Cancer Runs in the Family

MY TWO DAUGHTERS were in college when I was diagnosed with breast cancer, and my husband drove down to their school to tell them. The girls talked a lot about it, and the school chaplain, who was a friend of my younger daughter's, was a great source of strength. I know their main concern was for me, but they were worried—rightly—about their future health too.

Then three years ago, at the age of thirty-three, my older daughter got breast cancer. Hers was very contained, but she had bilateral mastectomy and reconstruction.

My other daughter is now, of course, at very high risk. You

read about the new developments, how they can trace cancer genes, but they're not available yet. She expects to have that down the road. If she has that gene, she might have prophylactic mastectomy. Right now, her oncologist follows her twice a year, very carefully.

I think it's important to talk to daughters and granddaughters frankly. You don't want to scare them, but they should be made aware of their own responsibility in detecting any breast cancer as early as possible. The American Cancer Society has wonderful information about breast self-examination. Sometimes, particularly in managed care, you have to push, but women who have a strong family history of breast cancer should have mammograms much earlier than is recommended for the general public.

—Elizabeth Martin

CHAPTER FOURTEEN

Bad Hair Days

Why a chapter on looks? Because we found that during cancer therapy, there was a direct correlation between the way we looked and the way we felt. Whether we were in the hospital or at home, the clothes we dressed in, the tone of our skin, the weight we gained or lost, and the hair or lack of hair on our heads and bodies made a big difference in the way we felt and in our outlook on life and therapy.

The most traumatic experience for many of us was losing our hair. It came out in patches, in handfuls, in the shower, and in bed. Some of us chose a razor early on. Afterward, some of us went au naturel—after all, Michael Jordan has made it a fashion statement. Others of us fastidiously pursued the perfect hair rug and head glue, and many chose to sport hats and headbands. And then, of course, there were those of us who chose a piece only to find it far too tempting not to doff it in a bar or ice-cream parlor when the need for humor arose. One was nearly lost at sea.

No matter how we chose to deal with it, deal with it we did. We also tried to stay as fit as possible given the circumstances.

And when we could, we even dressed up and went out. In the end, we found that there definitely is truth to the old saying that if you look good, you feel good.

BEFORE MY HAIR started falling out, it hurt—like when you wear your hair in a ponytail all day and then let it out. I said to my nurse, "You're going to think this is so weird, but my hair hurts." She said, "That's a sign that it's going to fall out. It will probably start in a couple weeks." And it did.

I had incredibly thick hair, so I probably lost half of it before anyone could tell. Some people say, "I was cooking, and it all fell out in the pan," but it didn't happen that way for me. It came out when I was taking a shower or when I was combing it or if I just pulled on it.

—*Kristina Matsch*

MY REACTION TO the fact that I would lose my hair was probably what should have been my reaction to having cancer. I cried for days. I felt sorry for myself. I wallowed in self-pity about my *hair*.

I was told to start looking for a suitable wig before my hair fell out. I went with my family to buy the wig. The wig guy advised me to cut my hair short so that when it did start to come out, it would be less of a mess. I got a funky boy cut, which I had never had the guts to do in the past. This is the one time to really take a chance on a cut because you don't have to worry about trying to grow it out!

I had had curly hair all my life, and I had always wanted straight hair. Since I could choose whatever hair I wanted, I decided to take advantage of the situation. I chose a stick-straight, shoulder-length brown wig with bangs (although I never wore it because I ended up preferring hats and scarves instead).

I wondered if I would just wake up bald one day, or if my hair would come out in handfuls or clusters. I had no idea what to expect. When it finally began to come out, it was really slow. You wake up and there are a few strands on your pillow. There is hair on your back and shoulders. It clings to the car upholstery, falls in your plate when you eat, lands on exam papers when you're trying to concentrate. It clogs the drain when you ever-so-carefully attempt to wash it. Within a few days, you can tug on clumps, and they come right out.

On my twenty-fifth birthday, my mother and I combed out the remainder of my hair to avoid further mess and clogs. In retrospect, I would have shaved my entire head the first day it started to fall out. Shaving would have given me the power to choose when I would be bald and would have saved a whole lot of vacuuming! After we finished removing the last of my hair, I put on a scarf. Then my mother and my boyfriend both put scarves on their heads for moral support. The three of us walked around Ann Arbor, Michigan, like that for the entire day.

—*Karen Manheimer*

I STARTED FEELING my scalp tingle, and I knew that was the beginning. It was very uncomfortable, and my hair wasn't that clean at this point because I didn't want to wash it too much—God forbid you pull out more than is actually going to come out.

I guess I was in a state of denial at that point, because one night I was lying in bed, and I discovered that my hair was starting to mat. It was actually coming out of the scalp—my hair is sort of long and curly—and getting stuck in the other hairs that were still there. It was really gross. I wanted to run into the shower right then—in the middle of the night—and pull out whatever I could, but I thought, "That's a little dramatic. Let's just wait until the morning."

I didn't sleep the rest of the night. I was just waiting until the sun came up so it could seem like a normal thing to do: get up and take a shower. I got up and got a plastic bag and walked up to my mother and said, "I'm going into the shower and taking it all out, and we're not going to take it to the next level. Whatever I look like when I'm done, just look at me and do whatever you have to do. This is what I'm doing." My mother was a wreck. I told her to just go in the other room and leave me alone.

I went into the shower with this plastic bag, and I just washed, pulling out whatever I could, and I tried not to get too emotional. I knew I needed to get through this physically disgusting thing. It was disgusting—there's no other word for it—and I put my hair in the bag.

There were some strands left on the sides, a thin covering on my whole scalp. I wouldn't go out in public like that, but I could put on a hat and it looked like I had thin hair. And I didn't lose much body hair. I still had my eyebrows and eyelashes.

But the hair loss is a huge thing. People say all the time, "Well, at least it grows back," but no matter how many times you tell yourself that it grows back, it's still not there now, and it's not there next week, and it sucks being bald. It's a much bigger deal than people are led to believe. Just because it's going to grow back eventually does not make it okay now.

You may feel fine, but you have to put on a hat or a wig to go out in public. And there were days when I didn't feel bad— physically or emotionally—but I'd look in the mirror and think, "I look sick. I look like a patient."

—*Jodi Levy*

I GOT A wig before I was totally bald. I went the cheap route at first. Wigs are so expensive. My husband went with me, and we got one for $150. I took it to this guy who was very good with wigs. He was used to working with cancer patients and actually set up the Look Good . . . Feel Better program in Delaware. It was nice because you go to a real salon where everyone else is getting their own head of hair done and manicures and every-thing, and you go into a nice little room in the back, and no one knows what you're doing.

This guy tried and tried to fix this absolutely incredibly cheap wig. The more he cut, the more disgusted I got. I kept looking at it, thinking, "There is no way I'm going to wear this thing." Finally I said to him, "This is the worst wig in the world, isn't it?"

He said, "I'm so sorry, but I can't do anything with it."

I thought, "Okay. There goes $150."

He had all these gorgeous wigs in his little room, and I ended up getting one that cost almost $400. It was hard to pick a color. I grew up being a natural blonde, but my hair had been gradually getting darker. I went for a dark brown wig. Don't ask me why. It was nice, but I just couldn't handle it. I only wore it for a week. I just didn't like it. I didn't like the style. I didn't like the color. It was uncomfortable. I just did not like it at all.

I decided that I was just going to wear hats. I went up to Cape Cod for the summer, and I found the cutest flowered baseball caps. They had a big bow in the back out of the same material, so they really covered my head. I loved them so much that I found the address of the woman who made them and wrote to her. I told her what I was going through and thanked her. About a month later, she sent a whole carton of these hats. My sister said I should write to Chanel and tell them I was wearing handbags on my head!

—*Kristina Matsch*

HAIR LOSS WAS a major trauma for me. I had just taken about ten years to grow my hair. I had this beautiful long curly hair, and when I was told that I was going to lose it, I was not a happy camper. The way I handled it was to cut it short a week or two before they told me it would come out. I got a wig, but I hated it so much that I got rid of it and just walked around with a quarter inch of hair. I was brave. I felt better because I didn't feel like I was being phony. I was being myself.

—*Charlene Sloane*

CANCER CELLS ARE fast-growing, and you obviously want to kill them, so chemo goes after fast-growing cells. But your hair cells are fast-growing too, and this is why people lose their hair. I considered a wig; I got measured for it, but I finally decided, "I will shave my head, and I'll go with it. This is how I will handle it. I'll make it a look, an attitude."

My wife was very helpful. She suggested that I could try headbands. She made it a fashion thing. Being the wife or the husband or the immediate family is hard. They have a ringside seat. They have the anxiety or the worry of the thing without the adrenaline rush you get when it's your fight. So they're in a peculiar position. Jeannie was able to discharge some of that anxiety by helping me with my fashion statements.

I had trouble hailing cabs during those months when I was bald, because I'm six feet four. One night we were going to a concert, and I was wearing this leather motorcycle jacket that I'm very fond of and have worn numerous times and gotten in dozens and dozens of cabs in without any trouble. But this night—and this was during the Los Angeles riots, actually—the cabs were zooming past. I figured they must be thinking, "What? I'm going to pick up this white skinhead the night of the Los Angeles riots? Forget it!" My wife, who's sixteen inches shorter than I am, stepped out and got one without any trouble. That was amusing. Humor, if you can summon it, is very important, and I do have a morbid sense of humor.

—*Richard Brookhiser*

WHEN I KNEW that I was going to lose my hair, I went out and got a wig that was very close to what my own hair was like. I knew my hair would grow back when the treatment was over, and I just refused to let my hair loss knock me down. Sure, I dreaded losing my hair, but once I lost it and I had this wig, I found it reasonably okay. I just refused to make myself miserable about that.

I had a couple of people say to me, "I can deal with anything, but I can't bear the loss of hair." But I never let that become an issue for me. Actually, it was kind of amusing because I didn't have hair for most of the thirteen months of my treatment, and during those thirteen months when I was wearing a wig, I must have had fifteen or twenty people—strangers on the street—stop me and say, "Where did you get your hair cut? That's such a great haircut. Who's your hairdresser?"

—*Toni Zavistovski*

MY HAIR LOSS was never traumatic because I was able to focus on the true enemy—the cancer. A few days after my first chemo treatment, I went to a wig shop with my sister and a few coworkers. I wanted their company and their advice, even though the final decision would be mine. We had a blast trying on different wigs—matching wigs, rock-and-roll-singer wigs, old-lady wigs, you name it. I finally went the conservative route and picked the one that came closest to my own hair. We all went to lunch together afterward. It was actually a fun experience, one I will never forget.

—*Monica Ko*

EVENTUALLY I CUT off whatever little long hairs were left because it started looking ridiculous. I went from wearing hats pretty much all the time to wearing wigs a lot more. I got to the point where I was comfortable enough in my own home to not wear anything, but it definitely took a while. One of the first mornings, I got up and I was brushing my teeth and wondering whether I should put on a hat to go in and eat breakfast with my father. He hadn't seen me bald yet, and I knew it would freak him out, but I figured, "He's gotta see it—he's my father. I'm going to just go in there. If he has a problem with it, he'll get over it." And that's exactly what happened. He didn't pretend not to notice; he just said, "Wow." There are no words, I guess, when you see your daughter bald.

I got pretty used to my bald head after a few months, and I showed it to a friend of mine. I know she wanted to say that it was no big deal, but I could see the horror on her face. I felt bad—not because it bothered me that she was horrified—but because I had flipped her out. I felt like I should have been a little more graceful about it. People can be very uncomfortable when they see something that shocking.

—*Jodi Levy*

THE BEST WAY I found to deal with hair loss was to try to develop a sense of humor about it. My wig never fit well and actually blew off on the beach one day so that I had to chase after it, completely mortified. It took some time, but I did learn to laugh at the ridiculousness of the scene. Once when a woman kept pressing me on where I had had my hair cut, I finally said, "If you like it that much, you can have it," and handed her my wig.

—*Tali Havazelet*

I REMEMBER SCRATCHING my head and the first few strands dropping onto my journal. I had told myself that I didn't care about going bald, that it was not important in the overall scheme of things, but when I saw the strands of hair on the pages of my notebook, I have to confess that I did care. But then I reminded myself that the hair loss was only temporary, that the chemotherapy was doing its job, and that losing one's hair is the most insignificant of inconveniences compared to the big picture.

When I felt my worst, I still made a point of taking a shower every day. It was in response to the ever-present urge I had to throw up my hands and say, "What's the point of doing anything if I might die in a week?" I also shaved as often as possible even though due to the chemo, I didn't grow much more than a light fuzz. The doctors weren't too crazy about my shaving because low platelet counts made me more vulnerable to bleeding, but I was willing to accept the risk in the interest of bolstering what was left of my personal pride. It was something I could do to improve the way I looked, and more importantly, it allowed me to participate in what is considered a normal morning routine for healthy men. If I stopped shaving, soon after I might stop showering. If it came to that, it would mean I had stopped caring, and then how long would it be before I gave in and stopped fighting?

—*Jonathan Pearlroth*

ABOUT EIGHT WEEKS after my first treatment, I was really at my lowest. I was tired. I felt ugly. I had sores in my mouth. I had aches in every bone in my body. I was really a basket case. Someone sent me an article from *Town & Country* magazine about a program called Look Good . . . Feel Better, to help women undergoing chemo and radiation deal with hair loss, change of skin tone, et cetera, so I signed up for it.

It's a great program. You spend two hours with other women, and all you do is makeup and wigs and scarves and turbans, and you don't talk about what's wrong with you. The leading cosmetic companies donate makeup, and everybody gets a free bagful. It reminded me of when I was in a sorority and we all exchanged makeup. The camaraderie was really terrific. The women ranged in age from their early twenties to their seventies. That's how important it is for a woman to look good, no matter what age she is.

You come in haggard-looking, unhappy, and you leave feeling like a million dollars. It's a one-shot deal, but you don't need it more than once because you go home with an uplifting feeling, and you keep it with you forever. Those two hours gave me back my life. My husband picked me up, and I said, "We're going out to dinner tonight." That's what it did for me.

My hospital didn't offer Look Good . . . Feel Better, so I had to do it at another one. I said, "If I get better—*when* I get better—

I'm going to bring it to my hospital." And I did. I'm a volunteer now, and I help run this program once a month for women who are undergoing chemo and radiation.

—*Bev Yaffe*

How to Look Your Best When You Feel Your Worst

Look Good . . . Feel Better® is a program sponsored by the American Cancer Society, the National Cosmetology Association, and the Cosmetic, Toiletry, and Fragrance Association. In each session, trained volunteers spend two hours coaching women cancer patients about creative makeup techniques, nail care, how to buy and style wigs, and how to cover the head with colorful scarves and turbans. For information about the nearest Look Good . . . Feel Better program, call 800-395-5665. Here are some of the program's best tips:

1. Shop for a wig before treatment starts. It's much easier to match your natural hair color before it falls out. Later, take note of your skin tone. If it grows paler, you might need to switch to a lighter wig. (Tip: Some insurance companies cover wig costs. If your doctor prescribes a "cranial prosthesis for alopecia"—a scientific way of saying a "wig for baldness"—you'll stand a better chance of receiving reimbursement. Also, some American Cancer Society offices sponsor wig banks that offer "gently used" wigs free of charge. Call your local chapter for more information.)

2. Be tender with tender scalps. Use a wig liner or wig cap under the wig, but make sure the liner fits properly. If it is too tight, it will cut off the circulation.

3. Consider using synthetic wigs. Human-hair wigs look great but often require salon care, and if you are perspiring into a wig every day, that might mean a couple of trips each week for a shampoo and set.

4. Have your wig cut by a professional. Because they can be difficult to trim with scissors, synthetic wigs often require a barber's razor. Besides, with a wig you only get one chance. If you slip with the shears, it won't grow back.

5. Use cotton or rayon scarves for head wraps. They hold better than silk ones, which tend to slide off the scalp.

6. Make your own low-cost turban. Buy T-shirt material, which is sold by the yard at fabric stores (ask for "tube material"). Using a third of a yard, stretch the material over your head, twist it, and loop it back over your head. Dress it up with a colorful scarf.

7. Fill it out. To give your wig or turban that full-head-of-hair look, tuck a foam shoulder pad (or two) underneath. To keep them attached to the turban or wig, sew on a strip of Velcro, which you can buy at fabric or five-and-dime stores. Another inexpensive scarf-stuffer is cotton quilt batting, sold in bags at fabric stores. (One cancer patient we know had her own idea: She takes a maxi pad, pulls off the adhesive strip, and puts it on her head.)

8. Brush on new eyebrows. Use two tones of colored pencils and short, light strokes to draw what look like fine pieces of hair, which gives a more natural look than one thick line. If your eyelashes are gone too, use a little eye shadow, drawn in at the base, to give the appearance of a lash. Because cancer patients are especially susceptible to infection, try to avoid false lashes. The sticky surface can irritate the skin and create sores.

9. Moisten dry nails. Use creams and oils to keep nails from cracking, peeling, and getting sore. Soak them in warm water and bath oils regularly. Avoid false nails for the same reason as false lashes: The glue can irritate the skin and cause infection.

10. Wear bright colors when you're feeling dark. You'll look happier—and it might just rub off. When you're really down, put on your wildest shirt, your brightest-colored scarf, and big gaudy earrings. Push yourself to feel better.

—*Look Good . . . Feel Better State Coordinators*
Mary Burt of Texas and Theresa A. Masinelli of Illinois

I WILL SHARE a tip about wigs that I found helpful: They look more natural when they're a little messy. If you make the wig really neat, you can see the fake part, and it looks like plastic hair, but if you fluff up the top layer a little bit, it looks more real. Bangs also help because they can cover the wig line. But most wig stores have seen a lot of people going through chemo, so they can give you suggestions. For them it's old hat, so to speak.

—*Jodi Levy*

I WANTED TO find a way to make my appearance acceptable to everyone because I found that appearance affected the way people treated me. If I greeted my mother at the door with a bald head, she reacted very differently than if I greeted her with a head wrap or a wig. Looking good was especially important because I was dating the man who is now my husband. I needed to feel attractive.

I went to a cosmetics counter and asked the sales representative to help me to aesthetically handle the side effects of chemotherapy. She behaved as though she was going to catch the cancer from me. She had no idea what to do for me. So I began to seek out my own solutions.

When you go to a restaurant with a wig, don't scratch your head because it will make the wig go up and down. When you go through treatment, your skin will most likely become dehydrated, so don't use products with alcohol in them because they will dry your skin. Before treatment, cut your hair short because it's easier to go from long to short to no hair than directly from long to no hair. Also, save some of your hair so that you can take it as a sample when you go to get a wig. Don't use fragrant beauty products because the smell may give you nausea. Before treatment, go get a makeover or otherwise try to look your best, then have a picture taken of yourself. Use this as an example of what you want to look like when you go to the cosmetics counter after you've begun your treatments.

Having found these tips for myself, I have since organized them—and more—into a book called *Beauty and Cancer* and into seminars of the same name.

—*Diane Noyes*

WHEN THEY TOLD me I had cancer, the first thing I thought was "I'm going to lose my hair. I can't lose my hair." After I lost it, I kept thinking, "When is my hair going to start growing?" I had my bone marrow transplant on September 21, and by Thanksgiving, I was still bald. It had grown in a little bit and totally fallen back out. I asked my doctor, and he said it would come in around Christmas. About a week before Christmas, I started to see a little bit. It came in brown, and I'm a blonde, but it came in evenly, and fortunately, you can do anything with a bottle.

Around that time, my husband and I were planning a trip to Hawaii. He had found an estate-planning seminar in Maui. I doubted that my bone marrow doctor would let me go. When it came time to buy the airplane tickets, I talked to my doctor, who is a wonderful man. He said, "Sure, you can go." I burst into tears. He said, "What's wrong?"

I said, "I didn't know I was well enough."

He said, "You are well. You are fine. Take that trip."

That week in Hawaii became my coming-out. I was a size smaller than I normally would be, so a friend of mine who has a wonderful wardrobe let me borrow anything I wanted from her closet instead of buying a bunch of things. That was kind of exciting. When we were there, I shed the wig and had my hair—it was only about an inch long—trimmed. That gave me time to get used to seeing myself without the wig, so I'd be able to face everyone else when I got home.

—*Karla McConnell*

ONCE I WENT to see a woman in the hospital who had towels draped over the mirrors. I put makeup and a fancy turban on her. She allowed me to remove the towels. She looked at herself and began to cry, explaining that it was the first time she was able to look at herself since she had lost her hair. Chemo is a very visual part of cancer. Looking well allows you to feel normal, not sick. It also allows other people to feel more comfortable around you because they see you and not a sick person. But most of all, it gives you a way to face yourself and to face what you are going through.

—*Diane Noyes*

CHAPTER FIFTEEN

Damn the Torpedoes: Life Doesn't Stop During Treatment

Okay, so yesterday you were sick as a dog from chemo, but today you're going into the office—and you're going in on time. And don't skip that wedding on Saturday—just buy a new hat to cover your thinning hair. We found it useful to continue with our normal routines as much as possible.

By and large we found bosses and office mates understanding. Sometimes those of us in very high-stress jobs, with tasks that needed constant attention, opted for a change in lifestyle, however. That usually worked for the better, but if you're in a comfortable job, be honest with your boss and colleagues and see if you can work out a schedule that fits with your therapy. Jobs continued to give us the satisfaction of small daily achievements and to provide us with companions outside the family who were valuable to our well-being. Our jobs also distracted us from our problems.

Exercise was another essential for many of us. In between chemo sessions, we walked, we ran, we biked, and we even played basketball. It didn't matter that we weren't up to par. It was the fact that the effort was made. The body responded as best as it could, but, hey, at least it responded.

As far as social engagements went, instead of canceling the whole slew of them, we took them one at a time. When you have a serious illness, people tend to be very understanding if you suddenly have to cancel, even if it's at the last minute.

Sex life? Why not? Sometimes circumstances made it tough, but there was usually no need to abandon the pleasures of life altogether. We simply had to communicate more and learn to adapt to a variety of new conditions. Quite frequently the renewed sense of honesty more than compensated for the new challenges.

I GOT THROUGH chemo and radiation by continuing my normal routine. I worked every day I was able, continued to exercise, and never gave myself time to feel sorry for myself. I did not take a sabbatical from life and did not think of myself as damaged goods. I filled my brain with all of these things, while maintaining a sense of humor, and there was little room left for fear or doubt.

—*Jerry Freundlich*

MY DOCTOR PRESCRIBED antidepressants for me at a time when I was having trouble getting out of bed. They were helpful because they got me started in the morning. They helped me take the first small steps, like opening the shades, drinking a glass of juice, and getting into the shower. Once I got going, I could do an errand, take a walk, or see a friend. The more I did, the better I felt, and the better I felt, the more I was able to do. It was a positive spiral.

—*Josh Malen*

MY DAUGHTER REALLY helped me get through this experience. I couldn't lie around and feel sorry for myself because I had a six-month-old who didn't understand what cancer was. It didn't frighten her when I lost my hair, but at the same time, she didn't cut me any slack. Sometimes I'd be tired from treatment, but I'd have to get my act together for her. You can't tell a little baby to just go out and play.

—*Leigh Abruscato*

JUST AS I was going through my battle with cancer, we had to move. We had just sold our house when I was diagnosed, and we had not found a new house, so first—between my lumpectomy and the lymph-node dissection—we moved from a three-bedroom house into an apartment and moved the rest of our stuff into storage. Then two days after my second-to-last round of chemotherapy, we moved from the apartment into our house.

So I'd say, don't underestimate what you can do if you need to. It was a great distraction. Friends helped—all I did was direct traffic. I certainly couldn't lift, especially after the surgery. Sometimes those bigger things that go on in your life can be the saviors for you, can help you get through even though you feel like, "Oh, God, I don't want to be thinking about *this* now." It's a relief to focus on those things and not always on being the cancer patient.

—*Lorraine Anderson*

I HAD BEEN friends with a guy named Chip for over a year. When he found out that I had a brain tumor, I got a dozen red roses and a dozen white roses with a note saying, "We still have to go out next year." While I was having all the tests, he called every day from St. Louis. When I was in the ICU, he sent love letters through the hospital fax machine, which you're not supposed to do. He faxed in a letter confessing his love for me and how he had always been in love with me. We were at different universities, but now he wasn't willing to wait anymore. A nurse read this to me at my bedside in the ICU.

He kept sending these giant bouquets of roses and filling up the rooms. They were really beautiful. It was a crazy and wonderful thing happening all at once while I was dealing with the cancer. It had, without a doubt, a huge bearing on my attitude—while I was going through what could have been the worst summer of my life, I was falling in love. He ended up coming to Philadelphia. We hadn't even kissed at this point, but he'd already confessed his love.

We had an intense and romantic love affair that summer, which made the whole thing so crazy and wonderful.

Four days out of surgery, I got on a plane and flew out to Wyoming, where he was on a dude ranch for a week. My stitches were fresh out of my head, and my parents were beside themselves. But they let me go. Looking back now, we laugh about it. It's hard to deprive your child of anything when she's having brain tumors and brain surgeries. At that point, nobody knew what my future was or if I was going to have one. My dad laughs now because he was so afraid that, with this big hole in my head, the pressure on the plane would drop and cause an explosion.

Part of the bargain with my parents was that I promised I'd never get on a horse. I just wanted to enjoy the gorgeous scenery. Well, out there I was basically racing horses. One day, Chip and I were racing along, and I was catching up about ten feet behind him, when his horse wiped out and sent him flying, which spooked my horse. My horse bucked and threw me. As I was falling off, I remember thinking that my head was an egg and that it was going to crack, but I managed to keep my head up as I landed. So the crack of the impact was on my arched back. I thought I had broken my back. I was screaming. I had never experienced so much pain and never have since.

We were in the middle of nowhere, and Chip was terrified. I was screaming and lying flat on my back, and he came over and said, "Wiggle your toes." I did, and he said, "I have good news and bad news. Good news first: You're not paralyzed. Bad news is you're lying in a huge pile of horseshit."

That kind of set the stage for the summer I had. My two brain surgeries were followed by a root canal and the removal of four impacted wisdom teeth. My dog of fifteen years died. It was a joke—like a *Far Side* cartoon.

That fall I transferred to the University of Pennsylvania, which was only thirty minutes from my parents' house, so they could see me often. I wanted to continue with school and try to maintain as normal a lifestyle as I could. I began classes and began my treatments, and Chip would walk me to my radiation every morning. Then from there I'd go to a class. After that I'd go home and sleep for a while and maybe make another class. It was great because everything was so close together, and I could do it all. I managed to get through Penn and graduated on time cum laude. It was a victory.

—*Katie Brant*

I VERY MUCH wanted to continue to work. I have four children, and I wanted my family to see that my illness was something temporary, that life was going to go on as usual. I wanted that for them and for myself. I think people can deal with cancer much better if they are very much involved in something. For me, what worked best was continuing with my regular schedule and not wallowing in the misery and the fear. It's very tempting to dwell on those things, on the unpleasant treatment and so on. I just didn't give myself a chance to dwell on the dark side of what was going on.

—*Toni Zavistovski*

I WAS WORKING in the Wilhelmina Agency in New York as a model when I noticed the swelling in my leg. Four days later, my right leg was amputated. I went in as a New York model and came out as a disabled person. This was how others perceived me, but I focused on the fight for my life, which meant living, not obsessing over my leg.

There was a movement at the time to use bald mannequins, so I dared to go into Saint Laurent, hoping that they would follow the trend with a live model. They did. Five months after I lost my leg, I was back in front of the camera for Yves Saint Laurent, this time with a prosthesis.

After some time spent seeking out interested photographers, I discovered a whole slew of them who found the purity and boldness of my bald head and missing eyebrows intriguing. Eventually everyone wanted to take advantage of my baldness. Using wigs worked for me as well. I got more work that year than I ever had in the past because I was able to drastically change my looks by removing and alternating wigs. I made the situation work for me.

Working in between treatments turned that period into one of the greatest years of my life. I have since used the whole experience to my advantage, making exercise videotapes for amputees, inspiring others to triumph over their illnesses and disabilities, and carrying the Olympic torch in Atlanta the day before the Games began.

—*Ivy! Gunter*

BIKING WAS MY metaphor for cancer. I had been in a race the year before with twenty guys and me, the only girl. I managed to climb to the top of the mountain in that race and beat some of the guys because I had called on resources that I didn't know I had. I saw the disease as another, newer and bigger hill to climb. A friend even wrote me a letter comparing the disease to a bike race, advising me to "Gear down, keep pedaling, get down for water when you're thirsty, and get back on." I took the "Hillclimb Hat," which I won in the race, everywhere throughout my treatment as a reminder.

When my doctor and I discovered that we had in common a love for biking, he recommended that I join the following year's fifty-mile fund-raising ride for cancer patients. He told me I would be the first person with leukemia to ever do it. This became my goal: I would get rehabilitated enough to go do this race and raise research money for my doctor. I raised $13,000 and was so happy to be able to give something back. I did the ride again the next summer and raised even more—$14,000. Then they asked me to be on M. D. Anderson's board of directors.

—*Janice Thomas*

GETTING A PAGER has probably given me more freedom than anything else we've done during my husband's illness. I can go anywhere now. There was a time when Brian was under heavy chemo—dexamethasone, a very strong steroid. He was on four-day pulses and then off. He had mood swings, which are very typical with that, but he got to the point where he couldn't stand us being out of his sight, especially me. I was nervous no matter where I went because I felt I needed to be in contact with him, but my business requires me to run around—and there isn't anybody with a family who doesn't need to run around.

Finally, I got a pager. He could contact me no matter where I was, and it cut his anxiety by about ninety percent. I have also found it extremely useful with our children. I gave the number to the schools so at any moment they can contact me immediately. From a working parent's perspective, it's been a blessing. I wouldn't be without one now.

—Peggy Schmidt

I MANAGED TO graduate from business school at the University of Michigan on time. I even came out with decent grades. It was crucial for me, in my recovery from cancer, to be able to focus on my studies and my normal life, instead of my illness.

To make life easier, I went to the Department of Motor Vehicles and got a handicap parking permit. Being on chemotherapy is considered a temporary handicap. My permit allowed me to park on campus at school, and I always got a great spot at the mall, movie theater, and supermarket. With the handicap sticker, I was also exempt from paying at parking meters. It's amazing the amount of pleasure you can get from the little things in life.

—Karen Manheimer

INSTEAD OF TRAVELING three hundred and fifty miles each way to the hospital in Memphis, Tennessee, to receive my chemotherapy, I arranged to have the medicine sent to my home so that a friend of mine who used to be a doctor could administer it. My friend, who still had his license, had been shot and paralyzed and had quit practicing medicine. I didn't want to quit everything for the chemotherapy. I wanted to keep on coaching and doing everything I had always done. So after basketball practice, my friend would come to my home and give me the chemotherapy.

The experience helped us both. I got better, and he saw that even though he was in a wheelchair, he could help other people. He developed a new outlook, and since that time, he's started his practice back up.

—Danny Johnson

INSTEAD OF GOING to self-help sessions, which depressed me, I took cooking classes and gardening classes. That was me. I had to be the person I always had been.

—Diane Noyes

I READ AS much as I could, but with the chemo, I had a hard time concentrating. My memory retention was really bad. I would read something and have to read it again and again. I later learned that this was a side effect of the chemo. My parents would rent movies for me to watch, but what really helped was listening to music. It didn't require any thought. I'd sit there nauseated and make tapes.

I had started collecting oldies albums when I was in college, and that's when I became interested in classical music and jazz. Every time I went into Mobile for chemo, I'd make my parents stop at the record store, and I'd go in and buy records. Then I'd come home and make tapes, ninety-minute cassettes. I was very obsessive about the labels.

I made all these great tapes and sent them back to my friends at LSU, which was my way of staying connected with them. It was kind of like saying, "You have to call me now because you have to tell me what a great tape I made for you." I was so far from my friends at LSU, and not having them near was a big loss. Life went on for them. For a while, I resented having been robbed of those relationships, resented not being able to go back and finish the rest of my college years at LSU. The making of the tapes, the music, really helped. It became a bridge to the life I wanted to return to.

—*Lisa Hollingsworth*

I KEPT UP with the things that I'd always been interested in, although my perspective changed somewhat. For instance, I like all kinds of classical music, but when I was in the hospital, I just didn't want to hear certain composers, especially the romantics— Beethoven, for example. They made me feel like, what's all this fuss about? So I found myself listening to the Goldberg Variations and Louis Armstrong.

I saw *Wayne's World,* which my wife would never have gone to see, but I made her. It's a stupid, stupid movie, but it was funny to me at the time. I found the cartoonist John Callahan, who is a quadriplegic, very funny. It seemed appropriate. I read the letters of Evelyn Waugh to Lady Diana Cooper, and they were just the right tone. Slash and burn, take no prisoners. They were very funny—the type of humor that acknowledges that life is dark and there are dark things that happen. Something really awful is happening to you, and you have to recognize that. Maybe that's not where you end up, but you have to start there.

One friend of mine, a young woman graduate student in English, gave me recordings of poets reading their own poetry. It was interesting to hear these famous guys interpreting their own stuff. But there was this one poem by William Ebsom, and the refrain was, "Slowly with poison, the bloodstream fills. The waste remains, the waste remains, kills." This line kept coming up; this was after my surgery when I was looking at chemotherapy. I first thought, "Holy shit, what have you done?" But then I thought, "No, I'm going to listen to this and see what this poem is about." The waste that remains and kills in the poem is all the little things you leave undone, the opportunities you miss, so that turned out to be a useful thing to hear.

—*Richard Brookhiser*

FOR WHATEVER REASON, I did unbelievably well through all the chemo. One of the things that kept me sane was volunteer work. I worked at a soup kitchen. I worked for a while at a women's shelter, and I taught computer skills to young girls. I mostly wanted to spend time with kids, so I volunteered at a pediatric oncology clinic and worked at the Ronald McDonald Summer Camp.

Because I was diagnosed at age eighteen, I was—and still am—treated by pediatric oncologists and surgeons, so that gave me a chance to spend time with kids getting chemo. I loved these kids. They all had stuffed animals that they brought to the hospital. Everything that happened to them, the doctors would do to the stuffed animals too. My favorite was this little boy who held his Kermit the Frog by the leg. Meanwhile, Kermit had IVs hanging out of him and Band-Aids on him. It broke my heart.

I represented hope for these kids and their families—I looked so good and so healthy and normal. I would walk into the clinic, and they'd ask me the name of my child. I liked that part of being there, that I was able to give them hope, but being around them also helped me. After my first surgery, I was in a room recovering with five little girls. It was the greatest thing that could have happened to me. They'd wake me up at about five-thirty in the morning and would climb up on my bed. They wanted to brush my long hair. They were wonderful.

—*Katie Brant*

THROUGHOUT THE CHEMO, I tried to have as much fun with it as I could and to keep my head on straight through it all. I still ran when I could and got a lot out of it. It's great therapy and a great stress reliever and balancer. It's not all about competitiveness and running fast. It reinforced all the reasons why I chose to be a runner in the first place and helped me to deal with everything.

I think doing things that you're familiar with is important, going on with your normal routine. I'd still go out and have a few beers. Having cancer is a unique experience—you're part of a select club. It's not necessarily a bad thing; it's another growing experience. I tried to look at it that way and to have fun with it.

I was with a friend at a bar one night, and we were talking to these two women. I pulled out a big clump of my hair and said, "Boy, I've got to quit my job. I'm under way too much stress."

One of the women said, "God, what do you do?" I told her what was going on, and she started opening up and telling me about her ovarian cysts. People perk up their ears and listen to you when you've gone through something like this, and you can deliver a positive message.

What else can you do? It's not healthy to just sit on the couch all the time and wallow in self-pity, so I'd go out and walk around, and I didn't care if I didn't have any eyebrows or whatever. Big deal. Having cancer was just the way my life's course had taken me at the time.

—*Mark Conover*

Maintaining a Sex Life

I WAS TWENTY-FOUR years old and had a girlfriend I was crazy about. And in the hospital there was no thought given to the fact that we might want to get turned on together or do whatever we might want to do. Lord knows, there were twelve people per hour coming into the room without knocking. At a certain point, we decided that if they felt there was no need to knock on the door, then it wouldn't be our responsibility to protect them from anything they might find inside. Of course, the interruptions were so frequent it wouldn't even have been possible. So we wound up having sex all the time in the bathroom of the hospital room.

It's essential to bring all the things that you love about life into the hospital with you so that you're constantly reminded of what it is you want to get back to. I discovered that the systems and routines of the hospital—although some are better than others—are in place to keep that system running smoothly, not to help any particular individual. I was amazed to find that cooperation with the norm was more desired than my excelling as an individual. I got really hooked into all that stuff and my anger about it, and I actually found that anger a great energizer.

—*Evan Handler*

I HAVE NEVER felt as ugly and as unsexual and unappealing as after having ten different people poke around inside me over a two-month period. That's pretty awful. It took a long time for me to want to be with anyone sexually and to feel like I could be. Sex was really frightening. The cervix contains a lot of the glands that lubricate a woman's vagina and that also allow the sperm to travel up to the egg. You cut out parts of the cervix, you cut out those glands; that's how the fertility is compromised. So not only is my fertility compromised, but so is my sexuality in that I can't really lubricate to have sex.

That change was really hard to deal with, mentally and emotionally. I wasn't in a relationship, and I couldn't understand how you could negotiate that loss. I didn't know if I was brave enough to. It seemed so weird to me that after the surgery, sex was never going to feel the same again. Even your ability to have an orgasm is compromised. In terms of external orgasms, everything is fine, but internal orgasms are a result of the cervix having spasms and being prodded, and now I can't have them because I don't have a cervix—or much of one.

But the physical problems haven't made a big difference. And maybe that's why I found the person I'm going to marry—because I started looking at dating and relationships very differently. I was always pretty serious—during the last five years I've had two or three boyfriends, each one for a year or two—but I was uninvolved when I got cancer. Honestly, I was thinking that if sex isn't going to be any fun, and I'm not going to have kids, then why don't I just not have boyfriends? Just give up relationships?

As it turned out, I talked to men differently, gave out fewer sexual signals so I ended up getting involved with somebody I was already very comfortable and friendly with. I had to be in a position where I could talk openly. He knew me for eight months before we started dating, and he knew about my cancer.

My fiancé happens to be very comfortable talking about emotions and touchy issues. We talk very specifically about my physical problems. We also go and get lubricants together. We've got to use them, so we try to make it enjoyable and part of a good thing, as opposed to something that has to be done. Still, I get frustrated sometimes when we're making love and I'm not responding enough for us to start having intercourse. I feel kind of guilty about it, but I'm also relieved that I can feel frustrated and angry or feel sorry for myself, and he's okay with my feelings.

It's important to express how you feel. In the beginning I'd shelve my emotions because I didn't want to make him feel bad. That doesn't work. My advice is: One, there are solutions to physical problems. There are a lot of people who can't lubricate who still have sex, and it's okay. To solve the problem, communicate. Two, understand that to problem-solve doesn't mean you won't still be frustrated sometimes.

A year ago I hadn't resolved a lot of this—the permanency of it is so frustrating—but now I have. Communication is the key. If I had had to keep it all to myself, dealing with it would have been harder. I'm fortunate that I found him.

—*Rachel Kaul*

AFTER SURGERY, RADIATION, and chemo, I had no libido. It was gone. I had had a very strong libido for a long time, so I recognized the difference. Everyone kept saying, "When people are going through cancer and chemo, they often lose it. They don't feel attractive, and they don't have energy."

I kept saying, "This is different. It's not about feeling attractive or having energy. My libido is just gone."

I also lost my periods. They stopped entirely after my surgery. They now think that my pituitary gland got a lot of extra radiation and maybe that's why I wasn't producing the right combination of hormones. My libido was gone overnight too. I was incredibly sexual about six months before my treatment began. I had felt like I was in overdrive, like a twelve-year-old boy. So when, all of a sudden, it was gone one day, it was shocking to me. It was such a loss and such a sadness.

I was in a new relationship. We'd been going out only two months when the chemo started. I tried to convince myself that we were just so comfortable already, saying, "Oh, sex can't stay like the first few weeks in a relationship." But it was more than that. The change felt chemical. I wasn't producing any hormones. I was so vaginally dry, intercourse was impossible. It was terrible. So I would use K-Y.

We were tremendously close and intimate. Not being able to express those feelings sexually broke my heart. At night I'd be physically tired anyway, but we were very affectionate and hugging and kissing, and this man who so loved me and would never dream of pushing or even asking me obviously wanted to have sex, and so even though I had not an ounce in me that wanted to make love, I would have sex with him—as a gift. I pretended that I enjoyed it, and the deception was so terrible. I was caught in this gigantic dilemma. I never felt like having sex, but this man was someone I adored and wanted to *want* to have sex with. So I was living a lie. Months down the road I confessed to the lie, and it was so terribly hard and sad.

He was amazing. He was sweet and thoughtful. His attitude all along—ours really—was, "Well, we have a lifetime together. This bad time won't last forever." We got through it, and our sex life is much better now.

—*Anonymous*

SEX IS AN issue during the year of chemotherapy because your libido completely goes. Especially when you're losing body hair and you're feeling sick and you're gaining weight. I was married, so it wasn't, "Oh, my God, nobody is going to fall in love with me." It was, "Oh, God, go away."

I think that when someone is going through treatment for

cancer, the sexual aspect of the relationship probably changes and becomes more about tenderness and comfort and touching and cuddling rather than actual sexual encounters. That kind of thing is really important for someone who is feeling the way people feel about themselves when they have cancer. There's a lot of self-blame in this culture about cancer—you're responsible for your disease, that kind of thing—which is not particularly useful and can become very destructive.

If you're trying to help your partner get through treatment, talk a lot. Be very romantic—in a courtship mode. It helps the self-esteem of the person who is going through it. And if you're the patient, you have to overcome your reluctance and your apathy. When you're feeling better—because there are times when you feel okay—set up dates, situations where you do something special. Be generous with each other.

Everything does come back. Treatment is temporary. You aren't going to live like this the rest of your life; it's just a rocky spell.

—*Leslie Kaul*

WITH THE FIRST treatment regimen of six months, I lost some libido, and it was very hard to talk about it to others. With the second treatment, with the cisplatin, I lost a lot of libido. But the real issue is that I'm alive, and I didn't lose my libido totally.

Sure, the frequency of our sexual relationship is down. Far down. From a male point of view, I don't have the confidence and the strength that I used to have. But sex is much more meaningful and more loving on my wife's part. It's almost as if we took the relationship that we discovered in sickness and tried to express it physically: It's supportive and sensitive, patient and understanding; it's more meaningful, more choosing to come together. My wife and I hold hands. It's a most profound spiritual, sexual, physical, sensitive, sensual, an incredible thing just to hold hands and walk down the street.

Our relationship is profound, almost as if we are sharing something more eternal. Those words sound funny to some people. It's like going away on retreat and not having distractions. It's pure relationship.

—*Frank Sheridan*

Sex During Cancer

While you shouldn't torture yourself if you feel too lousy to have sex—it's not going to permanently damage your sex life—if possible, you should try to maintain an active sex life during treatment. If you feel well enough to stay sexually active, it's certainly a healthy thing. If you don't feel well enough to have intercourse, you might feel well enough to cuddle or to have a more gentle or gradual form of sexual activity.

Start slowly with sensual touching and backrubs. Try to bring each other to orgasm through means besides intercourse, because intercourse tends to be the most performance-oriented situation. During intercourse, the emphasis is often on the man's erection, and some forms of treatment interfere with a man's stamina. Chemotherapy can decrease testosterone production. Radiation to the pelvic area can harden the arteries that create an erection. And removal of the bladder, prostate, seminal vessels, or rectum can damage the nerves that control blood flow to the penis. In the case of women, intercourse might be painful to those who have had genital cancer or surgery. Radiation therapy can damage the walls of the vagina. Both radiation and chemotherapy can cause premature menopause, which leads to hot flashes and vaginal dryness.

Couples often wait for sex to be spontaneous, but when you're recovering from cancer and treatment, you need to plan more than usual. Find times when you're feeling as good as possible, when you're not exhausted or, if you're still on pain medication, when you're not too drowsy. If you're going through chemotherapy, take advantage of the window of time in between courses of the treatment. If you've also got kids at home and you're

working, sex tends to be at the bottom of the priority list,
so you need to give it some quality time.

Leslie R. Schover, Ph.D.,
Staff Psychologist, Cleveland Clinic Foundation,
Author, Sexuality and Fertility After Cancer
Cleveland, Ohio

CHAPTER SIXTEEN

Complementary Treatments, Conventional and Otherwise

In recent years complementary or alternative healing has been receiving more and more attention. In 1992 the National Institutes of Health established the Office of Alternative Health to study seven categories of alternative medical practices. These include: diet, nutrition, and lifestyle changes; mind/body interventions; manual healing methods; and herbal medicines. Among other things, they are funding research into the value of such herbal remedies as essiac, the Hoxsey treatment, and mistletoe.

On the whole, we put our confidence solidly behind Western medicine, but we did venture out in other directions as well. When it came to beating cancer, we wanted the best that science has to offer, but we also wanted to better address pain and stress management and quality-of-life issues, as well as to complement chemotherapy and radiation therapy with natural and traditional remedies. We wanted to explore a more all-encompassing route back to good health, and that encouraged us sometimes to test unknown waters.

Currently, despite positive anecdotal evidence for some of these methods and programs, there is little concrete evidence of their efficacy—hence the word "alternative"—and interest tends to be highly individualistic. If you're interested, you'll have to search around and explore the possibilities to figure out what you might be open to.

Mental Imaging, Meditation, and Visualization

I USED GUIDED-IMAGERY techniques to reduce stress and help me relax. I would put on relaxing music, sit in a comfortable chair, close my eyes, and begin to breathe slowly and deeply. I would create a beautiful place in my mind, a meadow full of trees and flowers, and would imagine myself carefree and at peace in that meadow. Once I had created that place solidly in my mind, I was able to call it up more quickly each time until I reached the point where, moments after I began, I would get to the meadow and almost immediately feel the stress and fear dissipate. The imagery restored my body, relaxed my mind, and gave hope—which is so necessary in fighting cancer—a chance to shine through.

—*Blythe Ritchfield*

I DISCOVERED SOMETHING called psychoneuroimmunology, which is a fancy way of saying mind over body. I visualized my healthy killer cells devouring the cancer, and I learned to relax through meditation.

Every morning on my train commute to work, I meditated. I would take a seat, get into a comfortable position, and close my eyes. Most people thought that I was catching a few winks, but I was actually wide awake. I would repeat my mantra—my favorite one was the word "peace"—over and over again in my head. I would inhale for ten seconds and say "peace," then exhale for the same amount of time. Peace. Thoughts would come and go, and I would let them pass, without dwelling on them, always returning to the word "peace."

What did it do for me? Well, I'm a type A person. With meditation, I became an A− or maybe a B+. In other words, I'm a pretty energetic, sometimes nervous guy. Meditation calmed me down and helped me to focus. Having some clarity was essential because I felt overwhelmed at times by the amount of information I was receiving from doctors, nurses, family, and friends. I knew I had to sift through it all and make the right decision for myself without wasting too much time trying too many different approaches. By clearing my mind of clutter, meditation helped me focus on what I needed to do. In the end, it gave me just what I asked for: peace.

—*Maurice Chesney*

WHEN I WAS released from the hospital, I was frightened to do anything or exert myself in any way. A psychiatrist whom I was seeing at the time said, "Do whatever you feel like doing." And I remember walking across Central Park and realizing that it was going to be up to me to just grab life back in any way I was willing and able to, instead of waiting for some pronouncement of my ability to do that.

I worked with psychic healers, psychiatrists, massage therapists, aromatherapists, nutritionists, hypnotherapists. I went to a psychiatrist who specialized in end-of-life issues and life-threatening illnesses and who I came to refer to as my death therapist. I did anything that made any sense to me, and I saw everyone. I kind of embraced and abandoned things as they impressed me along the way.

I went through the gamut of believing and not believing. I felt that even if these therapists and healers had no inherent power, there was power in the gesture of the search. Anything that I did became a message I was sending to myself—to my body and soul—about how much I wanted to get life back. Action versus inaction. My attitude was: I'm going to do anything that might be possible rather than just taking some medicine and then sitting back to see if it works or not.

I went out to the Simonton Cancer Center and spent the week doing all kinds of visualizations and techniques and designing get-well plans. One of the things that was promoted there was assigning oneself a guide, a personal guide, whether imaginary or real. I had long conversations and spent many meditation sessions speaking with someone who I imagined to be myself twenty years down the line. I felt it was a great device. Not only did he give me a part of my psyche to talk with and bounce things off of, but every encounter with this image was vivid proof of the inevitability of my recovery because this guide, who again and again assured me that we would meet one day, was me, well, twenty years into the future.

—*Evan Handler*

I PICTURED RADIATION as a healing light—a lot of people do that—but when it came to my tumor, I pictured the light frying it. I also put in smells and sounds and other things to help me really focus on it. Once I was at a restaurant and heard fajitas being cooked, and I decided to add that to my visualization. I also used the smell of burnt hair. It became a multimedia thing going on in my head.

Having this burnt-hair fried-up thing inside of me wasn't exactly comforting, so I'd always try to add a piece of something that was cleansing afterward. For me, water is cleansing and relaxing, so I would picture waves or rivers and fish and sort of making peace with this thing in my head.

—*Sheri Sobrato*

I USED IMAGING techniques, which I learned from Bernie Siegel's book *Love, Medicine and Miracles,* to help with the nausea of chemo. I found a comfortable place in my living room where there was absolute silence (which has always been difficult to find because I come from a family of musicians). I would lie on the couch with my eyes closed, and I would attempt to fill my head with the vision of a white light. It took a week before I was able to get the white light into my head for more than a minute, but with practice I was able to keep the vision for longer periods of time. Then I tried to make the light expand and move to my left lung, where the disease was. I tried to keep it there for as long as possible. With practice, I got better and was able to picture the light throughout my left lung for at least twenty minutes. The white light made me feel like I was doing my part to help the chemo. I called my chemo and the white light the SWAT team, whose mission was to blow the cancer out of my lungs.

—*Genya Ravan*

I COUNSELED WITH a woman who wrote a book on mental imaging. Her specialty is cancer patients, and she gave me cassettes of what I call "soft talk." They were lectures and poetry. The idea was to distract your mind and occupy your thought processes with something distant and removed from your ailments. On more than one occasion when I was feeling lousy physically, I would lie on the floor and listen to those cassettes. They were very effective. It was a mind game, obviously, an escape from the body. The whole thing happened so quickly—being diagnosed and the same day going to the hospital and then surgery a few days later—that I needed time to catch up.

—*John Hall*

I WAS HIGHLY influenced by Norman Cousins's book *Anatomy of an Illness,* which I read early on. He persuaded me of the benefits of trying to be happy. So I tried to make myself happier. I tried to let bad things roll off me a little bit more than they normally would have. And this may sound funny, but I practiced smiling.

I read an article in *Science News* about a study by some psychologist on the effect of facial expressions on your mood. Normally you think that your face expresses what you're feeling. They had people put expressions on their faces, and then they measured the physiological responses to those expressions. What they found was that the physiology followed the expression almost as much as or as much as the expression followed the physiology.

If you're depressed and your mouth turns down, there are some measurable effects on your body, some of which involve the immune system. So basically what that article says is that your face and bodily responses are hard-wired, and the messages run in both directions. If you feel happy, you smile, and if you smile, you feel happy. And if you feel happy, that's good for your immune system. So I tried smiling a lot, and there's no way you can measure the benefit of that, except that it makes you feel better. You just feel good.

When I took that on as part of my program, I would do it whenever I thought about it. You can't smile all the time, but every time I'd think about it, I'd smile. I often smiled when people were around, and they must have wondered what on earth I was smiling about, but you have to get into it. You have to make your eyes crinkle up. If you just put on a smile without your eyes being part of it, I don't think you're doing any good.

What effect it has on your cancer is impossible to know. The median survival time for people with my level of metastatic prostate cancer and the treatment I've had is a little less than five years. I have doubled that. Is it me? Is it just my physiology and my body and my response to the drugs, or is it some of the things that I've added to the drugs? There's no way to know.

Norman Cousins developed a serious illness (not cancer), and he went to the hospital. They weren't doing him any good, so he checked out. Somehow he found out that vitamin C might help him, so he took massive amounts of vitamin C. But he also rationalized that since it was known that negative emotions affect your health negatively, positive emotions probably affect it positively. So he tried to make his life emotionally positive. He found that when he watched a funny movie and laughed for a while, it would relieve his pain for some period of time.

He later became an adjunct professor in the school of medicine at UCLA, to try, among other things, to research the effects of emotions on cancer survival. In his book he talks about one experiment he performed on himself. He had a sample of his blood drawn and then spent five minutes thinking positive thoughts. This was back in the mid-eighties, and he imagined how wonderful it would be if the United States and Russia were friends instead of enemies in the Cold War. He really got into it. His face got red, and he was enthusiastic. They drew another sample of blood after, and he had the two samples of blood assayed for their immune-system components, of which there are a number, and the average increase in the number of immune-system components was fifty-three percent. Some had gone up as much as two hundred percent. The question is, can that make a difference with cancer?

There is no definitive answer to that question, but it seems reasonable to think that being happy would be beneficial. It made a huge difference in his immune-system components, and I think it made a difference in mine.

—*Damon Phinney*

The Paintbrush Is Mightier

People feel out of control when they get diagnosed with cancer, and art is really useful for regaining some of that control. Before, during, and after chemotherapy, I go to patients' rooms or to the treatment waiting rooms with a huge basket of art materials on a luggage caddy. I have chalks, oils, pastels, watercolors, felt pens, glitter, glue, clay, crayons, and pencils. Instead of being told that something's going to be done to them, the patients get to pick and choose. They choose sizes, textures, and colors of paper and do whatever they want with their hands. They remember being a kid.

You don't have to consider yourself an artist. This is process art, not product art. Whether it's writing or movement or music, there is power in creativity. It's about using art to express how you're feeling, when words aren't enough. It helps people come up with images and metaphors of security. For instance, some people have made shields—literally shields of protection—and hung them on their doors. There was one young man who was very scared. He was having nightmares and was really jumpy. I asked him to draw that fear and look at it head-on. So he drew this scary-looking face, and he started laughing. He brought the fear to light, and it had less power over him.

Some people say that the only time they're not in physical pain is while they're making art. They say it makes them feel less scared, more grounded. Art taps into the subconscious—the place where our dreams come from—and brings to light things that we didn't even know we were thinking. It helps us pay attention to what needs healing.

Get a big pad of paper. Get some big fat crayons or bright paints or anything that delights you, and use it to chronicle your experience. Use your nondominant hand to short-circuit that place that says, "I can't draw a person." Draw stick figures. Use the colors and materials you like. Give yourself that gift.

—Wendy Traber,
Director, Art for Healing, Stanford University Hospital
(and a veteran of Hodgkin's disease and breast cancer),
Stanford, California

SINCE I'VE BEEN sick, I've been seeing a massage therapist who also does holistic healing. I found out about her through a friend who is a massage therapist and went to school with her. This woman went to another year-long program to learn the techniques of holistic healing.

When I get there, I lie down on a massage table and close my eyes. She makes me very comfortable. Before she starts, she puts her hands on my shoulders, because I have a lot of tension there, and tries to have me release the tension. She then proceeds to talk in a very soothing tone, while I concentrate on what she's saying. It's a guided meditation. She tells me, "Think of a peaceful place, and then put yourself in a healing warmth, a light. Imagine a light surrounding you. It's warm, and it's healing you. Imagine this light is penetrating every inch of your body. The light is healing you. You're being freed of all of the leukemia." At times when I needed my blood counts to come up, she would say, "Imagine that the light is working on increasing the levels of your blood counts."

Then she works on the channels in your body, which she says can get blocked. She imagines the channels being opened to release the negative energy from the illness. I don't know how helpful all this really is, but I have an open mind toward what she does. My point of view is that it can't hurt me. I know there are a lot of doctors who think that it is really good for you. At this point, I am willing to try anything, and I think it's helping me. When I leave there, I feel really good and very relaxed.

For me, it's important not just to stick with the conventional methods of treatment but also to explore what else is out there. I would never use only these guided meditations and support groups as a treatment for leukemia. But the fact that I am leaving this lady's house and feeling relaxed and tension-free is helping me. Even after my transplant and when I'm in remission, I'll probably continue to do it.

—*Michele Fox*

I WANTED TO do other things to try to help myself besides the surgery and chemo and radiation, so in November of 1990 when I finished the radiation, I spent a week at the Maharishi Ayurveda Health Center in Lancaster, Massachusetts. Deepak Chopra was the medical director there at the time.

I didn't know very much about Dr. Chopra before I went. When I was recuperating from my surgery, I saw him on television talking about how your mind affects your body, and then somebody else mentioned his book, *Quantum Healing*, which I actually found hard to get into. Anyway, he just kept popping up. My son sent me an article on reducing stress from *Longevity* magazine, and this Maharishi Ayurveda Health Center was listed as one of the spas that was good for stress reduction. I called them to see if they took cancer patients, and they said they did as long as your blood count was high enough that you wouldn't be too susceptible to anything. So I tentatively made a reservation to go for a week, and strangely enough, my blood count was high enough that week.

There were twelve of us there—three cancer patients, a businessman from Mississippi, a husband and wife from New York who came to reduce stress, a girl from Connecticut—different people from all walks of life. It was fairly expensive, kind of spa-like, but I thought, "What better thing could I spend my money on?"

They feel if you can get your life back into balance, your body can help you heal yourself. They prescribed a lot of massages—long, wonderful massages that they feel help rid you of toxins. The food was very fresh, vegetarian. And we learned some simple yoga exercises and transcendental meditation. There's no religious aspect to it, but you can do the meditation with your own mantra, something appropriate to your religion. I had learned TM years before, but I found it hard to do on my own. Getting into a routine for a week at the center made it easier to continue, and they were very positive. "You really are doing well and have a strong physiology." They make you feel like you will be around to come back.

I was meditating twice a day for a while, and then I got down to once a day. I really do think it reduces stress, which can have such a big effect on your immune system. When your adrenaline is flowing and it doesn't have any way to be spent, it hurts your body. Meditation helps you imagine peaceful things. It relaxes you and rids you of that frantic feeling.

—Kay Chenoweth

Coping with Pain

BEFORE THE SURGERY, I went to see a professional hypnotist— he's an M.D., but he does hypnosis. I was told that people who had seen him before surgery tended to get out of recovery much more quickly. That certainly proved to be true for me. I don't know how much of this was him, but I didn't spend any time in a recovery unit. I was in an immediate postsurgery room, but then I went straight to my room in the hospital.

What he did was teach me to put myself into a trance by telling myself, "Yes, you're going to have this surgery. These people are going to be cutting you open with a knife, but they're not muggers. They're here to do a job. Relax and let them do the job."

For the chemotherapy visualization, we figured out a fantasy that the chemicals themselves were a boisterous, obnoxious crew of street cleaners who came into Manhattan every night. My blood vessels and arteries were the streets of Manhattan, and they cleaned them out. They played boom boxes and made this terrible racket, and their chemicals stank, but they did the job and then went back to Brooklyn every night.

I don't know how deep this was. I wasn't unconscious. I could hear an ambulance passing in the street. It felt almost like being really tired, like just before falling asleep, but not quite. It was something you induced in yourself, like taking a deep breath and counting to three and closing your eyes and imagining yourself thinking down. Time seemed to pass more slowly. I would think that I'd been doing it for a couple of minutes and it was more like five. Hypnosis doesn't make a huge difference, but a definite one.

—Richard Brookhiser

Easing Pain Through Hypnosis

Pain is a signal. When you bang your arm, you feel the pain and say, "Oh, my God, I just banged my arm. It's bleeding. It's bruising. I have to take care of it." During surgery, pain doesn't serve any purpose, so we anesthetize to eliminate the signal. When you undergo cancer treatment, you know exactly what's causing the pain, and there's nothing you can do with that information. Through hypnosis, we cut off the signal. With one patient, for example, we created an elaborate "castle." Through a very focused state of inward concentration, he moved away from the painful treatment to the castle, where he could go and leave his body behind to withstand the treatment.

We can also create an acceptance of chemotherapy to overcome nausea, even anticipated nausea. The chemo comes into your body through the bloodstream, but the body treats it as if it has entered the stomach. The body's response to a poison, which is what chemo is, is to get rid of it. Instead, you should picture the chemicals as your mercenary army, if you will, or as a sweep-out team or clean-up crew, coming in to help your body rid itself of malignant cells. You want your body to support this intrusion and work with it. The body's tendency is to fight back, which is the worst thing it can do. It needs to flow along, to accept the treatments. You can do this by focusing inward using any one of several techniques—meditation, self-hypnosis, Zen.

One way is to sit quietly, or lie quietly, close your eyes, and focus on your breathing. Become aware of your breath moving in and out of your body, and let your body go completely. Relax every muscle, every inch of skin. Make yourself as comfortable as you can, letting the chair or the bed support you. It's in that state of focused concentration that you now can use your imagination to flow with the chemotherapy. Or if you're in a painful situation, like a bone marrow biopsy, you can take yourself to another place. Imagine a place where you've been or want to be, and use your imagination to fill in all the details—what it looks like, how it feels, the smells, and the sounds.

Success depends on the individual. Some are good at communicating with their bodies, and others can hardly do it. But even people of low capacity can do it well if they are truly motivated. For a referral to a professional hypnotist, send a self-addressed, stamped business-sized envelope to: American Society of Clinical Hypnosis, 2200 East Devon Avenue, Suite 291, Des Plaines, IL 60018. The society will send you a list of hypnotists in your state.

—Stanley Fisher, Ph.D.,
Clinical Psychologist, Author of Discovering the Power of Self-Hypnosis,
New York, New York

WHEN I HAD my treatment, they had just brought out the antinausea drug Zofran, which was pretty good. The first two times I went into the hospital I did not actually throw up, but I felt like the next time I was going to. So then my wife became a criminal, and she brought me some marijuana. After the third course of chemotherapy, if I hadn't had it, I would have been sick. There's no question in my mind. None of my doctors or nurses discouraged me from using it. They said, "Just do it in the bathroom." They were very good about it. But I thought it was outrageous that this had to be done criminally. I'm in New York, a cosmopolitan place, and I'm a journalist and sort of in the elite by virtue of that fact. If I hadn't lived here, I could have gotten in trouble. This is terribly unfair. As a result, I've become a crusader for medical marijuana.

I had smoked a few times in college, and, unlike the President, I'd inhaled, but I had not done any in years and years. I don't like to smoke—I don't even like being drunk—and I would never touch it again. Now I'm the perfect citizen of drug-free America—except that I want to make marijuana legal.

The one time this affected my work negatively was at an editorial conference to decide whether we should favor dumping Quayle from the ticket or not. I thought it was a stupid idea, not because I was fond of Quayle, but I thought it looked desperate. It wouldn't work. However, I'd just gotten out of the hospital, and I was still smoking pot because the nausea lasted a day or two after the treatment. I just sat at the conference listening to the debate in that sort of pot-induced passivity, and I didn't say anything. *National Review* called for dumping Quayle. I don't know if I could have prevailed, but I certainly would have said it was madness.

—*Richard Brookhiser*

Complementary Medicines

A FRIEND TOLD me about shark cartilage, and I decided to try it because I wanted to help with my treatment rather than just let my doctor do all the work. Shark cartilage was originally given to people who had severe arthritis, and they discovered accidentally that it also shrinks tumors. You can take it in combination with any conventional treatment—chemo, radiation, or surgery. Commonly the powder is more effective, but I take capsules because it's easier for me. I take ten capsules a day. At the very least, maybe it will keep me from having arthritis.

—*Bev Yaffe*

I WENT TO a nutritionist who was an M.D. He did a blood chemistry on me and suggested a number of vitamins. I'd been taking vitamins anyway for a number of years, but he suggested some other vitamins that would be helpful during chemotherapy. He also gave me some dietary suggestions. My oncologist asked for a list of everything I was taking. He said, "As far as I'm concerned, with the exception of one," which was folic acid, a vitamin that apparently works against the chemotherapy drugs, "I completely approve of your taking these vitamins." Most doctors don't give much credence to vitamins, but I think they were very helpful to my system in dealing with the toxic effect of the chemotherapy drugs. I think that is one of the reasons why I didn't battle nausea. I believe it helped keep my blood counts up as well. I never missed a treatment because of a low count.

—*Toni Zavistovski*

Considering Complementary Care

The focus of complementary care is on improving treatment outcomes. Through the use of complementary modalities, we help individuals prepare for and get through their surgery, as well as prevent further complications or illnesses. All of our modalities are safe, noninvasive techniques that we believe will help patients improve their quality of life and regain optimal health. We use aromatherapy, guided imagery, hypnosis, massage, meditation, music therapy, relaxation tapes, t'ai chi/qi gong, therapeutic touch, and yoga. T'ai chi/qi gong, for instance, has been deemed walking meditation. A person is instructed in slow, rhythmic postures to elicit the relaxation response. It is practiced throughout China—about twenty million Chinese do it daily to increase the mobility of their joints, stimulate their immune response, and prevent illness.

The reason we have such a smorgasbord of complementary modalities is that no one therapy can satisfy all patients. If you say "yoga" to someone, and they have a preconceived notion that we're going to dress them in orange and shave their head, they're not going to embrace it. We have a consultant meet with the patient to find out what they know and don't know about some of these buzzwords. That way we can prescribe the best modality treatment program specifically for them.

Success really depends on what point of reference the person is coming from. Do they feel they can take an active part in their healing process? Or do they feel that it's an act of God? These modalities may work best for open-minded individuals, who feel that other things can complement their medical or surgical treatment (although only clinical research can determine whether complementary care is more successful with somebody who believes it will work).

Complementary care is growing across the United States at a rapid rate, but we are far behind other parts of the world, where many of these modalities have been practiced for thousands of years. Ayurvedic medicine, the oldest known medical system still in use, is based on the theory that health depends on the balance of a person's body, mind, emotions, and spirit. Here in the States, this belief is just catching on.

If you're interested in complementary care, you should look for a qualified individual to act as a guide or advocate. It should be someone who is open to criticism and who will allow a dialogue, which is very important to the success of the treatment. Begin by looking in the yellow pages for a holistic practitioner, preferably an M.D. or an N.D., a naturopathic doctor. Call the American Holistic Medical Association (919-787-5181) and ask for its directory of practitioners. Call a nearby medical center and ask if they have a complementary, alternative, or holistic care program. Many medical centers, including those at more than 130 colleges and universities, have started programs. Ask yourself if the therapies offered suit your needs. Most important, visit the practitioner and decide if you feel comfortable with him or her.

—*Jery Whitworth, R.N., C.C.P.,*
Executive Director/Cofounder, Complementary Care Center at
Columbia-Presbyterian Medical Center,
New York, New York

I USED CHINESE remedies to help my body fight the cancer and the side effects of chemotherapy. My mom used traditional Chinese herbs and roots to make concoctions for me—things like a bitter-melon shake, shark's fin soup, and bird's nest soup, which is made from actual bird saliva. These drinks are considered very nutritious and are part of everyday Chinese culture. Although I never loved the way they tasted, I grew up on them, so they were comforting to me when I was sick. Besides, they made my mother happy. And maybe they actually did help because my nausea was never severe, and here I am, years later, happy and healthy.

—*Monica Ko*

MY SON, WHO was always doing a lot of research, wanted me to see an anthroposophic doctor—"anthroposophic" means wisdom of man—to complement my traditional therapy. So in February of 1991, I spent a few days at the Fellowship Community in Spring Valley, New York. A doctor there prescribed Iscador, a derivative of the mistletoe plant. It reduces tumor growth and boosts the immune system and was promoted by Rudolf Steiner, an Austrian philosopher who lived from the 1860s to the 1920s and practiced what is called spiritual science.

Steiner had a lot of ideas about biodynamic gardening and healing plants. He gave around six thousand lectures on his ideas about science, education, art, and so on, and there are people who study them. One thing he believed was that certain plants have relationships with certain parts of the body, and the use of Iscador grew out of that. It's manufactured by a company called Institut Hiscia in Arlesheim, Switzerland. They grow the mistletoe on different trees. The one you take depends on the kind of cancer you have. Mine is mistletoe that grows on the apple tree.

The anthroposophic doctors are Western doctors who have had traditional training but are interested in Steiner's ideas. My doctor at home was aware that I was trying some other things. He said it was fine as long as I didn't do something that would hurt me. I took him some information on Iscador, but he didn't want to do the injections, so I have it sent directly to me from Switzerland, and I inject myself.

As time went on and I went back for checkups, my doctor

would say, "Are you still taking that Iscador?" I think he became more and more interested because only a very small percentage of patients survive pancreatic cancer with lymph nodes involved. I believe the Iscador has been really helpful.

—*Kay Chenoweth*

ONE OF THE alternative treatments I used was something called Russian tea. It tasted like vinegar and apple juice. It's made from a fungus that grows like a mushroom in water. You mix it with sugar and yeast, and you grow it and keep it in the fridge. As soon as you use up the tea, you move the mushroom into a new container and grow it again. It just keeps on growing. I found out about it through some relatives in Arizona, who had a friend who used it for cancer treatment. Supposedly there's an area in Russia where the people drink this stuff daily, and they apparently have no cancer. I drank it for about six months.

—*Brian Schmidt*

THERE'S A GERMAN doctor, Johanna Budwig—she's a seven-time Nobel Prize nominee—who has treated cancer patients with flaxseed oil, an essential fatty acid. She took some cancer patients who were literally at death's door and gave them nonfat cottage cheese mixed with flaxseed oil, and it changed something in their blood. A lot of them became much healthier.

Flaxseed oil is something you see in the health food magazines. Dr. Budwig has written a book about it called *Flax Oil as a True Aid Against Arthritis, Heart Infarction, Cancer and Other Diseases.* The idea is that nowadays we don't get a lot of the essential fatty acids. They take them out of food to give it a longer shelf life, and they're not in fruits or vegetables. So you buy flaxseed oil at the health food store. It's cold-pressed—not processed with heat like a lot of other oils—and it should be refrigerated. It has a life of about two or three months. For a while, I was eating flaxseed oil and cottage cheese every morning, but now I do it periodically.

I think you try different things, and you stay with the things you feel help, and the other things you let go. I had some herbs that they gave me at the Maharishi Health Center, but I only took those for a while, and the same with some homeopathic drops that a doctor in New York prescribed. I tried a macrobiotic diet, but it wasn't for me. I was already losing weight from radiation, and I thought, "I don't want to eat these weird things and lose more weight." You don't need to do it all. You have to see what works for you.

—*Kay Chenoweth*

AFTER I FINISHED up the chemo, I was back in remission. In the past I had not stayed in remission for more than three months. I went to a place called the Livingston Foundation Medical Center in San Diego. I wanted to explore every option—I didn't feel like I had too many chances left. I saved this one for what I thought was an appropriate time. When you go through chemotherapy, 99.9 percent of the cancer is killed, and it's up to your body to fight off the remaining cells. But your body is in a weakened state because of the chemotherapy. Your bone marrow is wiped out, so it's not producing red and white blood cells rapidly. That's when you really need something to give you a boost to recover. That was why I decided to go then.

The program was two weeks long. They put you on a special diet, which is not unlike other healthy diets—lots of fruits, grains, vegetables. I think they allow some dairy products, but they don't allow any meat. They also gave me megadoses of vitamin C through an intravenous drip. To help boost your immune system, they create a vaccine for you from your own body fluids. I also received units of whole blood on three different occasions. I was so wiped out from the chemo, and my white counts were so low that I needed blood. It's difficult for the body to recover if there's no fuel going through the veins, but during standard medical treatment, doctors won't give you blood. That really helped boost my energy level, and I think my body responded better.

I can't say the program cured me because at that point I was in remission. The vaccine is such a radical theory—I don't know whether they were right or not. But the treatment did help my feeling of well-being. I got out of there and went camping in the Sierras. I felt like a new man. Then I started the waiting game. To make a long story short, it didn't come back.

I took some of the vaccine home with me after the treatment

and gave myself injections for a number of months afterward. I also continued getting intravenous injections of vitamin C a couple of times a week for more than six months. A friend of mine's wife, who's a pediatrician, offered to do the injections, and, being a member of the American Medical Association, she was pretty skeptical about this place and their claims. Later, I was still doing well, and a friend of theirs had a relapse of some type of throat cancer. Doctors at the Stanford Medical Center told him he had three weeks before the mass would grow to block his throat, and he wouldn't be able to eat. So, my friends called me on a Friday night, looking for any option. I told them all the details about the Livingston Center, and they put their friend in the program on Monday morning. He went through the program, and his tumor went away. Incredible. It turned skeptics into believers.

—*George Clark*

Faith Healers

I WENT TO see a spiritual healer at the Meadowlands with five thousand other people. He was a priest who was very straightforward. He said that healing may come spontaneously through God—or if you stop smoking cigarettes. I viewed unconventional medicine as complementary—not as an alternative—to the regular stuff sanctioned by the American Medical Association, but I also believed in this kind of thing, that a spiritual healer could make the crippled walk. The priest did not know I had lung cancer, but when he laid his hands on me, I felt a burning sensation. It gave me a spiritual and emotional charge. It also convinced me to go for a second opinion, which showed that I had a different—and curable—type of lung cancer.

—*Maurice Chesney*

AFTER BEING TOLD by so many doctors that they had nothing for me, I decided I had to help myself. One day while I was having a liver biopsy, I told the doctor, "I really hope you can get it because I would do anything to stay alive. I would dance on top of this table with an umbrella if that's what somebody said it would take."

He said, "I'm going to tell you something, but if you ever tell anybody, I'll deny I said it. My wife has a friend who goes to a faith healer, and she is just wonderful. If you'd be interested in seeing her, call my wife, and she'll give you the name."

Well, I ended up going to the faith healer for a year and a half while I was looking for a doctor who would treat me. I knew that I wasn't really getting better, but I was doing something for myself and it was helping me to relax. It was kind of like spending money at the beauty parlor every week. Each time she would say, "Oh, you're really doing very well. You're doing very well."

And I would say to myself, "Bullshit. You're a liar, but I don't care. It's making my head feel better." I always thought of myself as intelligent and educated and all that, yet I sort of *fell* for this. I just wanted to do something for myself.

—*Bev Yaffe*

CHAPTER SEVENTEEN

Pushing the Envelope: Dealing with Recurrence, Chronic Cancer, Loss of a Limb, and Bad Days in the Hospital

The sobering fact is that, while overall cancer mortality has declined recently in men and women under the age of fifty-five, more than half a million people of all ages still die from cancer in the United States each year. And for many more people, beating cancer means losing a body part or taking the fight right to the outer edge in another way. For still others living with incurable cancer, it means extending the longevity envelope beyond what the law of averages has to say and living as happily as possible.

It doesn't feel good to take life right to the brink, and some days you might feel like you don't care anymore. But you have to summon the will to get through, to persevere. And you can.

Dealing with Chronic Cancer

WHEN YOU HAVE metastatic prostate cancer, first of all, it's not considered to be curable, although I'm not sure anybody stated it to me that baldly at the time. So you do not have radiation. What you do is try to get rid of as many of the male hormones in your body as you can, because they stimulate the growth of the cancer cells and of the normal prostate cells. If you can shut that off, then most men will go into a period of remission.

In the early eighties, in Canada, a drug causing you to stop making testosterone was proved to work. The common name of that drug is Lupron. An oncologist in Boulder told me my options and recommended Lupron. I wound up taking Lupron in the form of a little injection that I give myself every day.

I used bike riding as a way to prove to myself that I wasn't being devastated by cancer. I used it to offset the effects of not making male hormones, or having them blocked. Some of the effects include impotence, weight gain, body-hair loss. You lose muscle tone, and you have hot flashes. The list is a bit longer than that, but those are the bigger things. So how do you preserve your male identity? How do you protect your ego when you're losing some of your masculine characteristics?

Bike riding was my main way to deal with those problems. When I found out I had cancer, I set myself a goal of doing a tour called Ride the Rockies, which takes place every year in Colorado. It is a four-hundred-mile tour with about two thousand people that starts in the western part of the state and ends up usually in the Boulder area. I started riding in early April, and between then and mid-June, when Ride the Rockies started, I had ridden eighteen hundred and fifty miles, including several hundred-mile days.

The fact that I could still be strong on my bike and keep up with most of the people my age made me feel good. I was able to do that, and I've continued to do that for the past ten years. We live in a beautiful part of the country for bike riding, and I try to ride every other day.

Despite my cancer, the only pains I get from biking are the ones that come from overdoing it and getting tired and dehydrated. Those are the days when you do something strenuous and come home with the greatest sense of exaltation at having done something that nobody would have expected a person with cancer to be able to do. For the last five or six years, I've been on bike tours in the mountains of France, climbing the ascents of the Tour de France. It's wonderful to be over there doing those really tough rides.

A couple of years ago I noticed that I only needed another nine thousand miles in order to make forty thousand by my tenth anniversary of having cancer, so I set myself a goal of riding forty thousand miles in my first ten years with cancer, and I met it. That's been a rather big thing for me.

—*Damon Phinney*

MY REMISSION LASTED fifteen months, and then the cancer reappeared in my stomach. I had to go back on chemotherapy, and this time I got forty radiation treatments. The second time around was hard to take. I was given an appendectomy along with having my spleen removed. I went back into remission, but it only lasted about a year. More cancer. More treatments. I thought to myself, "Is it possible that every time I go for a checkup I'm going to get news of a recurrence? How much longer can I keep this up?"

I knew deep down that this was the hand I had been dealt and I had to accept it and learn how to deal with it. I became very close to my doctor and his staff and worked with them to do whatever it took to get well. But once again my cancer recurred, this time in my lungs and liver. The ten years from 1980 to 1990 had felt like twenty. In disgust, I told the doctor that I was not going to take any more treatments, and that I was prepared to let nature take its course. I had had enough. I left the hospital for good, I thought.

The doctor and hospital staff called my home to try to convince me to come in for an appointment. I didn't want to go back. Finally, because of the persistence of a nurse I liked, I relented. I was close enough to my doctor to ask the question everyone dreads asking: How long do I have? He told me two years, but he wanted me to talk to another doctor who did bone marrow transplants before I gave up.

"Why didn't we seek him out sooner?" I asked.

I was told that my age—fifty—was a big factor against me. The procedure was rough, to say the least, and younger patients had a better chance of getting through it. He said that they didn't give the transplant to anyone over forty.

"Why?" I screamed and cried at the same time. "Why? If someone wants the chance, wants so desperately to live?" I was outraged when I found out that the answer to my question had much more to do with politics than medicine.

My doctor wrote a letter to the bone marrow transplant doctor that stated all the reasons for my being an excellent candidate for a transplant, despite my age. I finally got an appointment with the transplant doctor, who had the nerve to try to talk me out of the procedure. I was enraged. I told him that I had the will to get through it and that my body could withstand any of the side effects. I had never smoked; I was an athlete; and I did hard physical work. He sent me for every stress test imaginable to disprove that I was fit enough, but I passed them all. I became a tremendous nuisance to him, and I never let up. Finally, my persistence paid off. One Friday night, my phone rang, and it was the doctor. He told me that if I wanted the transplant, I had to come down to the hospital the next morning because a patient who had been scheduled got a fever and had to be postponed.

At the time, I was the oldest patient to get a bone marrow transplant, and because I never gave up, I'm here today to say that I've reached the five-year remission mark.

—*Frank Narcisco*

Dealing with Recurrence

I CAME BACK to the Giants, and in the 1988 season, I started the first two games. The only major side effects that I had from the radiation were slightly decreased lung function and cotton mouth, which was probably the biggest problem. When I got to playing, my mouth would go dry. During the second game, one of my own players fell on me and tore the ligaments in my ankle, so I was out for about eight weeks. But when I returned, I wasn't playing as well as I could. It wasn't because of the surgeries for the cancer or the radiation treatment. It was because of an unrelated shoulder injury. I was not able to get my starting spot back.

I noticed near the end of the season I was really fatigued. Before the last game of the year, I had a regular three-month checkup, and I told the doctor I was really tired. One of the things the radiation treatments did was knock out my thyroid gland, so I was on a synthetic thyroid medication, and one other time I had been tired, and it was just because the drug needed to be increased. I thought that was probably what it was again, but when he examined me, he found a lump by my collarbone. He said, "Do you have a cold?"

I play football outside all winter, and I said, "I've always got a cold."

He said, "It might just be from the cold. Do some blood work, and come back next week."

If we had won the last game against the Jets, we would have made the playoffs. We ended up losing. That was on a Sunday, and on Tuesday, I went back to see the doctor. He told me he wanted to take the lump out. As soon as he told me that, I knew that the Hodgkin's was back. I started putting two and two together. I was having night sweats and hadn't really tied that in with the lump and feeling tired. The first time around, I'd had no symptoms whatsoever. I was in training camp and was healthy except for my shoulder problem as far as I knew.

It just so happened that that night we were having about a hundred people to the house for a Christmas party. My wife was in the ninth month of pregnancy, and I had to go home and tell her fifteen minutes before everybody showed up that I had Hodgkin's again.

When I went in to have that surgery done, every time I lay down, the lump would duck behind the collarbone. I'm lying there on the operating table, and I've got all the IVs and everything in me, and the doctor is searching for it and says, "I can't find it." He says, "Sit up for me, please." I'm sitting up with my arms out straight with all these IVs, and they have to lift me back up, and as soon as I lift up, the lump pops out again. They find it and lay me back down.

It was Hodgkin's again, but it was considered atypical Hodgkin's in that it didn't die off because of the radiation treatments. Maybe it's a little stronger. The first time through, football was my driving force. My goal was to get back to playing again. They said I was playing the dumb jock and basically kept asking, "How soon can I play?"

My wife kept saying, "Don't worry about that. I want to make sure I have a husband, a father for my kid." But I was very driven by football at that time. The second time around, I wised up, not giving a damn about football. The doctor asked me if I wanted to play again after he cured me. I said, "Sure, I'd like to."

He said, "That might make a difference in how I treat you."

I said, "No, it doesn't. I want you to give me everything you can to make sure that I don't have to do this again." The second time it was my family that was my driving force.

—*Karl Nelson*

WHEN I GOT the second diagnosis of cancer, I was in a very high-profile management position that required me to be a perfect employee. It's hard to be a perfect employee in a new job when you have cancer. You have to leave early a lot, and you have to go to doctors a lot, and you get upset when phone calls come that tell you you still have it. I kept trying to behave as if I weren't sick. The day after my surgery, I was on the phone with the managers I supervise. I thought my mother was going to kill people, she was so frustrated with me. I was trying to work. I wouldn't do that again. You get this wake-up call: "Hey, your ride on this planet is a temporary one." That doesn't have to be a bad thing. It's just a truth. So take advantage of that knowledge. Instead, I was obstinately refusing to.

My first Pap smear three months after that surgery came back clear, and everyone was really happy. Then I got another one three months later, and it came back with irregular cells. All I could think of was, "Oh, my God, here we go again, and this time it's going to mean chemo or radiation—or both. I don't know if I'm ready for that." I resigned the next day. I thought, "I really need to start taking responsibility for saving my life, here. I cannot work and have the kind of stress that I'm swallowing and pretend that I can do all of that and convince my body that it doesn't want to kill itself. It's okay to quit and not make a lot of money." But it was a hard decision to make.

Since then, I've gotten engaged, and I'm thinking about how I can have kids. My Pap smear following that one came back clear, but we're still watching. I'm on a very short leash with my doctor. But he's more optimistic now. He thinks the irregular Pap smear could have been from an infection.

—*Rachel Kaul*

I GREW UP in suburbia in the sixties. Like the crayon drawing of a happy child, my world had the bluest sky, the greenest grass, the prettiest flowers, and five happy, smiling people standing in front of a nice house. I didn't think about my life. Life was like a Doris Day movie. Bad things did not happen to "us," only to "them."

That ended in the summer of 1972, when we learned that my twelve-year-old sister, Robin, had Hodgkin's disease. That summer a relationship began between Robin and me that would take years of therapy and hard work to undo. I was sixteen, the responsible older sister. She relied on me for support, and I fell into the role as naturally as a bird takes to flight. The difficulty didn't come until after her body was healthy. Like most people who have never been personally threatened, I could not understand why she was unable to put it behind her and get on with life. It would take me almost twenty years and a bone marrow transplant to finally get it.

When I first learned that I, too, had lymphoma, I wasn't shocked, devastated, or self-pitying. Where everyone else was asking, "Why me?," I was thinking, "Why not me?" I was rooted in reality. I knew what had to be done and how to do it. After all, I was a survivor by association and had been preaching the right answers to Robin all those years.

I followed all the rules over the next several months: biopsy, second opinion, scans, chemotherapy, radiation, follow-up scans, finished. I went through the discomfort of all the side effects: nausea, vomiting, mouth sores, baldness, weight gain, to name a few. Throughout the process, one thought kept turning over in my mind: If Robin could do this at twelve, then I certainly can do it now, at thirty-five, with a wonderful husband by my side and a clear, strong self-image. I continued working and treated this as a bit of unpleasantness but nothing that was going to change my life drastically. I had cancer that summer and by fall was ready to get back to my life and forget about it.

Then the rules changed. It recurred. Now the stakes became higher and the odds smaller. I was still rooted in reality, but that reality had only three alternatives: Plan A and a bone marrow transplant. If that didn't work, Plan B and a bone marrow transplant. And if that didn't work, Plan C, which was to roll up in a ball and kiss my ass goodbye.

Bone marrow transplant is not actually a treatment. It is really more like a rescue mission. The treatment is seven days of intensive chemotherapy, a series of drugs at doses that far exceed anything the body can tolerate. The chemo kills the cancer, along with your entire immune system. In order to survive the treatment, new marrow has to be infused and given time to start functioning, approximately two weeks.

During my four-week hospital stay, I thought a lot about Robin and the puzzle and inspiration she has been for me over the years. Now I understand her feeling that you are set apart and defined by your illness. Now time has a value to me that it never had before. Come what may, my days are more beautiful, my relationships more meaningful than ever before, and this I have vowed: My cancer may kill me, but I will not let it ruin my life.
—*Jeanne Clair*

I HAD ADVANCED testicular cancer. It had spread through a good portion of my body, and I was having trouble getting food through my system because it was so clogged up with tumors. They had to remove a testicle, and I received a few months of chemotherapy—four rounds of five-day sessions. Three months after I stopped the chemo, I had a relapse.

Once again, I was back at my doctor's office talking about more surgery. There were remnants of tumors along the spine. They removed those, and then I had more chemotherapy. At this point things were looking pretty grim because the tumors seemed to be growing rapidly and spreading into my lungs. The cancer was popping up like wildfire. I was very scared. The chemo they give you for testicular cancer is extremely toxic stuff. I would go into the hospital for a period of five days, and each night they would put me to sleep while they injected the chemotherapy into me. They'd just drip it in, but they'd have to put me to sleep to keep me from going into convulsions. It wiped out my system to a point where I couldn't eat anything. I would throw up every morning whether I had any food in me or not.

After looking at the blood markers following two rounds of chemo, my doctor was ready to quit. He didn't think anything had happened, and he was reluctant to proceed because it was wiping me out so much. Then we saw some improvement in the blood markers, and he gave me the third round. I think he had pretty much decided that that was going to be it. They had to stop the treatment because my kidneys weren't going to take it anymore. That was a bad moment. I was down to about 129 pounds from 150 pounds. But it turned out that I was in remission.

Within three months, however, the cancer came back. My doctor said there was nothing he could do. At that point, I decided I had to go after it myself. I had been involved with a Cancer Support and Education Center since I first got sick, and one of the things that I had learned there is that even though doctors sometimes think they're gods, they're not always right. I was holding on to that. I took that to heart and went out looking for any other treatment that might help me. I tried a macrobiotic diet for a while, which was really difficult, because in my malnourished state, I was craving everything. I went down to Los Angeles to try some experimental treatments at the UCLA Medical Center. They hooked me up to a kidney dialysis machine, ran my blood through a filter, and removed one essential amino acid from my bloodstream. That kept my body from producing proteins and inhibited the production of cancer cells. It seemed to hold the cancer, to keep it from growing for a little while. But it didn't end up being a cure. By this time, the cancer had become slow-growing, no longer popping up like wildfire.

I was at the Stanford Medical School library doing some research on treatments, when I ran into a doctor who had treated me previously. He invited me to come into a Stanford clinic called the Oncology Daycare Clinic. Actually, he had invited me when I had the first relapse, and they had suggested doing surgery. At the time, I declined. The cancer was popping up everywhere, and I didn't see how they could go into my lungs and cut out these little tumors when five more were popping up every day.

Once again they suggested surgery to remove a tumor in my lung. At this point, it sounded like a good option. There weren't any other options. So I said, "Let's do it." They entered the side of my chest and took a wedge out of one of my lungs. I went through a different type of chemotherapy, and it worked.

—*George Clark*

Dealing with the Loss of a Limb

THERE WAS ANOTHER fellow about my age in intensive care when I was there, and he had lost much of his digestive system to cancer. He was in every six months to be monitored because he couldn't eat. Everything he took in had to be intravenous, and he used to joke about it. I'd think, "How can he joke about this?"

That's tough. He was a tough guy and had a good impact on me. His back was against the wall too.

He thought the situation I was in was hard. He didn't know if he could function without an arm. I've lost a limb, but that will only prevent me from doing a few functions. I thought what he had was much more serious than what I had.

It's funny, but I have noticed that people who really have been in some dire situations, like myself, seem to have a better attitude than some who are less involved or maybe have not had as dramatic a treatment. Maybe when your back is against the wall, you change, and you say, "Hey, this is the best deal we have, and these are the cards."

I'm not saying that one person's cancer is less important than someone else's, but where I was, we had people with no legs and a guy who had half his pelvis gone, and this guy, you'd think he'd won a million dollars or something, he was so glad to be alive. I've always thought that maybe because I lost my arm, people expect me to have this doom-and-gloom story. I don't. I've lost something, but I've gained some things too.

—*Dale Totty*

NOT LONG AFTER I lost my leg, my wife went to visit her parents. After she left, I was hopping on one leg through the house with a plate of food, and I slipped and fell. Food flew on the ceiling and all over me, and I was hurting. I took a pain pill, and before I knew it, I took another one, and I was still hurting, so I took another. I was sitting there kind of feeling sorry for myself, and all of a sudden I couldn't remember how many I'd taken. I started feeling numb. I thought, "Well, here I am by myself. I sent her away, and I've overdosed probably, and if I die, they'll think I've committed suicide." Finally, I went in and mixed some eggs and vinegar and made myself throw up.

After that, I just had a whole new outlook. I quit the pain medication, and I said, "Hey, I'm going to beat this, and I'm going to make the best I can out of it." I started going out. I didn't have the prosthesis then. Every day we went for a walk, and I walked on my crutches. I walked around the mall just to be around people. I had a little girl. She was about a year old at the time, and I spent a lot of time with her. To do things with her and to carry her in my arms again motivated me to get back on my feet. The fear of not being able to see her grow up probably inspired me more than anything.

—Danny Johnson

Waking Up on the Wrong Side of the Hospital Bed

I THINK YOU feel a common bond with other cancer patients. In my novel *The Keeper of the Moon,* I describe how when you're sitting there talking to these guys, you get to be friends. But there is also this kind of thing, like in combat, where you don't want to get too close to somebody because you don't know what's going to happen to them.

Also, when somebody comes down with a fever or an infection or somebody dies—it sounds bad to say it, but it's true—there is almost a sense of relief among the other patients. You know there is a certain percentage of people who are going to die, and when somebody hasn't died on the floor for a few weeks, then the odds are going up. When someone else gets it, it's not you. Even though you hate it for that person, you're glad it's not you. It's basic survival instinct.

—Tim McLaurin

THE TUMOR HAD been right above my lung, and in order to keep from destroying my lung during radiation, they did an experimental procedure where they deflated the lung. I think they did that years ago with TB patients, but this was the first time they had tried it recently. It worked for a while, but I wound up getting pneumonia. That was worse than the whole deal up to that point. I was in the hospital for three weeks. When I'd had my original surgery, I was home in nine days.

One moment really sticks in my mind from that hospital stay. I had woken up and slowly recovered over a couple of days. Finally, I was thinking a little more clearly, not quite as heavily sedated, and somebody right next to me was having a lot of trouble. That was a real eye-opener. That was when I made a change, when I got this new attitude: Let's get going here and go on into the future.

Here I was, twenty years old, and I just didn't feel I should be in there. It was suddenly like the surgery was a distant thought. I said, "I've got to get out of here." I was determined, and I was up all the time, putting in my rounds. I'd get up and walk, and the nurses would say, "You need to get back into bed."

And I'd say, "I need to get out of here."

—*Dale Totty*

IF YOU DON'T struggle, if you give up, I think it will have a negative effect on your healing processes. It's the opposite of the placebo effect. I feel sure that having hope and having a strong desire to live a little longer, to get out there and do something vigorous, will make a difference in how long you live, and it'll make a difference in how you feel about yourself.

One of the books that influenced me a lot early on was called *The Cancer Survivor* by Judith Glassman. She interviewed a bunch of people who lived for a long time with cancer and some of their doctors. She said the one common trait among all the people she talked to was an unquenchable desire to get better. She found that it's important to want to get better, to live for a long time, and if you don't have that, then the likelihood of your surviving longer than would be expected is reduced.

—*Damon Phinney*

PART THREE

Allies and Other Wartime Matters

CHAPTER EIGHTEEN

Eating to Win

It's easy for cancer therapy to spoil your appetite. Chemotherapy can throw off the taste buds, radiation can irritate the digestive tract, and steroids can make you eat voraciously and feel bloated. Just when it seems impossible to maintain a balanced diet, healthy eating habits become more important than ever.

What you want, of course, is an appetite for food that will help your body thrive. Many of us tried a variety of diets. Most of us felt cravings, some very strange. And we experienced a variety of aversions based on a temporary change in the taste buds. The American Institute for Cancer Research (800-843-8114), an organization that focuses on the role of diet with regard to cancer, offers a free booklet called "Nutrition of the Cancer Patient," which, among other things, looks at a variety of cancer-treatment side effects—such as dry mouth, constipation, sore throat, and taste changes—and gives suggestions for dealing with them.

Listen to your body. Seek help if you need it. As a reality check, here are some of our thoughts and experiences.

BEFORE MY DIAGNOSIS, I had given up red meat because of the animal fat, but my nutritionist—who generally says no red meat—recommended eating a steak once a week during chemotherapy.

—*Toni Zavistovski*

DURING MY TREATMENT I craved meat. I hadn't eaten much meat before, so it came as a surprise to me that I would even think about it. One day I had an intense desire to eat a piece of liver. I have no idea why. So I went to the market, bought some liver, and sautéed it with onions. It was delicious, and it made me feel good. I listened to what my body wanted and took care of my needs—even strange ones like eating liver.

—*Susan Fischer*

DURING MY CHEMOTHERAPY, sometimes I'd get hungry for very strange foods, and I would go for it. I'd eat pastrami sandwiches and potato knishes—much heavier foods than I'm used to eating. I didn't deprive myself.

—*Charlene Sloane*

I WENT TO see a nutritionist because my diet was one area that I felt I could control. She told me what kind of vitamins to take and advised me to get off white sugars and carbonated beverages and to concentrate on complex carbohydrates for energy reasons. I took vitamins and ate whole-grain foods, as opposed to empty-calorie foods, like white bread and white rice. I think I lived off brown rice, baked potatoes, and oatmeal. They were very soothing to my stomach and improved my stamina and energy. To me, food is fuel, and its purpose is to provide energy. You want to put the best gasoline in your tank, so you don't have any knocks and pings.

—*Lisa Hollingsworth*

Soy as a Cancer-Fighting Supplement

To support your body during chemotherapy, give it the best food possible—fresh vegetables, fruits, whole grains, and legumes, including soy-based foods. But because food can taste different during chemo and you can have cravings, you need to eat whatever helps you get through the process.

Certain kinds of foods support the immune system and even enhance chemotherapy. Soy-based foods—such as tofu, tempeh, and miso—contain plant chemicals called isoflavones that can help protect us from cancer, especially the sex-linked cancers, like prostate, ovarian, and breast cancer. For example, some say the isoflavone genistein can cut off the blood supply to tumors, stopping their growth.

Soy also helps maintain hormonal balance. For women, hot flashes are sometimes a side effect of treatment with tamoxifen and other drugs. Men with prostate cancer who are on Flutamide or other drugs sometimes get hot flashes too. Soy products reduce hot flashes by helping to balance out the hormones.

Instead of cow's milk, I encourage people to use soy milk. I recommend the kind that comes in unrefrigerated cartons (that you refrigerate after opening). It's delicious. It tastes like sweet cow's milk, but it doesn't have the antibiotics or hormones that are in cow's milk. I use it for cereal and baking—anytime I would use other milk.

—*Gloria Kubel,*
Certified Nutritionist and Wellness Educator
(and breast cancer survivor),
Denver, Colorado

AT TIMES DURING the radiation process, I didn't feel too much like eating, so I focused on getting high nutritional value each time I put forth the effort to eat. I ate more fresh foods and began snacking on sunflower seeds and nuts. I ate less restaurant food and cooked more at home, paying special mind to using fresh foods. I had to think of eating in terms of getting nutritious food, rather than as an act of pleasure. It became a lifestyle change.

—*Jerry Dunne*

MY DIETARY PHILOSOPHY took a turn opposite to that of most people who are diagnosed with cancer. All my life I had been strict in my holistic view of life and health, and my diet ruled out most foods. I ate raw vegetables, sprouts, and wheatgrass. I avoided meat and fats. Yet, in spite of this ultra health-conscious regime, I was diagnosed with cancer. I felt that the diet had somehow failed me, that all the macrobiotic stuff simply didn't work. I decided to eat whatever made me feel good.

Now, I still maintain a healthy diet, but if I want bacon and eggs for breakfast, then that's what I have. I call it emotional food. If it tastes good, feels good, and I want it, then it's the right food for me. In fact, right after my colon surgery, I ordered a plate of sushi to be delivered to my hospital room. My doctor nearly had a fit when he saw me with my chopsticks poised to spear a piece of succulent raw tuna. I explained to him that I loved sushi as much as any food in the world and that it was the only thing I wanted to eat right after my surgery. "I have to get nourishment somehow, don't I?" He gave me a funny look, but he knew I was right. After all, the sushi got me eating again.

—*Blythe Ritchfield*

THE DOCTOR TOLD me I might lose the ability to chew and swallow after my surgery for throat cancer. I had dreams in which I was sitting down to a meal of pasta with marinara sauce and meat on the side—gravy, as we Italian Americans say. Those dreams would turn to nightmares as my mouth could no longer chew and my throat was unable to swallow. I was determined not to lose the ability to eat the foods I loved. After the surgery, I slowly began to eat. I started with Jell-O and yogurt, moved on to salad and mashed potatoes and, with painstaking patience, worked my way up to my beloved pasta with marinara sauce and gravy on the side. That first meal was second only to the pasta my mother used to cook for me as a child.

—*Tony Dalo*

ONE OF MY favorite memories from the time I was on chemo-therapy was the night that my mother-in-law took my wife and her sister Rachel and me to John Clancey's Fish House, a restaurant that knows how to prepare a healthy serving of fish. After devouring my ample plate of grouper, I polished off my wife's red snapper, moved on to my mother-in-law's huge piece of pompano, and then squeezed down a thick hunk of Rachel's poached salmon. My body was so juiced up on steroids that I didn't even suffer later. Had I kept going at this rate, I probably could have played pro football in a couple of months, and considering the euphoria I felt on steroids, I might actually have considered it.

But the flip side also came into play. One time as I was tapering off steroids, I gorged just before my metabolism shifted into low gear. Although I did not get sick, my stomach was extremely distended, and it caused a night of great discomfort.

—*Dean King*

IF YOU'RE TAKING food to someone who is undergoing chemo, it's important to be sensitive to what they can and cannot eat. That was difficult for me. People would bring me food that would be the last thing I felt like eating, and I didn't want to have to lie and say, "Oh, I'm allergic to green peppers." Sometimes I'd say, "I'm just not in the mood to eat right now," and hope that I wasn't hurting their feelings.

There were friends who were really aware of what my children like, and that's what they focused on. They knew that I kind of fended for myself and that I was going to eat whatever I could stomach, but that providing a meal for my children was a problem. They brought so much that I had meals for six months. My fridge and freezer were stocked. I had a friend who coordinated it for me. She brought the meals over every other day and asked me what we needed. They made really fun meals for my kids, and that was the best help of all.

—*Charlotte Wells*

DURING CHEMO, I didn't even want to grocery-shop. All of a sudden my husband had to plan what we were going to eat and do the shopping. Since I had mouth ulcers after the first two treatments, I stayed away from spicy foods and avoided extremes of temperature, which is hard in the summer, especially since I'm a great ice-cream fan. When my mouth got that metallic taste from chemo, I used plastic spoons instead of metal ones. At times the metallic taste of a pop can would bother me, so I drank from a straw or poured the drink into a glass. I ate smaller meals and snacked more, and I looked for high-protein foods.

—*Lorraine Anderson*

ONE OF THE problems I found was that my doctors didn't educate me enough about what foods to eat and not eat. My stomach was upset all the time after breakfast. I ate bananas and yogurt every morning and wondered why my stomach felt so queasy.

I didn't find out why until the first time my white blood cell count plummeted, and I ended up in the hospital because the normal bacteria in my body were causing me to run a fever. While I was there, I started to eat a banana, and a nurse said, "No, you can't have a banana. You're taking procarbazine."

I said, "Why not?"

She told me that I shouldn't be eating any foods or beverages that contained tyramine, which is a normal chemical component of the body that helps sustain blood pressure. Combined with procarbazine, however, it can cause severe hypertensive reactions. Beer and wine were off-limits. Foods to be avoided included cheese, sour cream, chocolate, smoked meats, pickled fish, fava beans, plums, raspberries, and, of course, yogurt and bananas.

Be sure to ask about any food restrictions with the drugs you're taking. You should keep a log of what you eat and then how you feel because certain drugs will affect you differently. And certain foods will affect you differently.

—*Karl Nelson*

WHILE DEAN WAS going through chemotherapy, he was the editor of a publication called *The Southern Farmer's Almanac*, and I used to help him out on weekends and in the evenings after my regular editing job. One of my responsibilities was to test the recipes sent in by readers for the cooking section. One Sunday afternoon, I pulled out a recipe for chicken salad that called for an incredible number of eggs, fourteen in all—seven cooked ones in the salad and seven raw ones in the mayonnaise that went with it. I remarked to Dean that I'd never made a recipe that called for more than a dozen eggs, and he said, "I think I read somewhere that it's not safe to eat raw eggs."

"Oh, it's fine. How else can you make mayonnaise?" I said, in a bit of a role reversal. Usually I was the one sniffing suspiciously at leftovers and tossing them in the garbage while Dean would stand, fork in hand, proclaiming that a little mold never hurt anyone. My objection to the recipe was based more on taste than safety—it didn't sound very good. But we were short on recipes, so I made it anyway, and we ate it over the next few days.

About a week or so after we finished it, *The New York Times* ran a huge article on how dangerous raw eggs had become because of the risk of salmonella poisoning. Those most at risk, the article stated, were people (like us) living in the Northeast, where the highest number of salmonella cases had been discovered, and those whose immune systems were compromised by, for instance, cancer-killing drugs. I felt terrible. How long had those eggs been in the refrigerator? How long had I let them sit out while I was making the salad? I half expected Dean to keel over at any minute.

He was fine, but from then on, I was ultracautious. I scrupulously checked the date not only on each carton of eggs but on every food item that I bought. I never used an egg without washing it first, and I started scrubbing all our fruits and vegetables with a brush before serving them. When other people are in the kitchen with me while I'm cooking, I know they think I'm crazy. To this day, I still rinse off a banana before I peel it.

—Jessica King

I'VE ALWAYS DRUNK pretty hard. It's part of my culture and teaching. About a day after I got out of chemotherapy, I went back to drinking beer and wine. Nurses told me that people who drink do a lot better than people who don't. I'm not sure why— probably for the same reasons that smoking pot is helpful. It alleviates certain symptoms. Maybe people who drink have a tougher stomach and deal with the nausea better than people who don't. If you drink tequila, you get a pretty hard stomach. Drinking also relieves stress.

I wasn't someone who was going to totally stop everything I enjoyed just because I had had cancer. After I came back from having my bone marrow transplant, I wasn't going to stop drinking or enjoying an occasional cigarette. I wasn't going to live the life of a monk and eat bean sprouts to increase my chances of survival. I went back to my same lifestyle, healthy and happy and doing fine.

—*Tim McLaurin*

Beating an Upset Stomach

Cancer and its treatment can cause a variety of eating problems, at a time when your body needs nutrients for strength and healing. Because individual nutritional needs vary greatly, the first thing you should do is consult your doctor, nurse, or a registered dietitian to find out about the diet that best suits you. Two of the most common nutritional problems among cancer patients are nausea and diarrhea. Here are some solutions:

Nausea and Vomiting

1. Ask your doctor about medicine to help control nausea and vomiting.
2. Try foods that tend not to induce nausea: toast and crackers, clear liquids, skinned chicken, pretzels, sherbet, and angel

food cake. Avoid spicy, fatty, greasy, and very sweet foods, since they may exacerbate nausea.

3. Eat whenever you are hungry. You do not need to eat just three meals a day.

4. Keep healthy snacks handy. Taking a few bites of food every hour or so will not only combat nausea but can also help you get more nutrients and calories.

5. Sip liquids throughout the day. Using a straw might help.

6. To avoid feeling full or bloated, drink fewer liquids with meals.

7. Avoid eating in a room that's stuffy, too warm, or has cooking odors that might disagree with you.

8. Rest after meals because activity may slow digestion. It's best to rest sitting up for about an hour after meals.

9. If nausea occurs during radiation therapy or chemotherapy, avoid eating for an hour or two before the treatment.

10. If nausea is a problem in the morning, try eating toast or crackers before you get out of bed.

Diarrhea

1. Ask your doctor about controlling diarrhea with medications.

2. Try some of the following low-fiber foods: rice, noodles, mashed potatoes, eggs (cooked until the whites are solid), bananas, smooth peanut butter, white bread, skinned chicken (baked or broiled, not fried), and cream of wheat or rice. Avoid greasy, fatty, or spicy foods; high-fiber vegetables such as broccoli, corn, beans, onions, cabbage, peas, and cauliflower and other uncooked vegetables; raw fruits.

3. Drink liquids at room temperature.

4. Avoid very hot or very cold foods.

5. After sudden, short-term attacks of diarrhea, try a clear-liquid diet during the first twelve to fourteen hours. This lets the

bowels rest while replacing the important body fluids lost during diarrhea.

—Melanie Polk, R.D., M.M.Sc.,
Director of Nutrition Education,
American Institute for Cancer Research,
Washington, D.C.

CHAPTER NINETEEN

Family to the Front

When a person is diagnosed with cancer, it deeply affects all of the family members. Parents, children, siblings, spouses, all play a unique role in helping with the physical and mental battle the cancer patient is waging against this disease. In turn, they are affected in ways that can change their lives too. In particular, families must pay attention to the effects on young children when a parent has cancer.

For those helping a spouse or family member, the battle is hand-*in*-hand combat. No matter how you are related to the cancer patient, your role is an individual one determined by your personal relationship. You will share the good times and the tough times, and you will bear a portion of the stress. Part of that stress is caused by the many things you wish you could do but can't. Being willing to be there—in whatever role you might play, be it limited or more extensive—is the most important first step.

Here are some things we did to help in the healing process and to maintain our own health during the stressful times.

Spouses: From the Patient's Point of View

THE LONELINESS YOU feel when you're diagnosed with terminal cancer is incredible. My wife and I tried various kinds of unusual therapies. Full-body contact was one. At night, I would lie naked with my soulmate so that I would know through touch, smell, and sight that someone was there with me, as close as possible. Total and complete physical closeness with my wife was the only thing that relieved those intense feelings of loneliness. We worked as one. In addition to relieving my feelings of isolation, it made my marriage even stronger. It was the first time in my adult life that I was completely dependent on someone else. My wife appreciated my allowing her to help, instead of my always being independent and apart. So, if you normally wear pajamas to bed, don't anymore.

—*Bill Goss*

AT FIRST, MY cancer was hard on our marriage. My husband and I did not seem to be on the same wavelength. He went with me to my second bone scan, which was more traumatic for me than the first because I was really worried. I remember lying on the table with this machine going up and down my body, and he kept asking, "How much longer?" I was about to jump out of my skin. I wanted to kill him. He didn't go to my chemo sessions, and at the time, I thought that maybe it was better because he's so hyper. But looking back, I realize I needed that support. We were both in our own worlds, but we should have discussed these things.

Not only do you need to listen to the patient's fears, but you need to express your own fears. It helps the person who's sick not to feel so isolated. My husband was worried that I was going to die, but it took him a long time to tell me he was scared. I know it sounds silly now, but I thought he didn't care.

—*Leigh Abruscato*

SATURDAY NIGHT WAS our date night when I was in the hospital, even if I could barely hold my head up off the pillow. We let everyone know that. My husband asked the church to make an announcement and told our friends and family not to call or come by on Saturday nights. There was a VCR in the room, and

Rick would bring in a special movie, like *South Pacific*. He'd lie on the bed with me, and we'd snuggle and watch the movie. Half the time, I'd fall asleep, but I do that at home anyway.

Rick always brought me something, like my favorite Popsicle. But he really didn't have to bring anything: Having him there was all I needed. Although he must have been stressed-out when he came to see me, he was so supportive and never showed signs of stress. We had some very, very special times.

—*Karla McConnell*

AT FIRST I stayed in my bedroom a lot because I felt too weak to go downstairs. Eventually my boyfriend, Chuck (who's now my husband), would entice me to come down. He made me get up and exercise. He didn't feel sorry for me. I had too many people around feeling sorry for me, according to him. He was mighty good-looking, so I agreed.

—*Lisa Hollingsworth*

MY HUSBAND IS an attorney and has always worked a lot. I'm a stay-at-home mom, and I've always done everything for the kids and for him and taken care of the yard and the house. When I wasn't there, he had to step in. He learned to do a lot of things he didn't know how to do before, like the laundry and the dishes. He learned how to go through bookbags and help with homework. He spent a lot of time with our three kids. Afterward, he told me, "I really feel like I know our kids now. I never would have been so close to them if this hadn't happened."

A lot of good came out of my illness. My husband is a pretty serious guy, the kind who doesn't smile for pictures. That's always been a problem between us. I'd say, "Smile!" And he'd say, "I don't want to look goofy." The first time I came home from the hospital, he had bought me this really beautiful chaise longue for our porch. My best friend, Ruth Ann, said, "I want to take your picture." So he stood behind me, and she took our picture. We got the picture back, and I cried when I saw it. My husband was grinning from ear to ear. I treasure that picture so much because he was so happy to have me home and alive. Now he smiles all the time.

They say things like this either make or break a marriage, and it really made ours stronger.

—*Karla McConnell*

From Supporting Spouses

I ALWAYS BELIEVE that when you're going through a really tough time, you focus your energies on other people, in other words, on what you can do for them. That's not deflecting; that makes you feel good as well as helps you cope. But it's very important how you give your support, because you don't want it to come across as "I'm feeling sorry for you." I was particularly concerned about that with my husband. I wanted to show support, but I wanted to give him the space to work it out in his own mind too. So I didn't hound him about what he was thinking, touchy-feely, let's talk about it. That's not his style, and I didn't try to change his style just because we were going through a crisis. He needed his space. He was on an emotional roller coaster, and I just rode it with him. I was just there, present and supportive, maybe with a higher degree of intensity, but not overbearing. The best thing you can do is give that person respect and treat them the same way you've always treated them. At the same time, as a support person, you have to maintain a sense of balance and routine.

—*Lou Ann Sabatier*

ON THE DAYS when my husband had chemotherapy, I felt pretty helpless. I would accompany him to the doctor's office and try to stay quietly by his side after the treatment, but I found it frustrating not to be able to do anything for him. Usually by the evening, he felt a little better, but he didn't want anything to eat and needed to lie pretty still. So I hit upon the idea of giving him a foot massage. This he could enjoy, and it became something of a ritual. It made him—and me—feel a little better.

—*Jessica King*

THE WAY I coped with my husband having throat cancer was very interesting. I went into low gear: no emotion. I became very supportive and never cried, never got stressed out. I tried to learn about it rationally, and I felt I had to be really strong. I thought it would be selfish to show emotion or be really upset when he was going through it. This is in hindsight—it wasn't conscious. I was not overly positive, but I felt I needed to be steady, like the Rock of Gibraltar.

After my husband found out the treatment was successful and started getting back into normal gear mentally, I fell apart. It wasn't planned. But I finally let my guard down, and I really went into a depression. Even though he still had five years to wait, I felt that I could really tell him then how I felt and how scared I was. I didn't know why I was crying, but I cried, and it took a while to come out of it.

I had a similar experience with my sister. She was thirty-two, the spitting image of health, but had the same kind of freaky thing as my husband. One day she noticed a bruise on her leg, and that night she was in the hospital diagnosed with acute leukemia. Although she was literally a thousand miles away, I wanted to be a support for her too. I flew to see her a lot. She had a bone marrow transplant, and I felt very guilty because I was not a match. Fortunately, my brother was. But I did what I could to be really strong. Then after they found out she was going to be okay, the same thing happened: I went into a depression that was just bonkers.

These are two people both in their early thirties that I'm extremely close to who were fighting for their lives, and my feelings at the time just weren't that important. I put it in that perspective, and then I didn't feel guilty falling apart *after* they both knew they were on the road back. To me, you can't be wigged out when they need you because that is very selfish.

—*Lou Ann Sabatier*

About Parents

MY DOCTOR TOLD me and each of my parents—separately— that I only had a twenty to twenty-five percent chance of full recovery. Each of us hid this information to protect the others. We felt that we were being brave by keeping the bad news to ourselves, that in some way we were acting in the best interests of the others. But in the end, by not being treated as a family unit by the doctors, we did not act like a family unit among ourselves. We hid the truth, and our communication broke down. One night when my dad was up late with my mother and me, he began to cry, and it all came pouring out. After that we all felt better. It's essential to communicate with your family and to be honest about what's going on.

—*Kevin Shulman*

IT WAS VERY easy for me to deal with my immediate family— my husband and my children—but it was very difficult for me to deal with my mother, who also had had breast cancer. She became hysterical, to the point where I didn't even want to talk to her about it. The way I dealt with that was to say, "I'm fine. I'm getting the treatment that I need. I'm being very careful." I tried to minimize discussion about my cancer, to speak one or two sentences and then change the subject. If I had not responded that way, she really would have pulled me down, way down.

What worked for me was to quietly explain, "Though I know that this is really hard for you, I'm the patient right now, and I have to do what's going to work for me in a positive way, and one of the most important things for me is to guard against falling into a trap of being terrified and worried all the time. I need to keep thinking positively, and you're going to have to understand that as much as I want to be able to help you through this, I have to get through it myself first." That's a pretty blunt, honest approach, but when one member of your support system becomes hysterical and out of control, it's really important to guard against becoming entrapped by that.

—*Toni Zavistovski*

WHEN I WAS at my sickest, my mother went to hire a private nurse to be with me day and night. She told the administrator that she didn't want the best nurse they had—she figured that all the nurses would be technically competent—she wanted the best-looking nurse, the one who would make her son feel happy and alive just because she was so pretty. And believe you me, the nurse she got was not only gorgeous, but she administered those injections with enough TLC to cure anybody of cancer.

—*Kevin Shulman*

I'VE NEVER HAD children, but I can imagine that having your child sick, or having a child die, of course, must be the worst thing in the world. And I think it was harder on my parents than on me in some respects because I always knew what was happening to me. I always knew how I felt. But they were dealing with their own issues, and they could only guess, by my words and actions, how I was doing.

My mother and I handled it by talking about it pretty much every day. We made little jokes about things. We used to say that we'd better wear different clothes because we didn't want the imaging center to think we only had one outfit, things like that.

My father was a different story. He's very loving and very affectionate, but he's not a communicator, and it was awfully hard for him. He just wanted it to be done; he wanted me to be better and to have everything go away. So to make him feel better, I just had to make it clear that I was doing okay. The more I did that for him, the more it strengthened him. I would overhear him on the phone with his cousins saying things like, "I don't know how she does it, but she's doing really well." I needed him to know that I was going to be all right—or even if I was not going to be all right ultimately, that I was dealing with everything pretty well. That I liked my doctor, and that I wasn't feeling too shitty. It did eventually get to the point where we were able to make jokes about my hair and stuff, but in the beginning it was not possible.

One thing that made it easier for all of us was that my sister had had a baby four months before I was diagnosed. It was wonderful to have a baby around to make everyone laugh and smile, to create positive energy in the house.

—Jodi Levy

MY HUSBAND AND I believed that attitude was all-important. We had to be optimistic and aggressive in order to make the treatment successful. Anything that got in the way of a positive attitude had to go, whether that meant specific attitudes or specific people.

My dad tried to make me feel better by saying, "Think of your cancer as if you were pregnant. It's only a temporary state, and it will be over." But he was also a pessimist. As a doctor, he knew what could happen and probably wanted to prepare himself for the worst. My mother didn't know how to help or what to do. She was a wreck. She would pat me like a dog, with pity, acting as though I were doomed to death.

My husband, Bill, took charge by explaining to my dad that we didn't want to hear any more negativity and that if Mom couldn't handle it, maybe she shouldn't come around as much. Bill was blunt, direct, but it never caused any family friction. Mom and Dad both seemed to understand that the welfare of the patient was the most important thing.

—*Elsie Stone*

MY FAMILY AND friends had a harder time dealing with my cancer than I did. They seemed to be walking on eggshells, never knowing what to say and yet saying too much, trying too hard, always hovering over me. I felt like I was doing just fine, but my family, with their worries, made it harder than it had to be. My mother wanted to do my laundry, even though she hadn't done my laundry in years. My friends wanted to help, but they treated me like a baby or an invalid. When I explained that I wanted them to treat me the way they always had, they began to ease up.

—*Mark Biundo*

MY PARENTS WOULD sit in my hospital room all day long. They were wonderfully supportive, but at times they were too supportive. I guess they were fulfilling their own need to be good parents by being there for me all the time, but sometimes they overwhelmed me. One day, when it became too much for me, I told them to leave. "Mom, Dad," I said, "I need an hour to myself. Go home."

I realized that I had to speak up for myself. I could no longer shy away from articulating my fears and needs in order to protect everyone else. By keeping things in, I only felt more alone. I only created thicker barriers between me and my loved ones. Communication was the only way to break down those barriers.

—*Susan Fischer*

I WAS DIAGNOSED with cancer when I was only twenty-three. It was a difficult time for me because, like most young adults, I was trying to separate from my parents. I was working to save enough money to move out of their house, find a place, and begin a life of my own. The cancer put that process into a screeching reverse. Suddenly, I wanted nothing more than to be nurtured by my mother, to be held in her arms and lost in her boundless love. I felt like a piece of dirty laundry that had been thrown back in the hamper, back into my mother's care. I wanted to let my mother do the wash and have it all come out clean and smelling fresh.

We all need someone to help us share the burden. For me it was Mom and Dad. For others, it may be a husband or a wife, a sister, a brother, or a child. I learned through my illness how to share that burden by allowing myself to be needy and emotional. If I had to cry, I would cry and sometimes even scream with tears. My parents were there for me. I can't imagine what it would have been like without them.

—*Josh Malen*

MY MOTHER WAS my rock. Many nights I would lie awake in bed, afraid that if I fell asleep, I would never wake up again. My mom would hold me and hug me and listen to me through those dark nights. She didn't need to say anything or to respond to any of my doubts. Her presence, her hugs, and the fact that her ears were open helped more than I can put into words.

—*Donna Avacato*

From a Parent

ONE THING THAT was extraordinarily helpful, far more than I realized at the time, was a monthly newsletter that my husband and I sent out to close friends and family members. It was exhausting dealing with scores and scores of phone calls. Usually you're not home and have to return the calls, and everybody asks the same questions. They're well intended, but it can be very draining. So we started sending out a letter, telling people that we would communicate with them this way so that they didn't need to call. We would keep them up-to-date on our progress.

The newsletter got people really involved in Evan's treatment and his life and certainly helped in terms of contributions to the fund that we had set up to help pay for his medical bills and people's willingness to donate blood, to send him cards, and to be supportive in many ways. The letter let our friends and relatives know that they were an important part of the support system, that we wanted to share with them what was happening, and that their responses were welcome. But it contained their involvement in a way that was much easier for us to deal with than phone calls.

On yet another level, the writing of the letter was a good emotional outlet. It gave us a way of expressing ourselves without always having to hear the other person's reaction, which can be upsetting. We didn't always send out what we wrote. Sometimes it just helped to write it down, throw it away, and start over again.

—*Enid Handler*

About Children of a Parent with Cancer

THE SOCIAL WORKER told us, "You're going to teach your children how to deal with illness through this." As parents, it made us want to rise to the occasion and set a good example. We explained the situation to our six- and nine-year-old sons, and encouraged them to take an active part in their father's medical care. Much of Brian's chemotherapy was given at home, and the boys helped by putting heparin in the IVs. They seemed to gain a lot of confidence by helping out, even though each one dealt with the situation very differently. The six-year-old is very blunt, very forthright. He walks around the house and says, "Gee, I hope Dad doesn't die. How many more years before I'm thirteen? Dad, are you still going to be living then?" The nine-year-old, on the other hand, is very quiet and conservative. You ask if he's worried, and he'll say, "No." That's it. I keep having to talk to him about what's going on. They're polar opposites. I don't know if it's because of the age difference or simply a reflection of their personalities.

It's really hard with children. When they're misbehaving, you don't know if it's normal, developmental, or caused by their parent's illness. My kids misbehave, like all children, and I have found that I need to talk to other parents with kids the same age in order to see if it's normal. Mostly it is.

As part of the University of Arkansas's family counseling program, our children spent half a day with a counselor. She asked them to draw a picture of their dad's cancer. Our older son, who was eight at the time, drew a picture of a bone, with bad cells and good cells in it. While he was explaining the drawing to the counselor, his younger brother took it and counted more bad cells than good cells. The five-year-old then pushed the paper back to his brother and said, "Put more good cells in." Later, the counselor told me, "We were looking to see if they had a grasp of the cancer, of what it was. They understood it!"

Another thing she did for the kids was to take them through the entire transplant program. She took them into the chemo room, which on a good day is ugly at best. Although she had them put masks on for obvious reasons, she encouraged them to draw big nostrils and smiley faces on the masks. They thought that was just fabulous.

One thing that they counseled us on was arranging for someone to take care of our children when we were going to be in Arkansas. My husband would be gone sixty to ninety days that year and I would have to commute back and forth. The counselor told us our sons needed to know who was going to take care of them, who was going to do the spelling tests with them, who was going to take them to hockey practice, who was going to make their lunch. My sister and Brian's sister were both more than willing to have our kids live with them while we were gone, but our counselors kept telling us that it was best to keep our children in their home, in their routine, as normal as possible.

We had to leave in January, and we didn't come up with a solution until the day after Christmas. Our old nanny called to say that she and her husband had spent the entire holiday doing nothing but talking about our situation. She explained that they were willing to sell their house and move in with us to take care of the boys.

It was the best thing that had ever happened to us. They have their own son who is two, and he's fabulous. All I can say is that it was a godsend—He sent us this wonderful family. We made a year-and-a-half commitment to each other. She's finished up her third year in nursing school this year, and her husband works nights. He takes care of the boys some mornings when she goes off to clinicals. It's an absolutely great living situation, and our home could accommodate it. We were lucky there too. Now my kids don't care what we do. Their lives go on just as normal.

As I was following our kindergartner down the hall at school one day, he turned the corner before I did, and I heard the teacher's aide ask, "How are the counts?" Apparently he told his teachers how Brian's counts were doing every day. They knew. And when I came walking around the corner, one of the teachers said, "That kid is so well informed. You should be proud of him."

Making sure they're in their own home is very important, and we learned that from the counseling we got at Arkansas and other hospitals. Just as I would not use only one medical professional, I wouldn't use only one counselor either. I don't think you can learn all you need to know from one. We've had three, plus several support groups.

How are our kids going to be in the long term? The jury's out. It scares me, but we'll do everything we can to keep those kids home and keep ourselves home.

—*Peggy Schmidt*

THE HARDEST THING I had to do was to leave my two kids, sixteen and eighteen, alone in Colorado when I went to Nebraska for treatment, not knowing whether I'd ever be back. We were up-front with our kids about everything that was going on, though I tried to minimize how much I cried in front of them. They were aware that it was a life-or-death situation. We tried to make them more independent than we normally would have for children their ages, in case something happened. We got them checking accounts and credit cards for use in our absence. We encouraged our son to drive and both of them to cook more.

When we had to leave the state for treatment, they were really on their own. Although I advocated their independence, I also worried. During our absence, I had them call a neighbor every night. My sister, who lived five minutes away, brought them a meal every week. Yet, I preferred, as they did, that the kids stay in a familiar environment, rather than go live with a relative. The less change they faced, the more easily they would be able to handle the situation.

—*Elsie Stone*

I HAD A lot of things to get in order the day before I went into the hospital, so I left the house early in the morning. My son—who was only about ten or eleven at the time—cleaned up the entire kitchen while I was gone. He had never cleaned up the kitchen before (and he hasn't cleaned it up since either). He never said anything—"I love you," "I'm worried about you," or anything like that—but I thought that was the sweetest thing. I told him how much I loved him and how much I appreciated what he had done and how that had helped me more than anything I could think of.

—*Katherine Arthur*

Red Flags That Indicate Your Child Is Not Coping with Your Cancer

It's hard for parents to know how children are coping, because children tend to be really protective. I've had parents say to me, "My child is fine. He never asks questions. He really has a good understanding of what's going on." Then I meet with the child, and he or she is exhibiting a lot of anxiety. One four-year-old I met with was trying to figure out how to sell his toys to get money, because he had heard his mother crying about how expensive treatment was. He thought they were going to lose their house.

It is important to let the children's teachers know what's going on. Teachers are with the kids eight hours a day. If a child's going to act out, he may do it at school, because he doesn't want to upset things at home. Here are some signs that your child may not be coping well:

• Wetting the bed again
• Temper tantrums
• Not interacting with friends the way they used to

- A change in school function. That is, grades dip down or improve. If your child has always been a C kid, and all of a sudden he's bringing home A's, don't just be glad about the improvement. Take a step back and look at this. What's going on that your child suddenly feels he has to perform on that level?
- Staying out more
- Starting to drink
- Signs of drug use

—Karen Atkin,
Social Worker, Arkansas Cancer Research Center,
Little Rock, Arkansas

Siblings

WHEN MY SISTER, Karla McConnell, went into the Indiana University Medical Center to be treated for leukemia, I became a long-distance support person. I visited from Virginia and had Karla's children for a stay, but I wanted to have a daily presence as well. My tendency was the smothering thing, to call all the time or send something every day. But I was careful to pace it, to give her enough space. So I sent her these things in the hospital:

1. Home movies. I sent films of us that simply said, "Oh, hi, here's where we are. Here's what we're doing, everyday things, like taking the dog for a walk." I was not even trying necessarily to cheer her up because sometimes she felt so bad she didn't want that. But I wanted her to feel like we were there.

2. Cards. I didn't want something that said, "Keep up the fighting spirit." I wanted something that made her strong, but subtly. I would go into the Hallmark store and read cards for an hour. It had to be right on. And somehow, because I'm close to her, I felt like I was hitting it, the pacing of it. This is the right message for her, right now.

3. A book of postcards. So she could write back easily if she felt like it.

4. Books. I sent her *The Delaney Sisters,* and I inscribed in the front, "These old geezers made it, we can too." It wasn't sappy, but there was emotion and meaning to it. She read it and loved it.

5. Pajamas. They were kind of sexy-looking, even though she was losing her hair. They definitely weren't flannel.

6. A grab bag. I sent a bag of presents and told Karla to open one every week on a certain day. Sometimes it was something goofy, like a four-roll pack of real toilet paper or a big bag of peppermints. Other times it was something to make her feel special, like nice pajamas.

7. An angel. I sent her an angel to put over her bed to watch over her.

8. A song. One day toward the end, after I knew she would be all right, I was driving, and I popped in a tape. All of a sudden this song I always liked, some old Ricky Scaggs song, about somebody must be prayin' for me or angels are watching over me, connected, and it hit me, "Wow, this is her experience." I was driving, and the tears were just rolling down my cheeks, and I thought, "I have to tape this for her." She called me and said, "You just know the right thing to do at the right time."

—*Lou Ann Sabatier*

MY SISTER AND I were very close growing up, but our relationship started getting rocky when she had her first bout with Hodgkin's disease. She was nineteen or twenty, and had moved away from home. I was in junior high school. I think that really split us because one, it was scary, and two, it made her very special and different and in need of a lot of attention. We stopped communicating, really, and that lasted for a long time. It lasted until I got cancer. It's not that we didn't get along when we were together—we were okay—but we weren't close, and there was a lot of unresolved resentment and hostility between us.

When I got cancer my sister was the only person I could talk to. She was my support group. She validated everything I did and pushed me to keep asking questions. She still does. She's also very funny. She's got a black sense of humor about the whole thing. Once I told her, "Sometimes it just pisses me off that I'm going to die of cancer." Her response was, "Everyone is going to die of cancer. We're just going to die of it first. What's your point?"

Cancer kind of tore us apart and then brought us back together again. She's my best friend now and my favorite person. I never would have thought that we could get this close again. We live so far away from each other, but we talk three or four times a week.

She has been a huge guide for me, but I think that I've helped her, too, by kind of refreshing her experience. As you get further away from cancer, you have to keep reminding yourself that as much as cancer requires and takes of you, it gives you something that most people don't have. In a sense, you're special in your knowledge of things.

I don't want to be the same person that I was before cancer. I want to be better than that, more knowledgeable, with a wider view than I had before. You need to be willing to take risks. For example, there are rules that we grow up with. Never quit a job until you have another one. Earn more money in your next job than you did in your last one. Have a goal. There are so many rules like that, and cancer means debunking those. It means saying, "Forget them. I need to quit this job. I don't like it, and I'm wasting time. I'm a talented person, and I could make an impact on people's lives somewhere. I'm not doing it where I am."

Battling cancer gives you that knowledge, but you have to work at retaining it. I think my cancer helped Leslie pick it up again.

—Rachel Kaul

Tapping Your Funny Bone

Obviously there are a lot of things about cancer that aren't funny, but this is a time—whenever possible—to intentionally seek out things that will make you laugh. It will make you feel better—and also help you relate to others. During treatment, family members and friends often aren't sure how to act, and if you can laugh at yourself, it opens the door for the people around you to be more natural and lower their guard, and thus be more available to you.

Try to see the absurdities in what is happening. Situations that don't seem funny now can be hilarious in retrospect. One woman who was bald from chemotherapy couldn't wait to take off her wig as soon as she got home. Forgetting that she was bald, she opened the door to the paper boy, who was dumbfounded at the sight of her shiny head.

It also helps to hang out with people who are funny. Laughter is contagious. A lot of times in support groups, someone comes in who is down, and they see survivors and others who are joking about treatment. You can see a transformation in these people. They think, "Gosh, they're laughing about this, and they seem to be enjoying life. Maybe I'm going to be okay, too."

Take note of funny things you hear and read. Collect funny props, video tapes, and books. Do something silly. Eat with your left hand instead of your right hand. When something bad happens, turn the negative stories into humorous ones. Say something like, "Well, that's the bad news, but the good news is. . . ." There's an old Chinese proverb that says, "You cannot prevent birds of sorrow from flying over your head, but you can prevent them from nesting in your hair."

—*Charlene Pennington, R.N., M.S.,*
Breast Cancer Outreach Coordinator,
Cancer Center of Southwest Washington,
Vancouver, Washington

Extended Family

EVERYBODY IN MY family came from Mississippi and Tennessee to Virginia for the operation. There were about twenty people—cousins, aunts, uncles, grandparents. They were all there during the operation, and when I woke up, my whole family was standing around my bed. I *know* that helped me get better.

—*Scott Cox*

EVEN THOUGH YOU think it's obvious, I can't stress enough the importance of telling the person in your life who has cancer that you still love her. Reinforce the fact that there is absolutely no difference in who she is. A body part, such as a breast, is not what makes a woman a woman. There is so much more to a person, so much more to life. It is essential to say things out loud, to communicate, to make an affirmation that your special person is loved, no matter how she may have changed in appearance.

—*Abby Drucker*

WHEN SOMEONE YOU love gets sick, you want to do everything you possibly can for her. Part of doing is, ironically, not doing. In other words, you can be most helpful by just being there. This can mean spending hours upon hours sitting in silent solidarity with your loved one.

I found that if I didn't take a break every once in a while to recharge my own batteries, I would feel like jumping out of my skin, and my company would not be any good for my aunt. I would take several laps around the parking lot or the hospital floor and come back ready for another shift in the room.

My talks with family and friends were open and honest exchanges about what was really going on in our lives. After spending several hours in the cancer world, you tend to have thoughts that are deeper and more introspective, and communication with others is usually more substantive. It brought me closer to my family.

—*Patty Aicher*

CHAPTER TWENTY

Companions in Arms: Making Friends Your Allies

Never is the kindness and generosity of people more apparent than when the chips are down. Friends and acquaintances rally around those fighting for their lives. All the sincere offers and all the goodwill and caring mean a great deal.

But sometimes it can be overwhelming. The offers pour in so fast you don't know how to handle them. You might not have the time or energy to return the phone calls, and you get tired of explaining things, and with a happy face at that. When you're focused on the fight, even expressing your appreciation can be difficult and stressful.

Still, your friends really want to help you, and, in fact, they need to. The trick is to make sure their help really is help and not a burden or nuisance. The first step you might want to take is to have a helper help the helpers. That way you can focus on yourself, as you should. A well-instructed front line—whether it's your mother, your brother, or your best friend—can make sure that all the friendly and sincere offers are put to good use. That person can weed out who actually gets through to you personally, determine which phone calls you take, and delegate chores to those who offer help. They can even make sure the cards you get from people are funny and not depressing.

Another good idea is to set up a formal or informal communications web so you don't have to repeat the same news over and over again. Let a close pal tell your friends, a work colleague tell people at your office, and so on.

Many entries in this section talk about things we really appreciated having done for us. When people ask you what they can do for you, keep these in mind. If they make a specific offer, these tips might help you refocus that offer. For instance, you might not feel like eating nacho casserole the day after chemo, but a meat loaf could make the kids very happy and keep you out of the kitchen. Refocus that offer and make your life easier. And you won't even have to lie about how good those jalapeños made your stomach feel.

There are, of course, the deadbeat friends, the ones who go MIA as soon as they find out. That's a whole different kettle of fish. You have to deal with it, but at the same time you have to realize there may be nothing you can do about it. It's their problem. It hurts, but you have much bigger issues to face.

By and large, remember, people really want to help you, and you should let them. Sometimes you just need to help them help you in the right way.

I REALIZED THAT it is up to those of us who have cancer to set the pace for how others treat us. Whatever attitude you put out is the attitude others will have about you, so I continued my life and didn't focus on my fear.

—*Ivy! Gunter*

STRENGTH DOES NOT mean doing everything by yourself without any help from others. To the contrary, it means, among other things, understanding that those who really care about you need to be allowed to do something, anything, to alleviate their feeling of helplessness. The ability to acknowledge that you need help is not only a sign of strength; it is also a sign of intelligence because it helps you survive.

—*Tali Havazelet*

MY FRIENDS HELPED to give me fighting strength. One of them made a meditation tape for me, on behalf of our group of friends. Initially, four of us held hands and listened to this tape in my room. Then we all agreed to stop for a few minutes at the same time every day and think positive thoughts about me. This was wonderfully uplifting.

One of my dear friends brought me a book early on, *The Cancer Conqueror,* by Greg Anderson. It had a profound effect. I recommend it to everyone who has cancer. Another friend brought a single rose every day. I learned to notice the particularities of each rose—how it smelled and unfurled—and I realized that each day is like a rose, unique in its beauty, and so I learned to take one day at a time, noticing the uniqueness of each one.

—*Janice Thomas*

MY FIANCÉE CAME to all my treatments with me. She'd be there, yet she wasn't pampering or freaked out, just levelheaded about it. I didn't want people treating me any differently than they usually did. And I had a good group of friends who didn't do that. That helped. Nobody ever acted like they were that freaked out by my illness, and that helped me realize that I was still the same guy to everybody, that I'd get over this thing. I just needed my friends to be there when I needed them, to be a phone call away, but also to realize that I'm strong and would get through this just like I'd gotten through other things in my life.

—*Mark Conover*

WHEN MY CANCER was diagnosed, the first thing I thought was, "My God, he's going to leave me. He doesn't want to be stuck with someone who is battling a life-threatening disease, who is going to lose her hair and her physical appearance." That was just my own problem, thinking that my boyfriend was that shallow. I thought, "He doesn't have to put up with this. He isn't engaged or married to me." In the beginning, it was really hard because I could barely talk to him without crying. He's the man that I want to marry and spend the rest of my life with—that's why it hit me so hard.

But he's been great. He's been there for me every time I go into the hospital. He comes to visit me and has been really wonderful. He tells me that he loves me and says, "Why would I not stick by you through this? It's something that we're going to go through together, and you're going to get better, and we'll move on."

—*Michele Fox*

I FOUND THAT I was happiest on my first two visits to the hospital because there were more people, more traffic, more nurses in and out, more patients. When I went to the bone marrow transplant floor, which holds only ten patients, I was kind of stuck at the end of the hall, where hardly anybody passed by. That was depressing for me because I'm a real people person. I think people were afraid to visit me because I was in isolation, but I really needed the company. During my first go-round, my nonstop visitors were what helped pull me through.

—*Karla McConnell*

ALL MY LIFE I've loved to read, so I was surprised to find that during Dean's illness, I could not concentrate on even the lightest magazine article. Instead, my husband and I craved the company of other people. We needed to feel connected to the rest of the world. Even talking to people who didn't know about my husband's cancer helped. Fortunately, we both felt the same way, and we let it be known to friends and family, who were more than willing to get together. We were comforted—and also distracted—by an endless stream of dinners, lunches, and other outings.

—*Jessica King*

I FOUND THAT one of the benefits of having cancer was that you could do what you wanted and people would understand. If you didn't feel like seeing your mother-in-law, it was okay. If you really didn't want to ruin your weekend at the beach for so-and-so's wedding, so-and-so would understand. If you wanted to eat in bed in front of the TV that night, well, sure, who's going to deny you that small comfort? When you're perfectly healthy, you have to make the right impression, and that means sometimes you have to do things you don't want to do. With cancer, you can do whatever you want and people understand.

—*Maurice Chesney*

AFTER MY SURGERY, my mother came and helped my husband with our three kids, and people from my Bible-study group brought dinner every night for six weeks. I received hundreds of cards and phone calls. In that sense, it was a wonderful experience because those kinds of things provided positive reinforcement. Knowing that people are so concerned encouraged me and, I think, helped me get well. I had always been on the giving end of doing things for people. This was my first real opportunity to be receiving from others, and I learned how unbelievably important it is to support people who are sick in any way. Even a card. Now I always send a note when someone is sick, and I try to get in touch with them to find out what I can do to help them the most.

—*Katherine Arthur*

THE PHONE CALLS were overwhelming. We'd get home, and there would be twenty or thirty messages. We felt that if people were making the effort to call, we needed to respond, but that's extremely difficult, especially when you have young children and you're trying to keep their lives on schedule. So I asked people to return phone calls for me. They'd drop by the house, take the phone calls off our machine, and then call people with a general update. It was a great gift.

—*Charlotte Wells*

AFTER THE FIRST treatment, when I realized what a stupor all the antinausea drugs put me in, I knew I would have to be accompanied to treatments. My friends wanted to help, and I was able to let them. I had a different person with me at almost every chemo treatment—volunteers on the "vomit brigade," as one of them dubbed it. The outpouring of love and support from my friends was overwhelming. My adolescence had been very painful, lonely, and isolated; it had taken me a long time to create a world of loving friends. My illness showed me that those days of loneliness were forever gone.

I drew on my friends constantly and without hesitation. This was a new feeling for me because I had never liked asking for help and hated feeling vulnerable. My illness swept those considerations away, however, and permitted me to enter into a tender and intimate relationship with my friends. They wiped my brow, emptied the bucket, entertained me, and kept the darkness at bay.

—Jacqueline Frank

MY SCHOOL PRINCIPAL single-handedly educated my entire school community as to what osteosarcoma was and what chemotherapy was. I didn't know it at the time, but when I was diagnosed, he went on the morning announcements and said, "As some of you may know, one of our students has been diagnosed with cancer. It's called osteogenic sarcoma—that means bone cancer." The whole time I was out of school—the last month of my freshman year in high school and the first semester of my sophomore year—about once a week he would go on and give an update.

My friends kept in touch the entire time. I got huge banners from the school. I went back to as many football games as I could. I had to be really careful about dampness and germs when I had chemo, so I only went to a couple of games. I wasn't even in school, and I was on the homecoming court my sophomore year, which was incredible.

It's funny because in the beginning, I remember saying to a friend of mine that I was really scared about going home. He said, "Melanie, the easiest thing is going home." And he was absolutely right.

I went back into school, and Mr. White got on the announcements and said, "Melanie's back." Everyone was really interested in my artificial limb and wanted to see it. In my science class, I did a little talk about my leg. It was really important for me to have people ask questions so that I could tell them about it. It wasn't a secret, and it wasn't a mystery, and therefore they didn't have to be afraid of it. The teachers were really supportive.

I was bald and wore a wig, and everybody knew it, but only my close friends saw me with the wig off. When my hair was fairly long—long enough to lie down—I stopped wearing the wig. The first day I went to school, I was terrified. I was walking in the door, and somebody I didn't even know ran up to me and gave me a hug and said, "Your hair looks great. I'm so excited to see you without your wig on!" I couldn't believe it. That set the stage for the rest of the day. I walked into class proudly. It was wonderful.

—*Melanie McElhinney*

Ask and You Shall Receive

As a social worker, I've found that the people who handle cancer diagnosis and treatment the best are the ones who learn how to live with it. I don't mean those who tolerate it, as in "I can live with it," but rather those who don't let cancer stop them from living. You accomplish this by being honest with your feelings and learning how to ask for help, a proposition that is difficult for people who are used to giving it. The easiest way to get used to it is to keep a list (mental or written) of favors you need done so that when people offer to help, you can take them up on it right away. It's a lot easier to say, "Thank you so much for offering. You could pick the kids up from school tomorrow," than to call back later and ask for a favor. Here are some other things you could ask friends and family members to do:

Drive you to a doctor's appointment.

Bring over a casserole.

Pick up your prescription at the drugstore.

Do your grocery shopping.

Baby-sit your children for a few hours.

Rake your yard.

Help you fill out your insurance forms.

Go with you to pick out a wig.

—*Harriet Mannheim,*
Director of Program Administration, Gilda's Club,
New York, New York

WE'RE PART OF a small community, and we have a great circle of friends and a big family, and I don't think we could have made it through this if it wasn't for them. The support that our church gave us was unbelievable. They announced one Sunday that I was ill, and they said, "If anyone wants to sign up to help out, come by after church." A hundred and eighty families signed up. They took over and allowed my husband, Rick, to cope with the kids. They just did everything.

They brought in food every night for four months, both when I was at home and when I was in the hospital. They cleaned the house, took the kids to Little League baseball games, swimming lessons, cheerleading practice, to youth group on Sunday night, anything that you can imagine for my three kids, so their lives could go on uninterrupted. It's just phenomenal what they did. You wouldn't believe it unless you were there.

We have a very large place, and they mowed our ten-acre yard every week. My grandparents live a mile down the road from us, and they're very active. Grandpa, who was eighty-three, took charge of the yard-mowing list and made arrangements and scheduled the different people. We have a big garden, and I can green beans and put corn up and do all that, and Grandma, who's seventy-nine years old, canned eighty-five quarts of green beans for me. A neighbor brought over a bunch of corn for the freezer. Another friend put up a bunch of fruit. People just poured their love out, did everything for us. We could never repay them.

I had people praying for me all over the country. I received letters from people I didn't know saying, "I've been there, and I know what you're going through. Our church is praying for you." Another thing that made my hospital stays much more bearable was that our church had people send me gifts, numbered one through thirty, so I could open one every day that I was in the hospital. People sent things like a box of candy, a box of Kleenex, a roll of Charmin—you know hospital toilet paper is the worst!

When I came home from the hospital, Grandpa stopped over to check on me, and all I had to do was call him if I needed a gallon of milk or anything else. They were so concerned, so helpful, and always there for anything I needed.

—*Karla McConnell*

HOW DO PEOPLE react to cancer?

- Some people just disappear.
- Some people can talk to you on the phone, mostly about the weather or movies.
- Some people can talk to you on the phone about anything but won't come to the hospital to visit.
- Some people come to the hospital to visit but can only talk about the weather or movies.
- Some people come to the hospital to visit and can talk about anything.
- Some people want to see your scars.
- And some people, the really special ones, come to visit you in the hospital, want to see your scars, and—and this is the key—can make cancer jokes. They can be real with you and at the same time make you laugh.

—*Kevin Shulman*

PEOPLE REACT TO someone else's illness in almost as many different ways as there are different people. No two people use the same means to express support or love, and none deal with their own fears of sickness and death in exactly the same way.

Most of my friends and family gathered around me, providing me with immeasurable comfort and security. There were also instances when formerly casual friends became close friends. My friend David, whom I had never been very close to, came to visit me in the hospital every day and even invited me to the seventh game of the World Series between the Mets and the Boston Red Sox. Conversely, there were a number of people—like my only aunt and uncle on my father's side—who reacted to my cancer in ways that can be described, most charitably, as strange. Their behavior baffled me, but I came to realize that some people just can't handle illness. I guess the lesson to be learned is that you can't expect everyone to be supportive, but you certainly have the right to tell people when they aren't being supportive.

—*Jonathan Pearlroth*

I ONCE WENT to visit a friend of mine who owned a store in Kennebunkport, Maine. It wasn't the best of times for me. I looked like I had just escaped from Auschwitz, the ninety-five-pound bald-headed, sallow-skinned guy that I was. When I arrived, I went directly to my friend's store in the center of town. He saw me as I approached the front door and ran out to greet me. We hugged for a good fifteen seconds, and he said gently in my ear, "It's great to see you, Kevin. I care about you a lot, but do me one favor: Please, please don't stand in front of my store for too long. I've got a business to run, and you're going to scare away all my customers!"

Strangely enough, that was just what I needed. He acknowledged what I was going through, and he did it with humor. He didn't lie to me by saying that I looked good or even by being silent. He connected with me by recognizing that if I looked like hell, then surely that meant I was going through hell. His honesty opened the door to meaningful discussion—the kind of discussion real friends have with each other.

—*Kevin Shulman*

I LEFT THE hospital with a catheter to drain urine from my bladder because some of my nerve endings had been severed during surgery. This problem, which occurs in approximately twenty-five percent of uterine cancer surgeries, prevented me from sensing when I needed to relieve myself. Fortunately, I only had to wear the bag for several weeks until the sensation returned. The most inconvenient part of it was having to empty the bag several times a day, but the funniest part was when a friend drew red and green stripes on it and told me not to despair. "Now you have your own Gucci bag," she said.

—*June Dressler*

WHEN I WAS diagnosed, I called one of my best friends to tell her the news, and she reacted as any good friend would. She came to see me right away, and we had lunch together. I never heard from her after that. It was baffling and quite hurtful, but after I had worked through my anger, I was able to let her go.

I learned not to be attached to her friendship because she hadn't acted like a friend to me. I tried to rationalize her behavior, surmising that she had her own fear of illness, that it must have been difficult for her to see me get sick. I don't believe that that's enough of a justification or an excuse. Times of illness test your friendships, and you have a window into a person's character. You learn who will truly be there for you, who accepts you with all your faults and shortcomings.

Truly good friends are a rare find. It may hurt to lose some, but you will be pleasantly surprised to find new ones come into your life. The blessing comes when you realize how much you have learned about people. You've basically gotten a crash course in human nature, and you have a much better idea who to invest your time with and who to let go of.

—*Josh Malen*

I HAD ONE friend in particular—I'll call him Bill—who avoided me completely. There were a few others too, but Bill and I had been very close friends for many years. He was someone I had been through other crises with before and who I thought could handle crisis situations. Of course, the other crises were his, and I was helping him.

I didn't hear from him when I was hearing from all of my other friends, and I went as far as mentioning it to my other friends, asking them why Bill hadn't called and what was up with him. They all told me that he knew and that he was kind of freaking out. He didn't really know what to say to me.

Most people realize that there isn't any magic word to say and you don't have to come up with some profound poetry or philosophy of life or advice or anything like that. You just have to say, "I am thinking about you. I care." You can even say, "I don't know what to say." It's the contact that matters. It's recognizing what's going on and being available to listen. I was hoping that that could be imparted to my friend, but he still didn't quite get it.

I suppose he was afraid of stumbling, of saying the wrong thing, so he didn't call at all. On a more serious note, I think he was afraid that I was going to die. He was afraid that I was going to leave him. I guess we all were, but you can't live your life like that.

After my surgery, I went back to Washington to visit my friends and get some of my belongings. I still had my hair. I still looked pretty good. A bunch of us went out to dinner. We had a table of about fifteen people, and when Bill walked in, he sat at the very opposite end of the table. This is somebody who's a big hugging friend of mine who would always sit by me, and now he couldn't even sit at the same end of the table. I thought, "I look healthy. I sound fine. I'm talking about it comfortably, but I won't harp on it all night. And he still can't deal with me."

Finally I decided that even though I certainly didn't have time for psychological counseling for anybody else right then, maybe I would just take the high road. I went over and said, "Hey. I know you haven't really been able to talk to me, but I just want to tell you that I'm doing all right, and I think everything's going to be okay. And I need you now. I need you to just be there and to recognize that I'm going through something huge. This is the hugest thing that ever happened to me. I want you to be aware of that and somehow connect with me."

His response—I'll never forget this—was, "Just tell me one thing: What are the numbers?" I wanted to throw something at him. He wanted statistics on whether I was going to live or die. That's Bill's personality. He's very black or white, and he isn't so skilled in the emotional gray area.

I looked at him and said, "Bill, it's not the numbers. You can't focus on numbers because they are misleading." He realized it, and I think it made him feel bad because he *had* stumbled, he *had* said something wrong. I didn't want to push him away by telling him he had done something wrong, but I also didn't want him to think of me as a number. I'm a person. I'm not a number. I said,

"Don't worry about it. Just call me when you can, and we'll talk more."

I tried not to focus on it too much because I couldn't deal with any negative energy, and if Bill wasn't going to hang with me on this, then I had other people who would. I could deal with Bill later. But it was definitely tough, and I know it's happened to a lot of other people.

We talked about it later, after my treatments were done. We were on a camping trip, and he admitted that he had been wrong and he told me he loved me and all that, but—I don't know if I'm childish—I think that there's a permanent scar. It's been such a tremendous part of my life, and we never connected on it. I think he recognizes that he did something wrong, but I don't think he really understands why or how or what he could have done, because it's not like he's talking about it now, and it's certainly still part of my life.

—*Jodi Levy*

I HAD WONDERFUL support from my friends and neighbors and so forth, but what moved me the most when I was going through all this was an experience that involved someone I did not know. My husband is a physician, and he has a long-time patient who comes in from an outlying town. My husband had no idea she knew I'd been sick, but when she came to see him, she said, "I just want you to know that all of us in our church are praying for your wife." I've heard many other cancer patients tell about things like that that meant a great deal to them. The support of others— friends, family, people you don't even know—is a huge factor. It keeps you up.

—*Elizabeth Martin*

MY BEST FRIEND, Max, was on vacation in Tahiti when I was diagnosed, so by the time he came to visit me, I was already bald from the chemo. When I opened the door to greet him, he beamed at me, wrapped me in a tight hug for thirty seconds, and then, stepping back but keeping his hands on my shoulders, stared at me for a good five seconds and then suddenly burst out laughing. After a few seconds, I smiled and broke into a chuckle.

My mother came in from the kitchen and, without really knowing what there was to laugh about, jumped right in with us. It
went on for about five minutes, and I got so involved in the joy of
the laughter that I almost forgot what had provoked it. Good old
honest Max. He wasn't going to pretend he didn't find my
baldness funny.

I remember thinking, "If it's true that laughter is one of the
best cures for illness, then Max's coming to see me, and the
contagious laughter he brought with him, must have knocked my
cancer clear out into the ionosphere."

—*Jonathan Pearlroth*

CHAPTER TWENTY-ONE

Psychological Support and Support Groups

There is no better place to learn about cancer treatment and to discuss the physical and emotional side effects you might be experiencing than with a group of peers who have been through the same thing. One of the mistakes that people make is to believe that their particular form or stage of cancer does not make them qualified to attend a support group. This is almost never the case. Unless the support group is specifically designated for a certain type of cancer, anyone dealing with cancer in any form is usually welcome.

No matter how strong the support of family and friends, support group meetings offer a complementary forum in which to express yourself and learn. They are also places where you realize that the hard lessons you have learned can be valuable to other people. You come to understand that you are now a part of another community with a special bond, and that can be a very valuable and rewarding discovery.

Another good way to address the many psychological, social, and physical repercussions of cancer and cancer therapy is with a licensed therapist. These professionals can provide invaluable insights into the way you are reacting to your cancer and can help you deal with negative feelings.

Making the Most of Support Groups

I PUT OFF going to a support group for a long time because I didn't feel like I deserved to go. I had had this really strange obscure experience that nobody my age has, and at this point, it wasn't life-threatening. It made me feel sort of unworthy. I thought most women in support groups had breast cancer or ovarian cancer. These kinds of cancer tend to be very serious, and my cervical cancer, at this point, was just life-altering.

Finding a support group that would meet my needs seemed hard, and I didn't want to deal with the hassle. I was so tired. I'd spent a year just researching treatment. I regret not trying harder, and I regret that I downgraded my own concerns and felt intimidated by the climate. I didn't give the cancer community an opportunity to talk to me, which was stupid. Cancer is not like a job you don't like, which, once you finally leave, is part of your past. It's a constant—a past, present, and future—and it makes you look at things differently, no matter what form of cancer you are fighting.

In a support group, there's a serious understanding of and respect for your individual experience and your right to the emotions that it has evoked. I wish I'd given that more of an opportunity right from the get-go.

—*Rachel Kaul*

IT WAS SO helpful to meet other people who were in my position and to realize that I wasn't alone, that what I was feeling was completely normal and that I would get through it just like the other women in the group had. I don't want to understate the help I got from my family and my doctor, but the women in my support group provided me with the hope, even the belief, that everything was going to turn out well. They became so important to my life that even years after my treatment, I continued to join in the monthly dinners we would prepare at each other's houses.

We were all from diverse backgrounds and at different phases of our lives, but we were bound to each other by the cancer and forced to open up and learn about each other from the inside out.
—*Karen Lawrence*

WHEN I WAS diagnosed, a friend whose mom had had cancer encouraged me to go to the same cancer education center her mother had gone to—the Cancer Support and Education Center, in Menlo Park, California, based on the work of O. Carl Simonton. It was phenomenal. It wasn't just a support group. Each week we'd go over several different ways of understanding cancer or different things people found helpful in terms of healing. I was exposed to a lot of information, some of which I grabbed onto and some of which I didn't.

For some people, resolving early family conflict was incredibly meaningful. That wasn't what I needed to change in my life. In order to release all the energy caught up in the fear of dying, we were encouraged to visualize our death. But I was in denial and couldn't do it. It was a healthy denial, though, one that kept me focused on getting better. It wasn't until years later that I went through the oh-my-God-I-could-have-died anxiety, and I think it was because by then it was safe for me to feel it. Denial has a purpose, and I don't think people should be pushed out of it unless they have something equally effective that will work for them.

What I did learn was helpful visualization techniques, like being able to picture myself in full health doing the things I wanted to be doing. I learned how to live authentically, how to do what's really important and live life with passion and purpose, rather than living life with "shoulds" and "oughts" and doing what people expect you to.

I learned the importance of expressing feelings and living in a way that was most helpful to my immune system. That does not mean being upbeat all the time. It means being positive but honest about your feelings, expressing all sorts of emotions on an ongoing basis rather than suppressing them. Improving communication skills was part of it—how to recognize my own needs, which I hadn't thought much about at the age of twenty-four, and communicate them to other people. It was also about structuring my life to meet my needs.

For example, I changed the work I was doing. I was a financial analyst on Wall Street, and now I'm finishing my training as a psychotherapist for youth and families. I am a creative person but had not given myself as many opportunities as I do now—through art and working with kids—to express my creativity.

—*Sheri Sobrato*

I GO TO a leukemia support group once a month through Georgetown University Hospital, but I wish we met more often, once a week or once every two weeks. I enjoy going to the meetings, and they help me deal with my leukemia.

My friends and my family and all the people around me are wonderfully supportive; however, sometimes it seems like all we ever talk about is my health and my problem and what's going to happen next. I get sick of talking about my problem. Sometimes it's nice to go to the group and hear others talk about their problems. For me to try to help them solve their problems, rather than always focusing on my own, makes me feel better.

There are other young people in the group too. When I was in the hospital, on the oncology floor, everyone I saw was older than I am, so when I first went to the support group, it was nice to run into people my age. One gentleman, who was in his early thirties and had had Hodgkin's disease, kept referring to his treatment as his "experience." He referred to it that way because he felt like it was something he had been through, something that was over and now he was moving on.

It's a good way of thinking. I adopted it. This was an experience for me—not an experience that everyone wants to go through—but it's my experience. It helps me to deal with the fact that there is hope and a future for me. If I say this is just an experience, I'm looking at the future. There will be other experiences; this is just one of them.

—*Michele Fox*

I WAS ONE of those idiots who thought I could take care of the emotional issues by myself. For a long time after the operation, I was trying to deal with the impact of having cancer on my own—emotionally being grouchy, thinking I could tough it out. I believe a lot of guys think that way. Originally, I went to the cancer support group at the New York Road Runners Club in New York City to help people out because I'd made it through.

When I got there, I met Jeff Berman, the founder and head of Cancer Support Services, who has chronic lymphocytic leukemia, and Fred Lebow, founder of the New York Road Runners Club, who later died of brain cancer in 1994, and all the other people in the club's cancer support group. I found out that I needed help as much as everybody else did. I think it happens a lot that you go through something and think everything is fine, and then bouts of depression hit because your life has been turned upside down. Talking to other people can help you through the hard times. Other times, when you're fine and other people are going through a rough patch, you can return the favor. It's a two-way street. If I can help people deal with what they're going through so that they don't have to feel alone, that's real important.

There are other people in the group who know exactly where people can go for financial help. As a teacher, I have good medical coverage—the few bills I had to pay were not unbearable. Some of the people who require continuous treatment have had more trouble. And that's where this support group has also been good.

Not everyone wins the battle. We've lost three people so far, but that's okay, because we're there with them and helping them through it, and at the same time, we're helping ourselves. Being together makes the victories sweeter, and mitigates the losses to some degree. It's important and powerful. We're an active, positive group. We're friends. We invite each other places. We run marathons together. We bring in speakers to talk about nutrition, attitude, and many other issues, and then sometimes we just cry and hold each other.

When I talk to people going through cancer, I tell them not to try to be superman or superwoman. You can't use your family for everything either. There's already a tremendous impact at home. Being able to get together with people who are going through it or have been through it to talk things out gives you perspective, so you can go back to your family and maybe be a little kinder, gentler, and more understanding.

—Rick Asselta

ONE OF THE hospitals in our city—Lafayette, Louisiana—sponsored Camp Bluebird, a cancer camp that's held twice a year for people undergoing treatment. It's a national program that was started by the Telephone Pioneers of America, a group sponsored by AT&T and some of the regional phone companies. We go out to a campsite in a beautiful natural setting for three days and two nights, and the hospital provides a lot of excellent staff support.

I attended nine of the camps and went back as a counselor after I got out of treatment. Then, when I found out I had a lung tumor, I went back as a camper for a while. Getting out in nature and spending time with people who know what I'm going through has made all the difference in the world. We built bluebird houses, had relaxation sessions, and took part in support groups, one for women and one for men.

We also had a lot of fun. On the last night we would always throw a costume party, with music. Everybody had such a good time. You would never believe that anyone there had cancer—you couldn't tell who was staff and who was a patient. On the last day, we would have a lunch that family members could come to. It was great.

—*Kay Chenoweth*

WHEN YOU'RE YOUNG and wild, you're usually not receptive to good advice, and not a good patient. I was hanging out at Max's Kansas City in its heyday, following Patti Smith, Blondie, the Talking Heads, the Ramones, and all the New York punk bands—the Dead Boys, Johnny Thunder and the Heartbreakers. There were a lot of Quaaludes, a lot of coke, and we spent lots of time in taxis, going from one after-hours club to another to continue whatever the hell we thought we were doing. A lot of time was spent falling down stairs and things.

The way I handled cancer was to pretend it was a role I was playing—okay, here's my Camille role—so I could fit it into my life that wasn't dealing with reality anyway. I didn't think of myself as somebody in a life-threatening position. I would go into my nine o'clock radiation session reeking of alcohol, having had two hours' sleep, and Millie, the technician, would say, "You should not drink!"

The radiation oncologist was Filipino and was very kind, but she would say, "Leslie, what am I going to do with you?" Well, tralala. Yeah, I wish somebody had sent a note home to my mother, you know. I would frequently miss my appointments.

During treatments, I had to lie with my head tilted back and my chin facing upward, since the tumor was in my neck. The rays hit through my chin straight back along my jaw to my ear. With radiation, the hair loss is due to direct irradiation of the follicles. It's not systemic. My hair was long, and I lost about two inches from my hairline in back, up into my scalp. So I sort of wore a fringe of hair. That was demoralizing.

The radiation to the middle of my body also made me quite ill. I got very thin and began to feel weepy. Counseling would have been very important at this stage. The best option would have been a peer support group, where I could sit around with people who were having the same kind of days that I was having and get really blackly humorous about it. Instead, I began to miss appointments. I was supposed to go five days a week for three months, but it took me about five months to complete my radiation.

I would strongly recommend that anyone who is in this position immediately seek counseling. I finally did years later, but I should have done it then. It would have helped me at least to deal realistically with the situation. You can carry on any lifestyle you choose, but I would strongly recommend deleting drugs and alcohol. It's only common sense. Think of the cancer as an opportunity to stop in your tracks and assess your life. That's the great gift that an illness of this magnitude can give you.

—*Leslie Kaul*

Take Advantage of Support Groups

Studies by David Spiegel and others have shown that social and emotional support is as statistically significant for an individual's longevity as not smoking. Support groups reduce isolation and normalize stress and mood swings. When you join a support group, you see that you are not crazy, that it is normal to be sad, upset, angry, that you are allowed to cry and you don't have to apologize for it. People in the support group understand your feelings because they have been there.

Support groups can be of any size or age mixture. It's helpful to talk to someone in a situation similar to your own, but since this isn't always possible, don't worry about the specific facts and try to identify with the feelings of others. I find that support groups that are led by the true experts— that is, people who have been through or are going through treatment—are the most effective.

Here is a list of some organizations that offer support groups for cancer patients:

American Brain Tumor Association: Offers support groups and a pen-pal program for patients with brain tumors. 800-886-2282.

American Cancer Society: Provides information for numerous support services, including CanSurmount, I Can Cope, Look Good . . . Feel Better, Reach to Recovery. 800-ACS-2345.

American Foundation for Urologic Disease: Support groups, including US TOO, for men with prostate cancer. 800-828-7866.

Cancer Care: Nonprofit social service agency that provides professional social work support and counseling. 800-813-HOPE or, in New York, New Jersey, or Connecticut, 212-302-2400.

CANSURVIVE: Offers support and advocacy for cancer survivors. 310-203-9232.

ChemoCare: Personal support for patients undergoing chemotherapy or radiation treatment, from trained volunteers who have been through cancer treatment. 800-55-CHEMO, or, in New Jersey, 908-233-1103.

International Myeloma Foundation: Information and support groups for myeloma patients. 800-452-CURE.

Leukemia Society of America: Support for leukemia patients. 800-955-4LSA.

National Brain Tumor Foundation: Support and education for brain tumor patients. 800-934-CURE.

National Coalition for Cancer Survivorship: Support for cancer survivors and their families. 301-650-8868.

United Ostomy Association: Support after ostomy surgery. 800-826-0826.

—*Randy Hale,*
Program Manager, Gilda's Club,
New York, New York

Seeing a Therapist

EARLY ON, I asked my HMO to send me to someone who could teach me how to use relaxation techniques during the chemotherapy treatments. I actually got more than I asked for. They have psychologists on staff who meet with oncology patients as frequently as the person needs. I saw one every two weeks all the way through chemotherapy, which lasted from February through July, and then beyond that until the end of the year.

I don't know if I could have done it without this help. Now I belong to a support group, but at the time, I needed individual attention, someone who would listen to what I was going through. I could say, "This is what I'm feeling this week," and she would make sense of it for me. It kept me sane the whole way through and kept me going spiritually, when I sometimes didn't have the energy or the motivation to participate in life.

Each week the psychologist and I would do a relaxation exercise for ten or fifteen minutes. She always taped the session so I could take it home and do it myself later. I used to get tension headaches from anxiety, but during treatment, I started having TMJ—when your jaw tightens up—and she helped me with that. She taught me breathing exercises and phrases that I should think about or say the minute I started feeling tension in my jaw. We did a relaxation exercise specifically designed to help me shift the pain and tension elsewhere so that I wouldn't end up with my jaw clenched again.

Seeing her really worked quite well to meet my relaxation needs at that point and to deal with what I was going through at the time.

—*Lorraine Anderson*

I HAD MANY procedures, including two bone marrow transplants, and I always found them to be comforting. Procedures are about moving forward, getting well, working toward the goal of cure. The day-to-day uncertainty, on the other hand, was much more difficult for me. I learned to cope by going to a therapist who helped me get in touch with what I was feeling and what I really wanted to do with my life. The path to finding a good therapist, however, was winding and at times quite scary.

Originally, I went to a Freudian psychotherapist who had no experience in crisis management. He blabbered on about my childhood and how it related to my illness and my relationship with my parents. He was an insightful man, but his approach was to slowly and painstakingly peel away the onionlike layers of my psyche in order to help me better understand myself. I didn't have the time or the psychological wherewithal to peel away the onion. I wanted a hatchet to chop right through it.

I needed to learn how to cope with a crisis and I needed to learn quickly, so I tried someone new, a hypnotherapist, who taught me how to relax and manage stress. That worked well, but something was missing. Finally, I found a woman whose specialty was helping people get through serious illness. Her credentials (besides the impressive degree on her wall): She had had a double mastectomy and was a cancer survivor.

She taught me many things over the course of my illness, but most importantly, she taught me how to live with the cancer. I had always wanted to buy a fancy guitar, and I figured I would get one as a reward after I got well. She made me realize that there was nothing to wait for, that I should go ahead and buy it if I could afford it and it was going to give me pleasure. She taught me how to live a concept that I had often heard: If not now, when?

—*Josh Malen*

I STARTED SEEING a psychologist when I was diagnosed, and I think it's helped me a lot. Some things are too hard to talk about with my family. The first thing I thought when I got sick was, "I'm going to die," and I wanted to talk about it with my husband and my mother, but I didn't want to scare them too. I felt isolated because I couldn't express my feelings. I could talk about these things with my psychologist. Another thing I'm doing now is keeping a journal where I can express things that are hard to talk about.

—*Leigh Abruscato*

AFTER MY RADICAL mastectomy, my doctor put me on tamoxifen, a hormone I have to take for the rest of my life to kill the estrogen cells. As it turns out, tamoxifen can cause a chemical imbalance and depression, but this was never presented as a possibility by the oncologist. So many times doctors take things for granted. I regarded my doctors as if they were God. If they told me to take something, I took it. Unfortunately, doctors often don't take the time to give people the information they need.

I really had a hard time with the depression. I could not pick myself up. Finally I went to a psychotherapist who solved the problem by prescribing an antidepressant, which I've been on for five years.

—*Charlene Sloane*

THERAPY, FOR ONE thing, helps you deal with the fact that you have the seeds of your own mortality within you. We all do. But most people gradually come to that realization later in life, not in early adulthood. The main thing I needed to work through and didn't, until fifteen years had passed, was a feeling of rage, a feeling of having been robbed of my sense of immortality at an age when you should feel that anything is possible.

It's not only what you go through; it's what you see other people go through. When I was in for a biopsy, I was on the head and neck ward of Memorial Sloan-Kettering, where people with smoking cancers—mouth, esophagus, tongue—tend to be. Suddenly, my whole worldview was changed from being twenty-one and running wild in the streets to being exposed to incredible suffering and fear of death. I think that pushed me into a self-destructive, fatalistic reaction, which therapy would have addressed and helped to counteract.

—*Leslie Kaul*

WHEN I WAS diagnosed with Hodgkin's in my early twenties, I didn't feel entitled to join a cancer encounter group. Since Hodgkin's is highly curable, I didn't want to be the prom queen who attends Overeaters Anonymous, extends her sleek legs, looks at a three-hundred-and-fifty-pound girl, and says, "I know just how you feel." All I did was crack jokes. I was damned if I was going to open up to anybody. I was all-powerful. I was in control. I was just going to get my treatment and not talk about it and not think about it and move back to New York and start my life again.

My advice is, find the nearest therapist and sign up. I did not, and I became very repressed and very funny and very witty and extremely controlled. It's actually surprising that I still have molars. There was hell to pay years later, when I moved back to New York and essentially stopped functioning. I had a real posttraumatic reaction. If I had spoken to somebody, I think I would have felt very differently about the whole thing.

So, in my opinion, seeing a therapist is vital. I would almost require it. Not talking about your feelings because they're too painful is no more valid than not taking your chemo because it makes you too nauseous. For me, it was also a question of being too mindful of how people around me were going to get through my illness. Now I say, forget what other people are going through. They're not the ones with cancer.

—*David Rakoff*

CHAPTER TWENTY-TWO

Getting Spiritual

A recent *Time*/CNN poll indicated that more than eighty percent of Americans believe in the healing power of prayer. In fact, some highly respectable scientific studies recently have shown that those who practice their religious beliefs have something extra going for them in the battle against illness. As anyone who has received the support of their church or synagogue or mosque during a time of need can attest, the mental boost provided by an outpouring of prayers can be enormously helpful.

In times of need, people tend to elevate their commitments to religious beliefs. And there is nothing wrong with that. After all, what could be more natural than for a person whose physical body is failing them in some way to turn to the spiritual, that which transcends the physical world. "With illness, someone who has drifted away from religion, roots, and community may find a yearning to be reconnected, although they may not know how to approach the issue," says the Reverend George Handzo, director of the Chaplaincy Service at Memorial Sloan-Kettering. "Illness may function as a bridge back to the community. If you haven't been to church in twenty years, you can go to the chapel in the hospital and begin the process of reconnecting. Nobody asks questions or wants to know what your religious practices were in the past. This is a time to think, get in touch with and focus on the path, the values, the people that are important to you."

In other words, if you're feeling the itch to get in touch with your place of worship, simply go, or pick up the phone and set up an appointment. If you're in a hospital, call the chaplaincy, or ask a nurse to do it for you. If in the past you lapsed in your attendance, put the years of neglect behind you. They aren't an issue. You'll be welcomed into the fold with open, unquestioning arms.

I TOOK TIME every day to read my Bible and to try to renew myself and my mind. I would only read little bits at a time, but I made sure that each day I had time to spend in quiet prayer and devotion. Even if the nurses were coming in and out, I didn't let that interfere.

—*Karla McConnell*

ALL MY LIFE I've been a very religious person. For seventeen years, I was a Roman Catholic monk. Then I left the monastery, married, and spent the last twenty-five years raising a family. But religion always has been a powerful support for me. Prayer has been an extraordinary part of our marriage. When I went to the hospital to have the operation or the treatment, I would hold hands with my wife and pray with her.

At one point during my treatment, I took a week off and went to a Trappist monastery in upstate New York. I spent four days in silence, chanting psalms with the monks—not as one of them but as a guest, a retreatant. It was a good break. One of the things about retreat—maybe the whole purpose of it—is that you have no distractions. You live in the guest house about seven-tenths of a mile from the abbey, where there are about forty monks and a monastery. The monks are vegetarians, so you eat simple, solid meals. The monastery supports itself by baking bread, so you have good bread. The rooms are very simple, but you do have a bed to sleep on. You don't need a car. So you remove all worldly distractions and face yourself. You come in touch with yourself and your relationship to God and your view of the eschatological questions. I cannot appreciate how anyone can go through cancer without contemplating the eschatological questions. Where do we come from? Where do we go? What's at the end? What happens after life?

I was challenged with those questions when I had cancer, but I answered to my own satisfaction that I am a believer. Once I discovered that, it was a tremendous consolation to me. I can't say I faced death, because you can't face your own death, but to some extent, I contemplated death. I remember one funny incident when I planned my funeral. I dealt with those issues, and I think anybody who is sick has to deal with those questions.

After the retreat, I felt as if four days were not enough. And at a later point—well after my treatment—I went back to the monastery for seven days.

—*Frank Sheridan*

GOD TELLS US in the Bible—in Philippians—"My grace is sufficient." I never really knew experientially what that meant, but I found out during my struggle with cancer. Breast cancer is one of the most difficult things a woman can go through, but the supernatural power of His spirit kept me from being afraid and from feeling alone.

A lot of people think it would be the most awful thing in the world to have cancer, but I don't have that fear anymore. I never feel anxious when I go for mammograms now. I don't hold my breath until they call and tell me that everything is fine. I had to have a spot watched for about six months before my doctor decided to biopsy it, but I didn't fret about it. I learned that whatever you have to go through, God will give you the grace that you need to get through it.

—*Katherine Arthur*

The Role of the Chaplain

As chaplains, we attempt to help patients gain strength from their own belief systems—whatever they may be. We try to support them in their strengths and reinforce what's right for them, without preaching or judging. We simply give people the opportunity to be heard and help them sort things out to arrive at answers on their own.

Chaplains, in that sense, are sorters of information, rather than providers of answers. Just as a satellite dish unscrambles a signal that is sent to it, so we, too, help to unscramble—make clear and more visible—the feelings and the yearnings of people who are confused and scared.

People have different coping mechanisms that are individual and special. I never impose my belief system or coping mechanisms on them. Rather, I help them discover their own mechanisms. I help them discover who they are, what they are, and what they believe.

I am reluctant to prescribe or endorse any particular way of acting or being as necessary to fighting cancer. I believe, for instance, that a positive attitude can help you recover, but I don't think that being positive necessarily means being involved in your treatment and constantly seeking information. People who don't want to know about their illness or their treatment are not necessarily in denial—they still may have positive attitudes. Prayer also is individual. I have heard many people say that you can't pray for God to make you well. I say, "Why not?"

—The Reverend George Handzo,
Lutheran Pastor,
Director, Chaplaincy Service,
Memorial Sloan-Kettering Cancer Center,
New York, New York

THERE WAS A priest named Peter who visited the patients on my floor. Usually he would stop by my room in the evening. We chatted a few times, and I found him to be a pleasant, friendly man. One day when he came by, I told him that I needed to speak to him. I said that I didn't know how to address him. "I don't feel comfortable calling you Father because you're not my father," I said. "I don't want to call you Priest because you're not my priest, and I don't feel comfortable talking to you about religion because I'm Jewish. So how do I address you?" He smiled and said, "Why don't you just call me Rabbi Peter?"

So each day I talked to Rabbi Peter, the Catholic priest. He told me what was in the news and gossiped with me about what was going on in life. Rabbi Peter helped me forget about where I was and what I had to face. He made me realize that life truly goes on and that good people may dress, talk, and pray differently, but underneath, they are all the same.

—*Rhoda Silverman*

A CLIENT I work with told me about her mother, who prays with people. She isn't a sister, but she works out of a Catholic convent, praying with people who have severe illnesses. My client said, "Someday you'll have to meet her." Somebody at our church also mentioned a lady they prayed with, and one of their friends was cured through the process. It ended up being the same lady. Like a lot of things that happened to us, people kept coming up with the same idea at the same time, indicating that it was something I should check out. Usually when you get information on cancer you think, "Oh, one more thing." You read it and set it aside. But the things that I ended up doing were the ones that kept coming back to me. This was one of them. For some reason, someone wanted me to talk to Virginia Russo.

It was amazing. Once my wife and I started this prayer process with her, we received a lot of messages. We'd walk out of a room where the doctor gave us terrible news about how soon I might pass away, and then, at a support meeting we'd meet a lady who had the same form of cancer and who had been clean for ten years. The timing and the way it happened convinced us that God is more active in our lives than most of us believe.

It also helped me to talk about how I felt emotionally. There were usually six or seven of us praying with this prayer leader every two weeks. We'd go in at nine o'clock in the morning and pray for about two hours. Through the process, some people praying with us started seeing events from my past. When I was nine years old, I was with a friend who was killed by a car. These people identified that I still felt bad about that situation. They saw it. They had a vision. It started when a guy in the prayer group said he kept seeing me in a red barn. This accident happened right near a big red barn. Then, somebody saw something else. It was a powerful and mysterious experience.

Some incidents that really affect you when you are little can stay with you throughout your life. The prayer group gave me an opportunity to deal with some of that baggage. I wrote a letter to apologize to that boy's parents, who are still good friends of my family's. I talked to them, met with them. Their reaction was favorable. The accident wasn't my fault, but for years I felt guilty. I was nine years old at the time, and we were biking by a busy street. Meeting with the boy's parents helped me get beyond my feelings of survivor's guilt. I felt much better about myself. All you have to do is ask for forgiveness.

Not only did going to the prayer group clear up the bad feelings I had about my friend's death, but it has had a profound spiritual effect on me. It has also made our marriage better. My wife and I feel better about our family and our kids and each other because of this experience.

—*Brian Schmidt*

ONE DAY MY girlfriend's uncle Baruch, an Orthodox rabbi, suggested I follow Jewish religious tradition and take a new name to mark the beginning of my new life as a cancer fighter. He told me it would make it more difficult for the Angel of Death to find me.

All things considered, I thought that was a pretty good idea. I asked him what sort of name I should choose. He suggested Chaim, which means "life," but I didn't want that name because it was too old-fashioned. I asked him for another possibility.

He came up with Alter and told me it was appropriate. "It signifies that you've gone through one life and are now starting a new life as an Elder," he said.

I was flattered that such a learned man would consider bestowing me with the title of Elder, but all I could think of was the term "Alter Cocker," which means, in its most literal sense, "old crapper," and even in its gentlest and most figurative sense, "grumpy old man." I didn't much care for it in either of its senses and pressed him for a third choice.

Finally he hit upon Raphael. It means "God has cured."

I liked it. Raphael had a nice, musical sound. It was biblical. It was modern. And together with my present name, Jonathan, it would give me a full Hebrew name meaning "God has cured what God has given." But my delight with my new name went beyond its novelty or its meaning. I was pleased because it was an expression of Baruch's confidence that I was on my way to beating the disease and beginning a new life. And with my new name, I felt I was.

—Jonathan Pearlroth

I DIDN'T CHECK the "religion" box when I filled out my hospital admissions sheet, so for a long time I didn't receive any visitors from the chaplaincy. One day a priest walked into my room, and the first thing that crossed my mind was that he had come to tell me I was going to die. After a few minutes of small talk, I realized that he hadn't come to recite the last rites for me. I told him that I appreciated his visit but that I was Jewish. He asked if he could say a prayer for me. I told him in the thickest Yiddish accent I could muster, "It couldn't hoit." We both broke out in full-throated laughter, and the afterglow of that visit—not to mention the prayer—stayed with me for days on end.

—Kevin Shulman

God at the Head of Your Bed

There is an exquisite Jewish teaching that I try to remember when visiting a very sick person. The Talmud prohibits sitting at the head of a patient's bed because, it says, "God's presence resides at the head of the sick person's bed."

The patient may be disabled, disfigured, and may feel

powerless, angry, and alone. Even if blessed with an optimistic mind-set, she may, after a long or frightening hospitalization, feel disregarded by the community she formerly felt her own. How can I break this isolation? How can I treat her so that she feels as valued as she was before?

First, I respect the intensely private nature of suffering. Jewish tradition and secular therapies encourage us to share feelings, but I can never know the immediacy of her pain. So I avoid speaking about illness in general, or about the illness of others, as this minimizes her suffering. Rather, I seek to restore a sense of connection with the human community in which she participated before the illness. What is happening in our local families, in the synagogue, in civic affairs? What does she remember? What may she hope to rejoin?

To reestablish this human connection requires that I meet the patient with total respect and no condescension. I am aided in doing so by the Talmudic insight, advising that I sit at the patient's side. I am there at her level, and at a reverential distance from the presence of God supporting her head—or her will. So situated, I am reminded of the sanctity of life that is equally hers and mine.

—Samuel H. Weintraub,
Rabbi, Kane Street Synagogue,
Brooklyn, New York

CHAPTER TWENTY-THREE

Hell's Bills

The last thing you need right now is to deal with the bills, but bills there are, and lots of them. They come from all directions—the hospital, the lab, the doctor's office. And then there are the collection agencies—surely the lowest form of life—with their threats when your insurance company is late paying the bill or sticks you with part of a charge they unilaterally deem excessive. It's one headache you just don't need.

When looking for financial assistance, there is only one way to find it, and that is to jump in with both feet. Don't fret, worry, grouse. Just start getting in touch with people who might be able to help you—your insurance company, social workers, the many cancer institutes that, although rarely and usually for very specific reasons, do sometimes offer assistance. For instance, the Leukemia Society of America (212-573-8484) will sometimes cover certain expenses, such as drugs, transfusions, transportation, and radiation treatment, for people with leukemia, preleukemia, lymphoma (including Hodgkin's disease), and multiple myeloma. They can also provide referrals to other sources of financial help.

You also might want to check out the American Cancer Society's (800-640-7101) Limited Financial Assistance program and RIG (Resource Information and Guidance) program, which lines you up with a volunteer who will provide information on federal, state, and local resources. The federal government's Hill Burton Free Hospital Care (800-638-0742) provides free care to those who qualify. Another potential gift horse is the Corporate Angel Network (914-328-1313), which can help you get to distant treatment centers via corporate flights, free of charge. No financial qualifications apply.

The key is simply not to give up. Don't stop looking and calling until you solve your problem. Even if you feel like you're groping in the dark, sooner or later you'll find the wall. Feel around the wall long enough, and you'll find the light switch. As Enid Handler prefaced some of her hints below, "Everything I'm telling you, I came up with by myself." She simply got started and found a way to get things done.

One place to check is at your hospital. If you can find a social worker who works within the institution most of your bills will be coming from, he or she can work wonders in negotiating fees and payment schedules.

As far as those debt collectors go, they are inevitable to some degree. Remember, they are simply gunslingers hired to collect money—coldly, callously. Don't waste a lot of breath on them. Avoid letting them bring you to tears whenever possible. Just politely inform them that you are working to resolve the situation with your insurer and hang up.

I HAD INCREDIBLE insurance coverage through two different unions. My mother managed the paperwork at first. The balancing act of keeping up with the forms and bills was practically a full-time job. The process was so overwhelming that she hired someone to organize and categorize the forms, to basically fight the hospitals to accept what the insurance companies paid for the procedures. That was a battle for a long time afterward.

My mother brilliantly took care of the finances and got me on

Social Security Disability, which required unbelievable documentation. It also required spending all my money so that I got below the poverty line. The ironic thing is that once I was in the program, it was just as hard to get out of it. I still get letters asking for documentation so they can continue to send me benefits. I haven't received benefits for seven years!

—*Evan Handler*

Getting the Most from Your Insurance Company

Don't let the health insurance struggle interfere with your number-one priority: winning the big fight against cancer. Here are some tips for collecting maximum benefits from your insurance company:

Make copies of all bills. Keep the originals and submit the copies, if your insurance company allows you to. Buy a bookkeeper's ledger and maintain a record of all bills (assign each a number) and claims filed, paid and outstanding.

Don't let claims pile up. Since most insurance companies have a time limit for submitting claims, you risk losing benefits. (Ask your company what its limit is.) Besides, this unpleasant task can quickly become an unmanageable one.

Avoid rejection. If your claim is rejected, carefully check the "explanation of benefits" (EOB), the form that explains the company's response to each claim you submit. Here are some of the common reasons why claims are rejected: You failed to call for precertification before a medical procedure (in the case of a managed-care policy); the insurance ID number is incorrect; the date the service was provided is missing; the patient's first name is missing; the superbill, or itemized statement of services, is not legible; multiple visits in a single day are not explained; the charges are not itemized; the diagnosis is missing or incomplete. Obviously, many of these omissions are easy to correct. Fill in the missing information, and resubmit the claim.

Ask for a claim review. If a claim is rejected because the company doesn't cover the procedure, write the following note on the EOB and return it: "Please review—I think you should have paid." If they still reject it, write on the next EOB: "I would like to request a review of this denial of coverage by the peer review physicians." Fifty percent of claims that are originally rejected are paid the second time around. Keep at them. It might even take four or five attempts.

Fight for the full payment allowed by your contract. If your insurance company only partially pays a claim—and your doctor does not agree to cover the difference—you might need to prove that the charge was, in their language, "reasonable and customary." Start by asking your doctor to write a letter to the insurance company justifying the charge. Make sure you get a copy for your files. If this fails, you might need to dig deeper. Call five to ten of the same specialists in your area and ask what they charge for the same procedure. Refer to the procedure code—a universally recognized five-digit number—on your doctor's bill (for example, the code for a subcutaneous mastectomy is 19182). Send your results in a clear and concise letter. Be sure to include your claim number and policy number.

Call for backup. If insurance matters overwhelm you, help is available. First, ask a hospital social worker to help you organize and submit claims (see "Seeking Financial Help from a Social Worker," on page 354). Or hire a claims-assistance professional, who will file claims for you for a fee—an hourly rate, a flat fee, or a percentage of each claim. Paying your hired help a percentage of each claim gives him or her the most incentive to fight for you. Look in the Yellow Pages under Insurance Claim Processing Services or contact the National Association of Claims Assistance Professionals (NACAP) for a referral: 708-963-3500.

—Irene C. Card,
President, Medical Insurance Claims, Inc.,
Kinnelon, New Jersey

IN TERMS OF financing, the basic starting point is to explore every avenue that's available—private insurance, Medicare, Medicaid, and any other areas, like employee benefits. Some companies have special funds for employees. One of the things I learned was that the Actors' Fund has money for actors stricken with catastrophic illness. I applied to the Actors' Fund, and they were extremely generous, helpful, and supportive, without a lot of red tape. They made it easy, which is not the case, of course, with government funding, but that, too, should be explored. Hospitals also sometimes offer assistance. Ask as many questions and explore as many avenues as you can think of.

I set up a fund for my son Evan, and we approached family members and friends. While it was not tax-deductible, people were willing to contribute anyway. A very close friend agreed to handle the fund for us—to accept donations, acknowledge them, handle the banking, and pay the bills. Organizations in many communities will provide publicity and help raise funds for something like a transplant, so those are other areas to explore.

Our main concern was whether Evan would be covered for the bone marrow transplant. At the time, it was highly experimental, and we had read of a number of instances where bone marrow transplants were not covered. It's an enormously expensive procedure. That's why we started the fund.

As it turned out, Evan's insurance policies did pay for a great deal of it, but there were other things that were not covered. For example, the sperm bank. Even though it was highly recommended medically that he store sperm—because he was only twenty-four and hoped to have a family and the treatment would almost certainly involve infertility—it was not covered. So that was paid for by the fund we set up. Evan had psychiatric sessions to deal with anxiety and to learn self-hypnosis so that he could better deal with the pain of treatments. That, too, was essentially not covered by his insurance.

His daily living expenses when he was not in the hospital were also not covered. He wasn't working, and being so young, he didn't have reserves to cover things like rent, electricity, and phone bills. So for ongoing expenses, we looked for help either from the Actors' Fund or the fund that we had set up.

—*Enid Handler*

MY INSURANCE COVERAGE under my father's medical plan had lapsed, and the hospital asked for $35,000, up front, before they would admit me for my bone marrow transplant. Thirty-five thousand dollars! Who the hell has that kind of cash?

Up to my twenty-fifth birthday, I had been covered for major medical and hospitalization under my father's policy. Even though my cancer wasn't discovered until two months after my twenty-fifth birthday, the insurance company had grudgingly agreed to continue my coverage because—luckily for me—they had never given me formal notice that my coverage was about to lapse. Then, in an obvious attempt to dump me so they wouldn't have to pay for the transplant, they took the position that my relapse and need for a transplant were not related to my original condition. How they arrived at that conclusion, I don't understand, but when the hospital was notified that my coverage was canceled, they demanded that I pay for the transplant up front and in full.

I got scared. What if, in the final analysis, I couldn't find the money? Would the hospital let me die? My father told me he was going to fight the insurance company's cockeyed ruling, and he believed that he could win. But in the meantime, I needed a bone marrow transplant, and the hospital wanted $35,000. I've heard it said countless times that it's impossible to put a price on a person's life. Well, it seemed it was not so impossible after all. Quite clearly, a price had been put on my life.

Fortunately, I learned that I was eligible to apply for Medicaid, which would cover the cost of the transplant. Medicaid is a joint federal- and state-funded medical insurance program for the indigent. In order to be eligible, the maximum you can earn in a year is something like $5,000, and you cannot own more than about $2,000 in assets. This is so low a threshold that people who own an old car or receive any kind of pension find themselves ineligible. Luckily—and it's weird using that word in this context—I had no trouble qualifying. I had been a student when I was first diagnosed, and the little money I made went toward paying off my college loans. My assets were zilch.

If I had been a minor, I would never have qualified because my parents made too much money, but since I was twenty-six and had been on my own for a few years, I could rightfully claim that I was independent.

—*Jonathan Pearlroth*

I HAD A student policy. I don't think people ever expect to use those, but that was the best insurance buy I ever made. They ended up covering a lot of my expenses. I was still saddled with twenty percent, though. Most of the doctors wrote it off because they were studying my cancer. Apparently where mine was located was very rare. I was fortunate to be at a teaching hospital. They followed me closely right through my therapy, taking pictures and all kinds of things. They were writing a book. I think I got better treatment than the average guy.

I also had a social worker at the hospital who was an amazing help. She got hold of all the itemized statements and found all kinds of duplicate charges. It's almost fraudulent what happens in these hospitals. If you have a catastrophic illness, you're talking about bills in the hundreds of thousands of dollars.

But I still paid a lot of money over close to ten years. I was in my twenties, and I was basically unemployed for two years trying to finish school and get back on my feet. I was able to get some disability payments from the government, but it wasn't a lot, because I hadn't paid anything in. I got the minimum amount. My wife and I had to show no assets. We wound up selling a car and doing a few other things to get in a certain category. It was tough. Most people my age were worrying about paying for their first house, and I was trying to buy a wing of the hospital. It changes your perspective. You either go crazy or you play the game the best you can.

—Dale Totty

Seeking Financial Help from a Social Worker

Because they are employed by hospitals for the patients' benefit, social workers are your allies on the inside. As financial counselors, they use their relationships with doctors, hospital administrators, and even insurance representatives to fight for your cause. Here's how to gain free, practical help from a social worker:

Drop negative preconceptions. Because social workers are traditionally associated with the needy, one of the biggest hurdles for some patients is agreeing to see one. Even if affording treatment is not an issue, a social worker can help you make sense of the financial chaos that accompanies cancer treatment. By acting as a liaison between you and the hospital's accounting office—to decipher bills, file insurance claims, arrange payment extensions—they take some of the pressure off you at a time when more pressure is the last thing you need.

Establish a relationship. Get to know your social worker. Be honest about your financial situation. The more you tell her about your needs, the better she can argue your case.

Don't be afraid to ask. People tend to think that what doctors say is the gospel truth, and that you can't

question them. You can—even when it involves fees.
And a social worker can help. Maybe you're
underinsured or you're a recent college grad setting out
on your own, and you need financial help. A social
worker arguing your case might ask a doctor to waive a
particular fee or to reduce the cost of another, or she
might negotiate a low monthly rate with the hospital's
accounts receivable office.

—*Peggy Conner,*
Social Worker,
Richmond, Virginia

WE WERE EXTREMELY fortunate that Evan had taken out quite a
bit of insurance coverage because he was eligible through unions
both as a stage and as a screen actor. He had coverage from two
private carriers. One paid eighty percent, and the next one paid
twenty percent, and I did not have any trouble with the insurance
companies.

However, I did find dealing with the medical bills from the
hospital and the doctors overwhelming. First of all, the bills were
almost indecipherable. I couldn't for the life of me figure out
what the charges related to, how they were arrived at, what was
being paid and what wasn't being paid, what was being paid at
eighty percent and what was being paid at twenty percent, and
what was being disallowed by the insurance company. Although
they say they will pay eighty percent, they have a cap on what
they consider reasonable for each test and procedure.

It was so painful to see all the procedures he was being sub-
jected to reduced to figures on a bill that I broke down in tears. I
decided that this was one job that I had to spare myself, and I
determined to hire somebody to relieve me of that responsibility.
I asked around, and first I tried a bookkeeper I knew, but she
didn't work out. She was not familiar with that kind of work, and
she wasn't good at it.

Then I found a young woman in the neighborhood, my
hairdresser's sister, who fit right into the slot. She worked for an
insurance company and could speak the language. I paid her $10

an hour, and she worked at home at her leisure. I met with her once a month to go over it, so I had a sense of where things stood. She was delighted to have the work, and for me, it was a tremendous emotional relief.

—Enid Handler

OUR INSURANCE WAS through an HMO, so for the most part we didn't have to deal with a lot of claims. But we would still get errant bills that kept coming back to us for no apparent reason. One day Dean called the HMO and somehow got through to the director of bill payment, who was actually a real person. He didn't even seem to be reading from a script! He was so helpful and nice that Dean got his name and extension, and from then on whenever we had a problem, we called him, and he would take care of it. I kept expecting him to say, "Look, it's not my job to be your personal bill payer. You'll have to go through the usual channels," but he never did. When you're dealing with a situation like this and you run across someone who is intelligent and caring—or, even better, powerful—I think you have to latch on to them and get as much help as you possibly can.

—Jessica King

I GOT CALLS all the time from bill collectors saying that they were taking me to judgment, all that sort of thing. It was very upsetting. Sometimes I would call and say that it was being processed and the insurance was going to pay or we'd get to it. Sometimes I would just turn it back on them: "My son is dying. The primary thing in my life right now is not paying bills. I'll get to it when I can."

After a while, you get hardened to it. I decided that it was not a high priority for me. Eventually the insurance company paid for it, or if the insurance company didn't pay for it, we got around to doing it.

—Enid Handler

MY INSURANCE COMPANY was fine at first. I had no problem with bills. They cover everything in the world—except a bone marrow transplant for multiple myeloma. They said they covered bone marrow transplants for leukemia and for other things, but they wouldn't cover it for myeloma because it was still considered experimental. So I was put in the situation of having to get a couple hundred thousand dollars, putting my family in debt for the rest of their lives. I really considered canning it.

But I had served with the Marine Corps right out of high school, and I found out there was a VA hospital in Seattle that was actually doing a test of bone marrow transplants for multiple myeloma and was looking for people who would fit the program. We gave them a call, and they said, "Get out here right away. We'll stick you in." It was a scrambled three weeks. We took off, went out there, and got the entire operation done for free.

I only paid the expenses of being out there for four months and my brother's salary while he was there; he's a trucker. But Lee Smith and a bunch of other writers and some members of the Red Clay Ramblers got together and had a benefit for me in Chapel Hill. They got a huge crowd and raised $15,000 in one night. It was wonderful.

Then when we got back, the insurance company refused to cover any of the aftercare, which could be in itself thousands and thousands of dollars. So we started talking to some lawyers. At the time, there were some other myeloma patients trying to sue the same company in order to get transplants. I know of two who died waiting. The lawyers told them, "We're going to put this all in the paper and make you guys look like a bunch of asses if you don't pay for his aftercare." They agreed to do it off the record if I didn't say anything to the media.

And they did for about four months, until the very first option on the insurance policy came up, and then they raised the premium so incredibly high that we had to switch to different coverage. Luckily we were able to do it through my wife's work. It's crazy the difference between what one insurance company will pay and another won't.

— *Tim McLaurin*

IF AN INSURANCE company isn't paying, it's up to you to jump in and start fighting. If you have to make that insurance company look bad, do it. I would never be averse to going to the media about a company that won't pay for medical treatment. If they say it's not customary and usual—that's the phrase they like to use—pressure them and don't accept what they first tell you. If you persevere, you can be successful.

The best thing to do is to find somebody who's willing to be your advocate and fight for you. At work, your personnel department will often step in and try to fight for you. Try and find somebody there—a contact you can be in touch with and speak to on a regular basis. At the insurance company, start with the benefits department, and if you get turned down there, gradually work your way up the line as if you had a complaint with a store that sold you a faulty product. A lot of times people accept no for an answer too soon. There is generally an appeals process.

After that, look to the federal government and your state and city government for any type of Medicaid or welfare. I would seek out an organization like Cancer Care, which offers grants to pay for transportation to and from treatments, as well as various places that will bring you meals.

—Jeff Berman

PART FOUR

After the War

CHAPTER TWENTY-FOUR

Rebounding and Rebuilding

This is one game where the fat lady never sings. Along with the battle scars, you've got a new outlook on life. What does that mean? It means you will carry your new perspective, along with a few fears, into the future. It means that you will have some additional considerations and challenges, as well as the joys of overcoming them.

First you must reconcile yourself to the realm of the healthy again. After you've been under the microscope for several years, this is not always easy. Believe it or not, there is often separation anxiety from the hospital/medical world, especially from the many compassionate souls who have taken such good care of you. Also, aches and pains are now measured by different standards. Yet you don't want to feel like a hypochondriac and call the doctor every time you sniffle.

Then you must move forward. Many of us noticed that one of the things that was damaged was our sense of mental and physical confidence, whether at work, at play, or on dates. After having battled the forces of nature, it took time to regain the will and desire to compete again in worldly matters. But sooner or later we rediscovered that spirit, whether it was feeling good about ourselves on a date or achieving new heights of physical fitness. In fact, many of us set very tough physical goals, including running marathons, and were able to meet them.

For others, having children became the single most burning issue. This is another area where science has made great leaps and bounds in recent years. Sometimes it simply took time to allow our bodies to regain their capacity to reproduce.

Indeed, time was the greatest healer and soother. The mental edge generally returned to full strength, though not as fast as we might have hoped. Physically, we had triumphs too. Many of us are in better shape than ever before, and others are flourishing even with what might seem like insurmountable physical challenges; but that, too, took time, effort, and desire.

As time passed and we were able to gain more and more perspective on the cancer recovery experience, certain advantages also became apparent. We generally feel as if we better understand what in life is valuable to us. We are better at channeling energy into meaningful activities, and we devote more time to the ones we love and who love us. In that sense, we are now blessed with more self-knowledge and better decision-making skills.

So, in many ways, the battle wasn't just to stay even; we got better.

Re-entering the Realm of the Healthy

THE THOUGHT OF undergoing radiation therapy had been extremely frightening to me—I had had no idea what to expect. But after a few treatments, the daily trips to the hospital became surprisingly routine. The six and a half weeks went by fairly quickly, and I was happy and excited when the last day of treatment arrived. I felt extremely relieved as I said goodbye to the nurses and left the radiology department, but as soon as I got outside—to my shock—I started to cry uncontrollably.

I was completely panicked. Who would watch over me every day to be sure I was okay? Was the cancer really all gone? How did I know I would live? As the questions raced through my mind, I thought, "I must be going crazy. Who in their right mind would want to prolong cancer treatments?"

Then I remembered something my surgeon had told me months before: "You may feel let down or frightened when the treatment is over. These are normal feelings. A lot of people have them." I am still grateful to him for those words because they are what helped me pull myself together on that street corner and face the future unafraid.

—Susan Fischer

I GOT SOME excellent advice from one of my doctor friends who happens to be on staff at the hospital where I had my surgery. He came by to visit, and he said, "I want to warn you about one thing. You're going to find, having had cancer, that for almost every little pain you experience from now on, the instinctive response is to say, 'Uh-oh, it's cancer. Bone cancer or this kind of cancer or that kind of cancer.' " He said, "Don't do it. You will continue, like every person on this earth, to have little pains here and there, and sometimes big pains, but they will most likely be for the same old ordinary reasons that everybody has aches and pains. Try your hardest not to worry if you don't have a reason to worry." He was right. Later, I had some pain in the bone of my arm and automatically I thought, "Uh-oh." But I stopped myself, and if I hadn't been given that advice I might not have known to stop myself.

—Toni Zavistovski

AS THE END of treatment grew near, I started to feel depressed, which my doctor had warned me about. He said that during treatment, most people feel safe, but once it ends, they can feel unprotected and afraid. I felt sorry for myself. There seemed to be nothing but more struggle ahead—struggle to find decent work, to pay the bills, to create a personal life. I felt like I had been a good girl—I fought the good fight, so where was my reward? The fact that my life was the reward didn't seem to be penetrating at that moment. I could practically hear the whining tone in my voice, which disgusted me, but there was no avoiding the way I felt.

I went to a therapist and also spent a lot of time talking to a friend who had had Hodgkin's disease three years before. With their help, I came to understand that getting my life back—and a deeper, more meaningful perspective—was indeed the reward for it all. But I had to go through a month or two of posttreatment depression before I reached that understanding.

—*Jacqueline Frank*

RIGHT AFTER YOU finish either chemo or radiation, you think, "Boy, I'm done, now I'll be back to normal, and I'll feel great." Well, both treatments have effects that recede slowly. The only time I got depressed was right after I finished, because I didn't pop right back. Don't be discouraged if you don't bounce back immediately—it can take six months or longer. I hit bottom. I finished my treatment in May and expected to feel better by my twenty-fifth wedding anniversary in June, but that was my worst month. I just didn't feel a lot better. I didn't have nausea anymore, but I had no energy, and my hair was slow growing back. I was discouraged.

I'm not somebody who spends a lot of time with her hair, but it threw me for a loop. I hated the wig, and I had to wear it all summer. I began to cheer up again in late June, but then I had a terrible experience at the beach. It was hot, and the water was calm, so I went in. There were about six young people on the beach and six more on the porch, including my four children, three of whom were in college and one of whom was in high school.

I went in, and the water felt wonderful. I was beginning to feel a little happier, when all of a sudden I turned around and a wave knocked me over completely. My hair went one way, and I went the other, and I couldn't see. I panicked and yelled for help, but nobody paid any attention. I finally saw this big seaweedy-looking stuff come up about two waves down. It was my wig. I went and got it, shook it out, plunked it backward on my head, and got out of the water.

You will bounce back, but try to be prepared for the waves that may briefly set you back.

—*Elizabeth Martin*

I THINK WHEN you're in the middle of a crisis situation, you're running on adrenaline. People kept telling me that I was so strong, and I *was* strong, because I had to be. I was concentrating on doing everything I could to help my husband get better, and I didn't allow myself to think about anything else. I remember when he came home from the sperm bank saying that they had told him that we only had enough sperm for two tries at conceiving (which turned out to be untrue: Don't get your conception information from your sperm bank), but even with this fairly devastating news, I remember saying, "That's not important now. We'll deal with that when the time comes." But, of course, after he got better, it was extremely important. It was our closest dream. Only then, when he was better, did I allow myself to relax and feel all the negative emotions, to consider what this cancer had done to our lives. Looking back on it, I realize that the year or so after Dean's illness was a very tough time.

—Jessica King

THERE HAVE BEEN many hypotheses about why people get Hodgkin's disease. Some studies say there is a correlation between the disease and people with affluent and well-educated parents. Some studies say that it is caused by Epstein-Barr virus or mononucleosis resurfacing due to immunosuppression or due to overuse of antibiotics as a child. My perspective is that if you need a cause, you must choose one that allows you to accept what has happened and move on. I attribute my cancer to immunosuppression due to a poor diet, environmental pollutants, drugs, and lack of exercise—all things I can control. Changing these things makes me feel better about myself because I know I am working to stay healthy and avoid future problems.

—Tim Batchelder

CERVICAL CANCER TENDS to be linked to or caused by a virus that is sexually transmitted. All the books say that women who've had a lot of sexual partners are at a high risk of getting this kind of cancer. What I found difficult was the amount of responsibility I felt in having it—as if, gosh, I must have done all of this wrong, and I caused it by being thirty and not married. But now I think that any number of things could have caused my cancer. And it's a big waste of emotional energy to sit around and try to ascribe responsibility for it.

—*Rachel Kaul*

I'M SINGLE, AND I never know how and when to tell the person I'm dating that I had cancer. If I tell him too soon, will it scare him away? If it scares him away, do I simply dismiss him as the wrong person anyway? Do I blurt it out, or wait for it to come up naturally? I'm not sure there is a right answer to these questions, but my rule is that before the relationship moves to a more intimate stage, I want the guy to know that I'm a cancer survivor. I don't want to be in the position of becoming intimate with someone who can't handle it or who is insensitive to a big part of who I am. As it turns out, I've received only positive responses. Most guys don't even flinch when I tell them. And with some, it seems to enhance the relationship because they feel they can be more open with me.

—*Karen Lawrence*

I HAD A laryngectomy, and therefore I speak with a heavy, almost mechanical-sounding voice. I've learned to write letters or get someone else to make a call for me, but when I do talk, I get some funny reactions from people. Most tell me that I should stop smoking. Some sympathize with how painful it must be for me to talk (it isn't). On the phone, people refer to me as Mr. Dwin because my voice is so deep. There was a point when I used a vibrator called a Servox to speak. Many businesspeople would hang up on me because they thought I was one of those mass-marketing robots trying to sell them something. But I just shrug it off, laugh, and keep on going.

—*Betty Dwin*

New Beginnings

THE DOCTORS WEREN'T able to remove all of my brain tumor, so I've tried to come to peace with the fact that I still have this growth inside my head. I realized that if I was going to stay well, I needed to make some changes in my life to strengthen my immune system. I needed to figure out what my needs were and to structure my life to meet those needs. For instance, I needed to communicate better and to learn how to say no.

Before I even finished my chemo, I started planning a trip to India, Nepal, and Thailand. I knew I couldn't go for a couple of years—until my immune system was ready—but I went to travel agents, collected brochures, and read a bunch of books by authors from those countries. What I learned helped motivate me to get well. And then I really did go. Just two years after I was diagnosed with a brain tumor, I biked around Asia for seven weeks.

Now I make sure I have plenty of time for sports, which I've always loved. I still have a partial balance impairment, but when my treatment was over, I decided to try to do the things I did before. The first time I played tennis, I threw back my arm to take a swing and fell over. Now I can rollerblade and windsurf, which are pretty hard even for people without problems. For me, it's important not to be afraid to accept challenges and to be proud of my accomplishments at whatever level.

Another goal I set for myself was to have a dinner party or cocktail party every other month. I even built a Caribbean-beach-bar party shack in my backyard. It's something I did to express myself and to have fun. I decided just to go ahead and do these things. I thought, "Why wait? The time is now."

—Sheri Sobrato

I HAVE AN M.S. in health education, and I worked for many years as a teacher until I decided I wanted to make more money. I got an M.B.A. in finance and worked on Wall Street. But after going through my breast cancer experience, I felt that the pendulum had swung too far toward money and that I needed to return to something more meaningful.

Today, I work at the Health Care Chaplaincy, which provides chaplains of every faith to hospitals throughout the country. We train students from all over the world and from Christian, Jewish, Muslim, Buddhist, Hindu, and Taoist traditions, to name just a few.

I was hired for many reasons: my M.B.A., my teaching career, and the fact that I was born Jewish but have recently been baptized a Protestant. But my experience as a cancer survivor gave me the best credentials for the job. It was at the cancer school of hard knocks that I learned about humility and faith and how to cope with life-and-death situations. God truly does work in mysterious ways. My life has been enriched by my cancer experience because it has led to a wonderful and meaningful new career.

—*Susan Fischer*

MY CANCER EXPERIENCE led me to ask my law firm if I could switch to part-time work. It wasn't an easy decision because basically it was an admission that becoming a partner was not a priority for me. They didn't really believe in that kind of setup, but since I had built up goodwill by working long hours in the past, they agreed to try it out.

I now work three days a week, and the other two days I have to myself. I set up a pottery studio in my apartment, where I spend hours making dinner sets, pitchers, and jars, and I've also learned to weave on a loom. I volunteer at several organizations. I help prepare hot meals for people with AIDS, record book tapes for blind people, and through the patient-to-patient program at Memorial Sloan-Kettering, I visit people who are undergoing treatment for cancer. The satisfaction I get from these different activities more than makes up for the salary cut I had to take at work.

—*Tali Havazelet*

Getting Back in Good Physical Shape

IT CAN TAKE a year—I've read even five years—for people to regain the energy and the stamina that they had before cancer treatment. And the older you are, the longer it takes. I've been finished with chemo and radiation for nine or ten months, and after going up two flights of stairs, I'm winded. I want to get back into an aerobics class, but my energy level isn't high enough yet. You really have to give yourself permission to let it come back gradually. Sleep a lot.

—*Lorraine Anderson*

I HAD BEEN running to get back in shape after my surgery, and one day I joked with the doctors about running the marathon. And then it dawned on me that it might be possible. I started running with friends who were serious runners, and we started training for the marathon and wound up running it. Eventually I started my own group, which is part of the Achilles Track Club. I work with troubled kids, and I've got them running too. It helps take their minds off their problems.

My way of dealing with this illness has been to use my body as well as my mind. It takes the pressure off. It helps you deal with pain. It helps you set goals and be a stronger person.

—*Rick Asselta*

REGAINING MY CONFIDENCE in competitive sports was a much longer and more involved process than I ever could have imagined. My Wednesday-night basketball game has been one of the few immutable dates on my calendar over the past seven years. I even played during my six months of chemo. It was humbling and emotional, because my body simply wouldn't respond, but I didn't want to use my illness as an excuse. Personally, I was pleased simply to be participating.

But long after my cancer went into remission, I was still not the same player I had been before. Even after having run a marathon, I was playing at a level far below my former capacity. That's when I learned how much my self-esteem depended upon my ability to compete and vice versa. The worse I played on the basketball court, the less freely I talked with my friends, the less naturally I could smile and laugh, the less moxie I had in my business dealings even. It became a descending spiral of self-loathing, and to avoid the embarrassment it was causing me, I regularly considered quitting an activity I truly loved.

Finally it dawned on me that it wasn't so much my physical condition. By running regularly, I had regained the conditioning in my lungs and legs. It was in my head. It was a reflection of my state of mind. I'll never forget the night after another disappointing outing, when afterward I told my good friend Nathaniel, "I don't know what's wrong with me. I'm just a freaking headcase." It was a low point. It was also the beginning of a change for the better.

Through the cancer experience, my goals and values had subtly changed. Competitive sports require a certain level of aggression, and I had lost some of that—the drive that would send me to the floor for loose balls and knowingly into a collision with a bigger player in order to retrieve a rebound. I was now more likely to stop and think before taking action. That's desirable in most of life's activities but not on the basketball court. Sports rely on instincts more than rational thought. The second you start to think about what *might* happen, you've missed the opportunity. I was no longer pushing players out of the lane on defense or driving instinctively to the hoop on offense.

It made me realize that dominating another guy on the court is all about confidence. I'm not necessarily stronger or quicker than the other guy, but if I have more confidence, I'm going to dominate that person anyway. I noticed that instead I allowed myself to be dominated—so much so that I even stopped calling fouls when I was fouled, which is a crucial aspect of the game. In my own mind, I didn't deserve to call a foul. I had lost my self-respect.

I could see that off the court as well. It really affected my self-esteem in the conversations after the games. I stopped talking. It was a big deal mentally.

Ultimately, it was about how I played the game. My state of mind—and game—had fundamentally changed. Once I realized that, I began to build a game that I could live with, and my fear of confrontation diminished.

—*Dean King*

AMPUTATION IS NOT the end of the world. I mountain-climb, I swim, I play basketball and softball. You can do everything you once did, though maybe not as quickly. I went back to coaching. I teach. Since then we've had a son. I've done everything I wanted to do. It just takes me a little longer.

After the surgery, you think it's the end of the world. But you can overcome anything if you strive for it and don't give up. You need to find something to do, something that can take your mind off your condition and make you stronger. You've got to believe in something. You have to have goals. My goal was walking. I was an athlete, and I still am.

At first, I just wanted to get my weight down, so I walked a couple of miles a day. Eventually, I developed a five-mile path that goes up and down the mountains. At first I walked without a cane, but I would fall, so I started using one. Then deep snows hit, and I started walking with two canes, and I still do. People began to walk with me, and it became fun. My goal is thirty miles a week, or fifteen hundred miles a year. I walk six days a week and rest one. I walk sometimes late at night, sometimes during the day, as long as I get in my five miles per day.

My son and a couple of friends and I are getting ready to walk the Appalachian Trail. It's going to take us a couple of years. We're going to walk in the summers, two months at a time. We'll start this summer in Georgia, and then we'll start back up the next summer. I've been on parts of the trail in the Smokies, but I'd like to do it all—just to say I accomplished it. To me, it's a matter of taking advantage of every second you can.

—*Danny Johnson*

Help for Getting Back on Your Feet

A lot of people are handicapped because of cancer, either from losing a limb or some other complication. I recommend the Achilles Track Club for people with disabilities and handicaps. The club, which was started in New York and has chapters around the country, operates workouts twice a week for people who have all kinds of disabilities. It gives you an opportunity to work out with people who are in a similar situation. It's a great organization in terms of prosthetics. (For instance, the people there give equipment advice—regarding fit, chafing, and wear and tear—to amputees who want to run on prosthetic legs.) Even if you're not feeling great, the Achilles people have something to offer you—an exercise program. You'll be surprised and amazed at what you can accomplish, no matter how great the challenge you face.

—Jeff Berman,
President, Cancer Support Services,
New York, New York

I'VE NEVER BEEN a runner. I'm six feet two inches and two hundred and sixty-five pounds. Even healthy, I could never run the marathon. But I could walk. The year before I got sick, I decided that I was going to walk the marathon as a challenge. And I did, although it took seven and a half hours.

The next year, I had cancer and couldn't join the marathon. I was looking for a support group, and I heard the Road Runners were thinking of starting one. So I joined the Road Runners Club. I was under treatment at that time—it was October and November of '92—and I couldn't do anything, so my niece, my wife, and I went over to Central Park and watched the race. We were spectators. That was the year that Fred Lebow, who started the New York Marathon and had brain cancer, ran the marathon with Grete Waitz. He was part of our support group.

After I finished my treatment, I wanted to prove that I was not on the way out, so the following year, I walked the marathon again. That was a great personal challenge for me. I did it with the Achilles Club, the handicapped group that walks the marathon. And even though it took me a half hour longer than the first time, the satisfaction of finishing—making a statement that I had conquered cancer—was wonderful.

—*Frank Sheridan*

WHEN MY CHEMO was over, my doctors said that things were coming along really well. They suggested radiation at Stanford, but my doctor here said it would definitely limit my ability to run again because they would have to radiate my lungs. Scar tissue would form in the lung lining, and the elasticity wouldn't be the same. So I vetoed the radiation and left it as an option if anything reappeared.

I challenged myself to get competitive again by trying to

qualify for the Olympic trials in 1996. I increased my training and started running some races. As the year progressed, I worked myself into marathon shape and qualified for the Olympic trials by running a marathon in Minnesota in June of 1995. It was about a year after I had finished my chemo. Then I kept training and ran in the Olympic trials marathon.

I'm not the elite that I used to be, but I'm fully competitive on a regional level. Of course, I'm almost thirty-six too. The guys I was competing with back four, eight years ago are also not running as fast as they were. The main thing is that I'm still out there and running pretty quick.

—*Mark Conover*

Making Babies

PRIOR TO GETTING cancer, I wasn't sure about kids or marriage, and now I couldn't be more sure. My career used to be so important to me. I was professionally successful, but I began to think, "If I'm diagnosed with this disease and end up dying in three years, I don't want my job to be the main thing I've had in my life." There are some jobs that I might feel differently about, but cancer underscored for me that I should be creating a life that makes me feel positive about what I'm giving. Having a family, volunteering with other cancer people, and finding a support group that works for me—these have become hugely important.

According to my doctors, the sooner I try to have a child the better. Jamie and I are getting married in a few months, and I'd like to start attempting to get pregnant right away, because the younger and healthier I am and the better shape I'm in, the better chance I have of carrying a baby. But I also want to build a marriage. I think they're two different things—building a family and building a marriage. But the bottom line is you can't necessarily plan what happens. Life doesn't work that way.

The first hurdle is, can I get pregnant? A cone biopsy really compromises your fertility because they remove part of the cervix, which is not only the muscle that holds the baby in while you're pregnant, it also contains lubricants that allow the sperm to travel up to the egg. Getting pregnant naturally can be difficult, but we're going to try before we go to any artificial methods. Then, I wonder if I can retain a fetus for nine months. Because I've had two procedures, chances are slim that I can carry a full-term pregnancy. As my doctor put it, "I wouldn't be really optimistic about it, but if I were young and healthy and had no children, I'd give it a shot."

That strikes me as fair. Quite frankly, I know a lot of people in the past few years who have had difficulty getting pregnant, and they've had no medical reason for it. I have the emotional advantage of knowing it's going to be difficult. I can start working on that now by getting myself geared up with my fiancé so that it doesn't pull us apart, but unites us. We know that it's going to be hard, and we're okay with that.

What frightens me is the concept of getting pregnant and carrying the baby for however many months only to suffer a miscarriage because my cervix can't handle it, even if it's been sutured shut. That experience would be very difficult. But I think I'd rather go through that and then deal with it than not try and wonder. That would be harder for me.

People love to tell you that there are other options. You can adopt. I know that, but that's a different experience. Yes, I want to raise a child, and I know I can do that, but I also want to *have* a child if possible. We're definitely going to give it a chance.

—*Rachel Kaul*

THE DOCTORS TOLD me that one of the long-term side effects of the chemo was infertility, but they said that girls who were older and had already started their periods when they began the chemo had less trouble than younger girls. Since I was nineteen and had been having my period since I was fifteen, they felt I had a better chance. Well, when the time came, I ended up getting pregnant pretty easily, believe it or not, but ironically, I had lots of problems with the pregnancy—breakthrough bleeding and placental abruption and preterm labor. The problems were unrelated to the chemo, though, and I ended up having a healthy baby boy.

—*Lisa Hollingsworth*

WE FOUND THAT people—even medical professionals—give you a lot of misinformation about the steps you might have to take to have a baby after undergoing cancer treatment. A nurse in the sperm lab that Dean went to told him that his four deposits would only provide enough sperm for two inseminations, with only a twenty-five- to forty-percent chance of success for each. That news not only was unwelcome in the frantic and confusing week between his diagnosis and beginning of treatment, but it also turned out to be untrue.

When we were trying to figure out how to best make use of our limited supply of frozen sperm, the first fertility specialist we went to said that it didn't make any difference whether we chose artificial insemination or in-vitro fertilization (IVF). He said that the amount of sperm used for each method was the same. Luckily, I had done some research, namely reading *How to Get Pregnant with the New Technology* by fertility expert Sherman J. Silber (Warner Books, 1991), and knew that IVF was the much more promising option in our case.

Obviously, the need for second opinions doesn't end with your treatment. The field of reproductive technology is booming, and new advances are made every day. For instance, just in the last few years, they have developed a way to separate a single, microscopic sperm and inject it into an egg, a pretty incredible feat when you consider that nature thought it necessary to shower an egg with a hundred million sperm, give or take a few.

The first step to take when you want to conceive after treatment is to consult with your oncologist or radiologist. Only your doctor can tell you when you have recovered enough from treatment to start on the task. It's hard to say who will have problems conceiving and who won't—and how long those problems will last. Chemotherapy can cause infertility in both men and women, but the likelihood of that depends on a lot of factors: your age when treated; the length of treatment; and the number, type, and dosage of drugs used in your treatment. Radiation to the pelvic region can also cause infertility for both sexes, again depending on the amount and length of treatment.

Unfortunately, for women, there are no egg banks as there are sperm banks for men. That's because it's impossible to freeze an unfertilized egg. You can freeze embryos (fertilized eggs), but the process involves taking fertility drugs for an entire menstrual cycle and then extracting the eggs for fertilization at just the right time. The month-long process (not to mention the extra hormones) is not really an option for most female cancer patients. But who knows? Doctors may come up with a solution to this problem soon. After all, they've only been doing in-vitro fertilization since the early eighties.

If you think your treatment has in fact impaired your fertility (for example, if you haven't been able to conceive after trying for six months), you should contact the American Society for Reproductive Medicine (1209 Montgomery Highway, Birmingham, AL 35216-2809; 205-978-5000) for the names of fertility specialists in your area. And don't despair: Even "hopeless" cases sometimes have happy endings!

—*Jessica King*

THEY TOLD ME it was likely that we couldn't have any more children because of the chemotherapy. We tried for a long time— naturally, that is. We didn't have any stored sperm or anything. Finally we kind of gave up. I told my wife we were trying too hard.

Then it just happened. We went to California to visit my wife's father. When we got back, my wife thought she was sick because she'd been traveling. She went to the doctor, and sure enough, she was pregnant. We had our son twelve years after our daughter.

Having another young one to work with has inspired me all over again. I coach him now in grade school and in baseball. I get out on the field and do all that stuff with him, and it's really motivated me again.

—*Danny Johnson*

A YEAR AND a half after my Hodgkin's disease went into remission, I ran the New York City marathon and felt like I was triumphantly putting bad health behind me. The next day my wife and I went to get the test results from my urologist, who I had gone to see because we had not been able to conceive during the past year.

Neither of us will ever forget his first words after we were seated in his office: "So you want to have children, but you have no sperm." That's how he broke the news to us that, based on these tests, he thought the chemotherapy had left me sterile. He had the verbal gifts of a loan officer. He recommended that I have a biopsy of the testicles to determine if, by chance, the lack of sperm was due to some kind of blockage. That turned out not to be the case. The doctor said, "You have less than a one-percent chance of ever being fertile. You should use the semen you have stored or adopt." It was the saddest news we had had since my diagnosis.

Then began the rounds of hormone injections and counting cycles and heart-stopping phone calls about the success or failure of each try that make up the world of in-vitro fertilization. Eighteen months later, thanks to the doctors and nurses at the Jones Institute in Norfolk, Virginia, and at Roosevelt Hospital in Manhattan, the efforts of many people paid off in Hazel, a beautiful baby girl.

She was a miracle of modern-day medicine—frozen sperm, harvested eggs, fertilization in a test tube. But the miracles weren't over. One morning just after Hazel's first birthday, Jess walked into Hazel's bedroom, where I was changing a diaper, and her hand was shaking. In it, she held a positive pregnancy test— the impossible positive pregnancy test. Eight months later, our second miracle baby, Grace, was delivered by the grace of God.

—*Dean King*

CHAPTER TWENTY-FIVE

Making Peace: Transcendental Moments, New Perspectives, Volunteering

Confronting and battling cancer is truly a profound, life-changing experience. Almost without exception, former patients agree that they are in many ways wiser, more sensitive, and stronger people for it. There is pain—emotional and physical—and there is grief, both personal and shared. But there is also humor and inspiration in the face of despair.

In a way, for patients and their support team, it's an initiation into a fuller understanding of what the human experience is all about. And when the smoke of the battle finally clears, a great deal of the experience—the pain and the suffering—fades mercifully into the back regions of our subconsciouses. Certain wonderful, life-affirming moments, however, remain like monuments in the battlefield.

Here, we share some of those transcendental moments, the events that had bigger meaning or were too funny to forget. They were hard-earned—only possible through our fights for recovery—and we're proud of them.

Finally, many of us feel compelled to return something, both for the care and kindness we received and because of our empathy for those now fighting cancer. Volunteering and visiting not only allow us to help others, but help us heal our own wounds. Giving back completes the process.

Transcendental Moments

NATIONAL REVIEW'S SCHEDULE, especially for the editorial people, or for me—I was a senior editor—was a part-time thing. I had to be in the office every other week to write the editorials and whatever else I was doing, but it was flexible. I was able to keep working during treatment. I even went to both conventions. The Democrats were in New York and the Republicans in Houston. I think my treatment had stopped by then, but I still didn't have any hair. And I did use it to my advantage once.

I was trying to interview President Bush for *The New York Times Magazine,* and his staff was blowing me off. So I was talking to Vic Gold, who is an old friend of mine and a very old friend of George Bush's—a kitchen-cabinet adviser—and I said, "Well, Vic, I'd really like to know when I can schedule this because I have to go into the hospital next week for chemotherapy." Ten minutes later, I got a call from Fitzwater: "You got the appointment." I guess that was a little sleazy, but I figured I'd make my cancer work for me.

—Richard Brookhiser

A FEW MONTHS into my treatment, my husband took me to the Canyon Ranch in Lenox, Massachusetts, for my birthday. At one of the after-dinner programs, the beauty specialist, a man, offered a makeup demonstration. All the women gathered in one room while the men went to watch a movie.

There were fifty women there, and the specialist came in and asked for a volunteer to make up. I raised my hand, along with forty other women. He picked me. I was wearing a black velvet turban with a scarf and bangs that were attached to the scarf by Velcro. He said to me, "Could you just brush your hair away?" I pulled the Velcro bangs off and said, "Are you ready for a challenge?" He said, "You're no challenge. You have high cheekbones. You're no challenge at all. But could you remove your hat? I want to do your whole face." So I did.

There wasn't a sound in the audience. There I was—with this big light shining down on me—totally bald except for maybe three little hairs. I said to him, "Well, I originally came in for a haircut," and everybody sort of gasped. He said, "Okay," and he took his scissors and snipped my three little hairs. More people were coming in from the dining room, and they were staring. I said, "You wouldn't believe it, but when I came in here I had such long hair, and look what this guy did to it." Everybody started to laugh.

"It's my birthday," I confessed. "That's why I'm here, and I want him to make me beautiful." Well, he did a lovely job, and people came up to me afterward with their cancer stories—about themselves, their mothers or sisters or friends. They all said I inspired them, and it was just wonderful. The next day, I went into the dining room, and all the men and women came over to our table to wish me a happy birthday.

—*Bev Yaffe*

I USED TO do snake shows at carnivals. I'd milk a rattlesnake, and then I'd drink some of the venom just to show people that it doesn't hurt you if it gets in your mouth. In fact, I had a snake show at Duke University after my third chemotherapy treatment. I had four days of intensive around-the-clock chemo, and the very next day, I did two programs back-to-back with fifty people in each group.

As part of the program, I'd take out a blacksnake, which is extremely aggressive, and let it bite my hand to show people that the bite of a nonpoisonous snake won't hurt you. So in the first program, when I took out the snake and stuck it up to my hand, he got a real good bite and drew some blood. After the show, I put him back in the bag and had a thirty-minute intermission before the next group came in. When it came time to do the blacksnake routine, I reached in and took him out of the bag, but he was stone-dead.

Reptiles are fragile, and my blood was so toxic that it had killed him. I got him behind the head and acted like he was alive and finished the program, but it just shows what that stuff is that they put into you. It's poison.

—*Tim McLaurin*

I REMEMBER BEING thrilled about taking a trip with a friend to visit another friend who lived on the Jersey shore. I dressed up, paying attention to my clothes, makeup, and, of course, my "hair." As my friend and I traveled down the parkway, I noticed the man driving next to us seemed to like what he saw. He started blowing kisses at me. I returned his kisses with a smile, and then, making sure I had his full attention, I whipped my wig off my head. His mouth, which had formed a kiss, suddenly hung open with horror as he screamed. His eyes were wide as he swerved right to exit the highway. It was a full ten minutes before my friend and I could speak. Our stomachs hurt from laughing. I thought, "Look out, construction workers, you're next!"

—*Kathleen Crowley*

ONE MORNING WHILE I was going through treatment, I ended up with a couple of hours of free time. I had taken part of the morning off work to go to a medical exam, but it was over in five minutes. I should have gone straight to work, but instead I went to City Island, New York, an island off the Bronx. As you cross the bridge onto the island, there's a little park. I sat there on a bench overlooking the water. The birds were flying, and the boats were rocking on their moorings.

It was very peaceful, and I was meditating. I was in touch with myself and the issues I had to deal with. Then I was distracted by a noise behind me. I turned around, and across the street from the park, a funeral procession was pulling up to a church. I thought, "A cheap way of saying prayers. I'll go over, and when they have a ceremony for this guy, I'll say some prayers." So I crossed the street and snuck into the back of the church.

I was back there, and they had a procession, and the deceased—apparently his name was Harold—came in with forty or fifty mourners and they had a mass for Harold. They started playing a hymn, and I thought, "My God, that's the most godawful hymn I've ever heard—they're not playing that at my funeral." So I sat there with a hymnal, and I picked out a hymn that was appropriate. Then they got up at the altar and started reading from the Scriptures. I said, "Jesus, that's the worst Scripture I've ever read. I'm not reading that at mine." So I crossed that off and chose some Scripture readings. This went on during the whole mass. Poor Harold, they buried him with the worst selection of prayers and hymns you could imagine. But by the end of the ceremony, I had planned out my whole funeral.

My wife and I were seeing a social worker for counseling. My wife was a nun for sixteen years, and she's a very spiritual person too. We have a spirituality that helps us deal with the major issues in life. So the same day that I attended Harold's funeral, my wife and I went to see our counselor, and he said, "Now, I usually don't do this, but because of the extent of Frank's cancer, I think we should introduce the topic of death. There is a possibility that you're going to die."

I said, "Let me tell you what happened to Harold." And we all had a good laugh.

—*Frank Sheridan*

I WAS GOING to the oncologist's office to meet my parents and discuss my latest MRI, which indicated another brain tumor. Somehow, I got on the wrong subway train, so I got off, ran upstairs, and hopped in a hotel cab that was supposed to be going to the airport. I said, "Could you take me to the Upper East Side?" I looked at his medallion. His name was Esperanza. I said, "Nice name. That means 'hope,' doesn't it?"

He said, "Yes."

I said, "I could use a little of that."

Looking in the rearview mirror, he said, somewhat coyly, "What, you? You're so beautiful. What could possibly be wrong in your life?"

I took that as something of a challenge. "Yeah, well, I'm going to the hospital to discuss my fourth brain surgery," I said. But that didn't faze him like I expected. He started asking me questions about my brain tumor. They were very intelligent questions. I answered them, and I said, "Esperanza, sounds like you know a lot about brain tumors."

He said, "I do."

I said, "Oh, my Lord, I hate to ask why."

He said, "Well, my little boy died of a brain tumor."

"I'm so sorry," I said. "You seem quite peaceful though."

He said, "I am peaceful, and I'll tell you why. My little boy died, and my wife and I were there. He'd been dead for two minutes and twenty seconds, and my wife and I called him back. My little boy—he was six years old—and when he came back, he looked at me and said with a smile on his face, 'Daddy, please let me die. It's so good.' "

I couldn't believe the coincidence of being on my way to Sloan-Kettering to discuss my brain tumor and getting in a random cab with a driver named Hope who was telling me about his son's peace. I took it as a positive sign.

—*Katie Brant*

MY BIGGEST FEAR was losing my leg. My doctor was quite straightforward about that. "I'm here to save your life," he said. "Your leg is second."

"Am I going to lose it?" I asked.

"I'll try my best to let you keep it, but it may have to go in order to save your life. Unfortunately, I won't know until I operate."

This news was not easy for me to take. In fact, losing a leg at the age of twenty-nine seemed like the worst possible thing. I was worried what people would think of me; I was worried about not being able to walk; I was worried about being ostracized and being thought of as "less than."

I forced myself to focus on what the doctor had said about wanting to save my life. If the leg had to go, then I would get a prosthesis. Maybe I wouldn't be able to walk as quickly as before, but at least I'd be around to take walks. I kept reminding myself of that fact, and it helped me to relax and to prepare myself for the surgery.

In the recovery room, I remember being nudged awake by my doctor. My mind was foggy from the drugs, but I clearly remember his words. "Can you wiggle your toes?" he asked.

"Yes," I said, as I moved them around under the blanket. Then it dawned on me what that meant. I pulled up the sheets and looked down. Yes, my leg was still there. I fell back on the pillow, and my eyes closed heavily as the drugs sent me back into a deep sleep. I woke up a few hours later with my lips creased upward in a deep, happy smile.

—*Mark Biundo*

TOWARD THE END of my treatment, my doctor and I could still feel some lumps deep in my neck, at the original site. He was pretty sure it was scar tissue, but the only way to know for certain was to have another biopsy. They couldn't schedule me for several weeks, and those next few weeks of waiting were the worst of the entire year. All the emotions I had been keeping rigidly in check erupted, and fear finally set in. What if they found something? I was terribly agitated, and I couldn't sleep. I tried to imagine what I would do if the news was bad, and my mind failed me. Instead, I had anxiety attacks. I shook and sweated and moaned, my stomach knotted. It was pure terror, unlike anything I had ever experienced. Sometimes I thought I would break apart. I burst into tears on the street, on the bus.

At other times, I would imagine my doctor telling me everything was okay. Then, I would weep tears of joy. I felt it in every cell in my body. It seemed like I could lift off the ground and fly for the happiness of being alive and well.

The biopsy day finally arrived. By then, I was quite out of my mind. I had called in the troops to help me. My friends took turns spending the night with me and were lined up to stay over during the waiting period afterward. On December 12, 1984, at 7:30 P.M., my doctor called. "It's normal," he said matter-of-factly.

"Say it again?"

"It's normal. It was scar tissue."

"You mean I don't have cancer anymore?" I asked, still unbelieving.

"Not that I know of. Not now."

"I love you," I declared with all my heart.

"You're not supposed to love your doctor." We were back to laughing, the sweetest, most welcome laughter I have ever experienced.

I ran across the street to my friend Janice, who had champagne cool and ready. Once again, I was crying on the phone to my mother and brother, but each of those teardrops contained indescribable joy. "It's all finished," I told them, "no more IVs, no more vomiting, it's all finished. I'm a healthy girl again." And I am.

—*Jacqueline Frank*

New Perspectives

IF I COULD say that any part of this was a fortunate experience for me, I would have to say that it put things into perspective in terms of what's important. I became infinitely more appreciative of the really wonderful things in life in a way that I was able to act on—not just "Oh, isn't everything wonderful? Aren't I a lucky person?" But I became much clearer of mind. I don't think I was a petty person before, but I sure discarded pettiness after. Although a certain amount of small-mindedness may be part of human nature, I have since found that those little things that people react to, say, a driver cutting you off, are so boring.

Something kicked in that made it easy for me to discard the uninteresting. Life actually became much more interesting because somehow I turned into this strange, positive person after having had what so easily could have been a thoroughly consuming negative experience. It was a deeply felt reaction that took shape gradually.

—Toni Zavistovski

IN A LOT of ways, I'm not sorry I got leukemia because it's made me more aware of life, what it means to see my children grow up and to have wonderful people in my life. I feel stronger because I got through a very difficult treatment and triumphed over the disease.

—Janice Thomas

ALTHOUGH I WOULDN'T wish the cancer experience on anyone, I felt I had been given a sort of gift, the rare opportunity for a young person not to take life for granted. I didn't tell this to many people—it sounded too melodramatic. But I started to feel it immediately and nourished it inside me. As the child of German-Jewish refugees, I had grown up hearing stories of heroism and survival. When I was young, I yearned to be put to the test. That part of me relished this opportunity to show that I, too, could be strong and courageous, that I, too, could be heroic.

After my battle with cancer, I learned to enjoy my life in many practical ways. I developed an active social life—going to movies, plays, operas, and concerts with my friends. My life became much less stressful, far simpler. I no longer needed to be a superwoman with my film-production career, relationships, and family. It was good enough to be alive and well and enjoying the moment.

—*Jacqueline Frank*

MY EXPERIENCE WITH cancer has made me make choices in my life a lot differently than I would have three years ago. Two weeks ago, I quit my job because I knew it wasn't good for me anymore. I wasn't happy going to work every day, and I felt I owed it to myself to be doing something that I'd enjoy.

Previously, I would have compromised myself, stuck it out and continued to be miserable, or waited for another job. I won't do that anymore. I know I've been given a second chance, and I have a very different mind-set. There's absolutely no reason for someone who's thirty years old to have gotten a mammogram, but I just thought it was the thing to do. Had I waited another six months, my doctor told me, the result would have been completely different.

That definitely put things in perspective. Although I'm still career-oriented and driven, I now control my life and my destiny a little bit more than if I were just going through the motions and doing what is expected. I still have to go to the oncologist every four months, and every four months, I still have that trepidation. But what's really important is that you can't stop living, that you don't take life for granted. I take more risks now.

—*Claire Noonan*

MY SISTER, WHO went through cancer throughout her twenties, was hugely helpful because she is a strong believer in the individuality of the experience—the license to feel however you feel. I think society and a lot of books, particularly a lot of books geared toward people with cancer, advocate an attitude like, "Oh, I had cancer and picked myself up by my bootstraps," or "I didn't let my life change" or whatever it is. A lot of the books made me feel kind of bad for feeling so devastated and confused and concerned by this.

The concept of going on and not changing your life because you have cancer is an odd one because the illness does change your life. Suddenly, you are different. Instead of being angry about it, I wanted to view it as a liberating experience. I'd gone through twenty-eight years of my life ruled by the fears and insecurities and uncertainties that we all have, and having cancer gave me permission and almost a mandate to look at things very differently, to reprioritize and decide what was important to me. It hasn't been a great experience, but it's given me the resolve to live as if I could get cancer again next year or next month—or not. Therefore, decisions that I'd been prolonging I'm not prolonging anymore. It really solidifies the fact that life is happening right now. And I want to act that way.

—Rachel Kaul

THE TERM "CANCER SURVIVOR" bothers me somewhat because I think of a survivor as someone clinging to a palm tree with everything gone except their life and their hanging-on. I don't think you should let cancer dominate your whole life afterward. I came out of there and didn't dwell on it. Eight months after my bone marrow transplant, I did a hundred-mile canoe trip down the Neuse River in the dead of winter.

In a sense, having cancer was a positive experience because it gave me an education that I otherwise would not have received. I received an education in the Marine Corps, an education at UNC, an education in the Peace Corps, but going through a bone marrow transplant was a totally unique experience and education. I saw a new side of life.

I'd like to say that I'm a cancer scholar instead of a cancer survivor. Given the choice, I'm not sure I would choose not to have cancer. It was an incredible experience. I learned a lot, and I got a lot of good writing out of it, and I'm alive to tell about it. There are other things that I've been through that were tougher, and I look at other people and see things that they've gone through that are incredibly more difficult.

On the plane home from Seattle after my bone marrow transplant, I read *All Quiet on the Western Front*. I had to wear a face mask to keep germs out. My face was all swollen up with steroids. I looked pretty much like a freak. But reading about those German soldiers living in the trenches of World War I for four years showed me that there are worse things you can go through and survive.

—*Tim McLaurin*

Volunteering

WHEN YOU'RE READY to give something back, then you've done your own healing. It's not what you have—it's what you do with it. That's true in every aspect of life. If you have money and you don't do something positive with it, what's the use of having it?

I look at cancer—and excuse me for saying this—as a gift, a learning experience, a wake-up call. It's something that says to you, "There's something more in your life that you need to do." It's up to you how you take it. You can say, "I'm going to work harder than I've ever worked at my job and put my nose to the grindstone and get more and more material things," or you can say, "How important is that? Where is that going to get me?" No one's last thought has been, "Gee, I should have spent more time in the office." It should be, "What can I do to make my life better, and what can I do to make the world around me a little bit better? Have I left a legacy?"

When Mark Conover, one of the volunteers at Cancer Support Services, qualified for the Olympic trials for the marathon after coming back from Hodgkin's disease, he said—and don't take this the wrong way—that everybody could use a tiny bit of cancer to get a little perspective in their lives. To realize how shiny your shoes are and how nice your cuff links are really means nothing compared to what you do with your life. You can have this happen and turn it into a learning experience. Or you can have this happen and pretend it was never there and just go right about your business. I think you miss the boat if you do the latter.

—*Jeff Berman*

I DO A lot of volunteering across the country with the American Cancer Society, mostly in the form of public speaking. It's really important for me to let people know that children or adolescents who have been diagnosed with cancer can live to become healthy, productive, contributing adults. When I was first diagnosed, it was important for me to demonstrate what could be accomplished when the human will refuses to accept defeat. I think one of the most powerful weapons we have in our arsenal against cancer is the human will. I have seen it time and time again. I have seen people not survive who were supposed to, who had very treatable diseases but would stay in a dark room and close their windows and feel sorry for themselves. We all go through that, but it's essential to rise above it.

—*Melanie McElhinney*

MY CANCERS WERE all related to cigarette smoking, so I decided to speak to schoolkids, young ones who haven't started yet. I warn them about the dangers of tobacco. I tell them my story, that I smoked from age seventeen until the day I woke up in a hospital postsurgery recovery room with tubes coming out of my body. I had lung cancer, and I was so addicted to nicotine that I had a cigarette right before—I mean *right* before—the surgery. I tell the kids that if they smoke, they can grow up to be just like me and, as a bonus, they can get heart disease. I show them all kinds of photos, charts, and graphs on the ill effects of smoking. The first question they usually ask is how they can get their parents to stop smoking. I see the fear in their eyes, and I believe that after seeing my lecture, most of them will never smoke.

—*Betty Dwin*

I VOLUNTEER WITH the Reach to Recovery Program, whose purpose is to aid women with breast cancer. We give information and assistance, including temporary prostheses, advice on getting a permanent prosthesis, and recommendations for exercises. But the main purpose is for people who have just been diagnosed or who have just had breast cancer surgery to see somebody who is a survivor and has gone on with her life. I think no matter what kind of cancer you have, that's one of the most important things you can do.

The women who volunteer in our program say they get more out of it than they put into it. They've all been out of treatment for at least a year and have completed an American Cancer Society training course to be able to participate in the program. It's hard to describe how rewarding it is to be able to give something back.

—*Elizabeth Martin*

IN MY DESPERATION during one of the dark moments of my illness, I went to see a rabbi.

"Rabbi," I asked, "Why? Why me? Why all of this?"

"There is no why," he responded. "And if there is a why, it is not for me to know." He continued, "But I can make a suggestion. When you're feeling better, do something for someone else. Try to help another human being. Give whatever you can. I promise that you will feel better for it."

Although I felt somewhat dissatisfied with the rabbi's suggestion—I wanted a hard answer to my question—I never forgot what he said, and years later when I started the Cure for Lymphoma Foundation, I came to understand what he meant. Last year, the foundation raised $250,000 for people who have lymphoma.

But more than the money I raise, it is the satisfaction I get from helping people that has made the rabbi's words so prophetic. I feel an indescribable spiritual reward when I tell someone who has lymphoma that I, too, was in the same hospital bed, getting the same chemo protocol, feeling the same fear and anxiety. I have been blessed by being able to give back, and at the same time, I get so much more for myself.

—*Jerry Freundlich*

The Importance of Teamwork

When I reflect on recent progress in the war against cancer, the concept of teamwork stands out as the key principle. *Cancer Combat*—an inspiring compendium of cancer-patient experiences—supports this concept by demonstrating, quite convincingly, that the cancer patient is an important team member in addition to being the focal point of this vital team.

At the beginning of my career in oncology, we called my field cancer surgery rather than surgical oncology. The emphasis of our work at that time was on increasing the survival statistics following treatment—the so-called cure rate. The other focus in those early days was the often mindless competition between the various medical disciplines dealing with cancer, i.e., surgery, radiation therapy, and the fledgling new specialty—chemotherapy. The emphasis then was on the patient's medical treatment and which member of the medical group could provide this treatment with optimal results.

Cancer care has clearly improved in the last half century, but not really in the way we envisaged some forty to fifty years ago. In my view, the major advances in cancer care over these years have been the development of an emphasis on the quality of life, rather than on the cure rate, and the vital importance of teamwork in accomplishing this goal. What is this "team" that is so important in achieving the goal of cancer care? Many chapters in *Cancer Combat* describe the major concerns and the important needs of the cancer patient at various stages of the discovery and the treatment process.

Some concerns are dealt with by the patient by taking personal control over the situation. Others are met by many specialized helpers. Some of these helpers are individuals with expertise in the medical disciplines, but there are many other advisers and helpers who provide nursing care, physical therapy, occupational therapy, counseling, social-work assistance, and other types of support that are so important to optimal patient care. Actually, this concept of the teamwork of multiple disciplines in cancer-patient care is the basis of a course in oncology that is offered to our medical students at the Medical College of Virginia.

What really stands out for me in the cancer-patient anecdotes appearing in this wonderful volume is the fact so often stated that the cancer patient is, and should be, a major player on this important team.

How should the patient actually view him or herself on the team? First of all, the dialogue in this volume clearly demonstrates the great value to the patient of being in control, to some degree. This extends from the discovery of this unexpected and unwanted diagnosis, to the acceptance of a treatment plan, and on to tolerance of the many adversities of effective treatments. From the people who have experienced those problems, the authors have collected valuable advice for the recently diagnosed cancer patient.

Several of the contributors are people whom I have had the privilege of knowing during these challenges that they have met so effectively. Suggestions from empathetic health-care personnel on the cancer-treatment team are presented also. The importance of the cancer patient's quality of life, as opposed to mere survival time, is clearly evident in all of these personal essays.

The things that really stand out, in my view, are the importance of the attitude of the cancer patient toward his or her disease, the attitudes of his health-care teammates, and the sense of control the newly diagnosed cancer patient has over his own situation. The message is loud and clear. The patient must retain a degree of personal control while at the same time being an effective member of the multifaceted team that is dealing with the many details of his or her cancer problem.

In the future, a focus on strategies for cancer prevention will surely have the most significant impact on cancer control nationwide. On the other hand, people of all ages will continue to develop cancers of various types, and each person will require diagnostic procedures, treatment, and rehabilitation. *Cancer Combat* tells each of us how we can contribute to our own welfare, our sanity, and our treatment process when that cancer patient is us.

—Walter Lawrence, Jr., M.D.,
Director Emeritus, Massey Cancer Center,
Richmond, Virginia, and
Former President of the American Cancer Society

RESOURCES

The American Association of Tissue Banks (AATB)
1350 Beverly Road, Suite 220-A
McLean, VA 22101
708-827-9582

American Brain Tumor Association
2720 River Road, Suite 146
Des Plaines, IL 60018
800-886-2282

American Cancer Society
National Office
1599 Clifton Road N.E.
Atlanta, GA 30329
Call to obtain the number for your local division and for information
about programs such as:

> **Reach to Recovery**—a peer/visitor program for women who have had
> breast cancer surgery, 800-ACS-2345.

Road to Recovery—a program that provides volunteers to drive patients to and from treatment, 800-ACS-2345.

Look Good . . . Feel Better—a program that provides techniques to overcome the aesthetic repercussions of cancer treatment (hair loss, cracked nails, etc.), 800-395-5665.

American Foundation for Urologic Disease
300 West Pratt Street, Suite 401
Baltimore, MD 21201-2463
800-828-7866

American Holistic Medical Association
919-787-5181
Call for a directory of complementary/alternative care practitioners.

American Institute for Cancer Research
800-843-8114
202-328-7744 in Washington, D.C.

The American Society of Clinical Hypnosis
220 East Devon Avenue, Suite 291
Des Plaines, IL 60018
Send a business-size SASE for referral to a professional hypnotist in your state.

The American Society for Reproductive Medicine (ASRM)
1209 Montgomery Highway
Birmingham, AL 35216-2809
205-978-5000
Provides a list of over 100 recommended sperm banks in the U.S. and Canada.

Bone Marrow Transplant Family Support Network
P.O. Box 845
Avon, CT 06001
800-826-9376
National telephone support network for patients and families.

Cancer Care, Inc.
1180 Avenue of the Americas
New York, NY 10036
212-302-2400
800-813-HOPE

CANSURVIVE
6500 Wilshire Boulevard
Los Angeles, CA 90048
310-203-9232

ChemoCare
231 North Avenue West
Westfield, NJ 07090-1428
800-55-CHEMO
908-233-1103 in New Jersey

Corporate Angel Network
914-328-1313 May provide free air transportation to distant treatment
centers via corporate jets.

Encore
212-614-2827
A YWCA-sponsored program for breast-cancer patients.

Hill Burton Free Hospital Care
800-638-0742 Run by the federal government, this program provides free
care to those who qualify.

International Myeloma Foundation
2120 Stanley Hills Drive
Los Angeles, CA 90046
800-452-CURE

Leukemia Society of America
600 Third Avenue
New York, NY 10016
800-955-4LSA (educational materials)
212-573-8484 (general information)

National Association of Claims Assistance Professionals
708-963-3500

National Brain Tumor Foundation
785 Market Street, Suite 1600
San Francisco, CA 94103
800-934-CURE

National Cancer Institute
800-4-CANCER
301-402-5874

The following materials are available through NCI's Cancer Information Service:

Physician Data Query—a list of the most current treatments

"Chemotherapy and You: A Guide to Self-Help During Treatment"

"Radiation Therapy and You: A Guide to Self-Help During Treatment"

A list of NCI cancer centers

National Coalition for Cancer Survivorship
1010 Wayne Avenue, Fifth Floor
Silver Spring, MD 20910
301-650-8868

United Ostomy Association, Inc.
36 Executive Park, Suite 120
Irvine, CA 92614
800-826-0826

Y-ME National Organization for Breast Cancer Information and Support
212 West Van Buren, Fourth Floor
Chicago, IL 60607
800-221-2141
312-986-8228 (24-hour hotline)
Provides telephone counseling, educational programs, and self-help meetings for breast cancer patients, their families, and friends.

BOOKS THAT HELPED US

Anatomy of an Illness as Perceived by the Patient by Norman Cousins (Bantam)

Beauty and Cancer by Diane Noyes (AC Press)

The Breast Cancer Companion: From Diagnosis Through Treatment to Recovery: Everything You Need to Know for Every Step Along the Way by Kathy LaTour (Avon)

Breast Cancer Journal: A Century of Petals by Juliet Wittman (Fulcrum)

Cancer and Vitamin C: A Discussion of the Nature, Causes, Prevention, and Treatment of Cancer with Special Reference to the Value of Vitamin C by Ewan Cameron and Linus Pauling (Linus Pauling Institute)

The Cancer Conqueror: An Incredible Journey to Wellness by Greg Anderson (Andrews & McMeel)

The Cancer Dictionary by Roberta Altman and Michael J. Sang, M.D. (Facts on File).

Chicken Soup for the Soul: 101 Stories to Open the Heart and Rekindle the Spirit by Jack Canfield and Mark V. Hansen (Health Communications)

Chicken Soup for the Surviving Soul: 101 Healing Stories of Courage and Inspiration by Jack Canfield, Mark Victor Hansen, Patty Aubery, and Nancy Mitchell, R.N. (Health Communications)

Discovering the Power of Self-Hypnosis: A New Approach for Enabling Change and Promoting Healing by Stanley Fisher, M.D. (HarperCollins)

Fighting Cancer: A Step-by-Step Guide to Helping Yourself Fight Cancer by Richard and Annette Bloch (Cancer Connection)

First, You Cry by Betty Rollin (Lippincott)

Flax Oil as a True Aid against Arthritis, Heart Infarction, Cancer and Other Diseases by Dr. Johanna Budwig (Apple Publishing Company)

From Victim to Victor: The Wellness Community Guide to Fighting for Recovery for Cancer Patients and Their Families by Harold H. Benjamin with Richard Trubo (Dell)

Getting Well Again: A Step-by-Step, Self-Help Guide to Overcoming Cancer for Patients and Their Families by O. Carl Simonton, M.D., Stephanie Matthews-Simonton, James Creighton (J.P. Tarcher)

Healing and the Mind by Bill D. Moyers (Doubleday)

How to Get Pregnant with the New Technology by Sherman J. Silber (Warner Books)

How to Live Longer and Feel Better by Linus Pauling (W. H. Freeman)

It's Always Something by Gilda Radner (Simon & Schuster)

The Keeper of the Moon: A Memoir of a Boyhood in the South by Tim McLaurin (Norton)

Life on the Line by Karl Nelson and Barry Stanton (WRS Group)

Listening to the Body: The Psychophysical Way to Health and Awareness by Jean Houston and Robert E. L. Masters (Delta)

Love, Medicine, and Miracles: Lessons Learned About Self-Healing from a Surgeon's Experience with Exceptional Patients by Bernie S. Siegel (Harper & Row)

The Merck Manual of Diagnosis and Therapy (Merck)

My Breast: One Woman's Cancer Story by Joyce Wadler (Addison-Wesley)

Quantum Healing: Exploring the Frontiers of Mind Body Medicine by Deepak Chopra (Bantam)

Recalled by Life: The Story of My Recovery from Cancer by Anthony J. Sattilaro, M.D., with Tom Monte (Houghton Mifflin)

Sexuality and Fertility After Cancer by Leslie R. Schover (John Wiley and Sons)

Superimmunity: Master Your Emotions and Improve Your Health by Paul Pearsall (McGraw-Hill)

Time on Fire: My Comedy of Terrors by Evan Handler (Little, Brown)

When Bad Things Happen to Good People by Harold S. Kushner (Schocken Books)

Where the Buffaloes Roam: Building a Team for Life Challenges by Bob Stone and Jenny Stone Humphries (Addison-Wesley)

INDEX

Abruscato, Leigh, and breast
    cancer, 8, 209–10, 214,
    234–35, 294, 336
Achilles Track Club, 369, 371
Actor's Fund, 352
Adriamycin, 10, 189, 209
Aicher, Patty, 9, 310–11
alternative or complementary
    treatments, 13, 16, 18, 249–
    68
American Brain Tumor
    Association, 333
American Cancer Society, 333
    Limited Financial Assistance
    Program and RIG (Resource
    Information and Guidance),
    348
    Reach for Recovery Program,
    207, 389–90
American Fertility Society, 376
American Foundation for
    Urologic Disease, 333
American Holistic Medical
    Association, 263
American Institute for Cancer
    Research, 118, 283
American Society of Clinical
    Hypnosis, 260
AML. See leukemia
amputation, 15, 18, 21, 34,

    188–95, 237–38, 277–79,
    317–18
    alternatives, 11, 89
    phantom pains, 195–96
    physical activity after, 370–71
Anatomy of an Illness (Cousins),
    253
Anderson, Lorraine, and breast
    cancer, 9, 115–16, 138–39,
    165–66, 205, 235, 288, 335,
    368
Andreef, Michael, 102
anger, 40, 54, 77
anthroposophic doctor, 264–65
Aquino, Elizabeth, 7
Arthur, Katherine, and breast
    cancer, 9, 210, 216, 305,
    316, 341
Asselta, Rick, and cancer of the
    esophagus, 10, 56–57, 182–
    83, 184–85, 187–88, 329–
    30, 369
Ativan, 142
Atkin, Karen, 75, 306
attitude. See also fear;
    perspectives
    at diagnosis, 43, 48, 49, 50, 56,
    57, 60, 63
    and doctor's manner, 97–98
    focusing on individual task, 78

attitude (*continued*)
positive, 85–86, 88–89, 278–80
and recovery, 188–95
relation to treatment, 43, 51, 53, 105, 276
releasing emotions, 81
Avacato, Donna, and osteosarcoma, 10, 89, 301

B
Baptist-Montclaire Hospital, Birmingham, AL, 20
Batchelder, Tim, and Hodgkin's disease, 10, 365
Baylor Hospital, Dallas, 19
Berman, Jeff, and chronic lymphocytic leukemia, 10, 330, 357–58, 372, 388
Beth Israel Medical Center, NY, 25
bilateral lymph node dissection, 31
Biundo, Mike, and sarcoma, 11, 83, 300, 383
blood tests, 108–9
bone cancer, 18. *See also* osteogenic sarcoma; osteosarcoma; sarcoma
bone marrow biopsy, 112, 113
bone marrow tests, 112–13
bone-marrow transplant, 3, 12, 14, 19, 22, 24, 25, 28, 33, 197–206, 271–72, 275–76, 335–36
Family Support Network, 198
financial/insurance concerns about, 351–53, 356–57
on-line chat sessions, 117
and pain control, 78
perspective on, 204–5, 387–88

stem cell transplant, 11, 33, 78, 141, 197
brachytherapy, 11
Brant, Katie, and brain tumor, 11, 57–59, 104–5, 147, 153, 167, 235–37, 241–42, 382–83
brain tumor, 11, 23, 28, 32, 57–60, 83–84, 85, 104–5, 185, 235–37, 366–67
breaking the news, 66–76
"cancer," using the word, 68, 69, 73
children, telling, 72–76
and cultural stigmas, 71
to dating partners, 366
delegating someone to tell for you, 65–66, 69
to immediate family, 66–68, 69
keeping silent, and emotional pain, 70
keeping silent, and family members, 70–71
openness, 71
sharing details, 68, 72
sharing fears, 70
at the workplace, 69–70, 71, 72
breast cancer, 8–9, 17, 23, 24, 25, 26, 27, 29, 31, 32, 34, 35, 49–51, 86, 92, 95, 115–16, 119–20, 140, 143, 207–19
and autologous bone marrow transplant, 197, 204, 207
dating/sex after, 212–13
effect of doctor choice on, 97–98, 99
and genetic risk of (runs in family), 218–19

hospital stay, 174
lumpectomy, 209
mastectomy, 208–13, 336
Reach for Recovery Program,
207, 389–90
and reconstructive surgery, 96–
97, 207, 213–18
support hot-lines, 207–8
survivability, 80, 207
Brigham and Women's Hospital,
Boston, 10
Bright's disease, 96
Brookhiser, Richard, and
testicular cancer, 11, 60–61,
108–9, 170, 224–25, 240–
41, 258, 260–61, 379
Budwig, Johanna, 265
Burt, Mary, 230

C
Camp Bluebird, Lafayette, LA,
331
Cancer Care, 333, 358
Cancer Dictionary, The (Altman
& Sarg), 106, 118
"Cancer Information: Where to
Find Help," 119
Cancer Support and Information
Center, Menlo Park, CA,
328
Cancer Survivor, The
(Glassman), 280
CANSURVIVE, 334
Card, Irene C., 351
CAT scans, 110–11
cervical cancer, 21, 53–56, 100–
101, 181–82, 274, 365–66,
373–74
ChemoCare, 334
chemotherapy, 137–57. *See also*
fertility concerns

appetite, maintaining, 154–55,
284, 287, 288–92
and courage, 137–38, 209–10
and fertility, 132–33, 134,
374–77
and life goes on, 155–57, 233–
48
and pain, 144
port-a-cath or Broviac catheter
for, 141
preparing yourself, 138–41
side effects, controlling nausea
and other, 2, 141–53, 240,
252, 261–62, 264, 290–
92
support/encouragement during
treatments, 81, 316–17
types of, 119, 143, 145, 150–
51, 209, 238, 276–77
and Zofran, 33, 78, 138, 143–
44, 155, 260
"Chemotherapy and You: A
Guide to Self-Help During
Treatment," 138
Chenoweth, Kay, and pancreatic
cancer, 12, 257–58, 264–66,
331
Chesney, Maurice, and lung
cancer, 12, 95, 250–51, 267,
315–16
children. *See also* fertility
concerns
born after cancer diagnosis and
treatment, 13, 14, 21, 23,
373–77
dealing with a parent's cancer,
302–6
red flags about trouble dealing
with parent's cancer, 305–6
telling about diagnosis, 72–76
and treatment choices, 104

Chopra, Deepak, 257–58
chronic cancer, dealing with, 269–72
Clair, Jeanne, and non-Hodgkin's lymphoma, 12, 142, 160, 202–3, 274–76
Clara Maass Medical Center, NJ, 14
Clark, George, and testicular cancer, 12, 266–67, 276–77
Clement, Ed, M.D., 7, 13
Clement, Jim, and testicular cancer, 13, 80
colon cancer, 13–14, 286
Columbia-Presbyterian Medical Center, NY, 31, 52
Community East Hospital, Indianapolis, 34
Compazine, 142–43, 145
cone biopsy, 55, 181–82, 373
Conner, Peggy, 355
Conover, Mark, and Hodgkin's disease, 13, 41–43, 69, 151, 242, 314, 372–73, 388
Cooper, Estelle, and lung cancer, 13, 93, 99
Cousins, Norman, 253–54
Cox, Scott, and colon cancer, 13–14, 142–43, 310
Crowley, Kathleen, and acute lymphoblastic leukemia, 14, 381
Cure for Lymphoma Foundation, 18, 390

D

Dalo, Tony, and cancer of the larynx, 14, 100, 286–87
Deaconess Hospital, Boston, 24
death rates, 4
denial, 70, 328

at diagnosis, 48
depression, 234
  and chemotherapy, 150
  after recovery, 363–64
  and tamoxifen, 336
diagnosis, response to, 39–60
  miminizing the sense of loss, 44–45
Dieppa, José M., 161
Dixon, Candace "Mamie," and Hodgkin's disease, 14–15, 42–43, 113, 156
doctors
  advice on being a good patient, 102
  anger at, 54
  assessing, 91
  attentive, 2–3, 54
  bedside manner, 91, 92–95, 119–20, 167
  and communication, 98–105
  compassion, 94, 189
  and control of treatment, 101
  differing competence of, 2, 46, 49, 56, 62
  insensitivity/arrogance of, 2, 40, 53, 92
  notebook, recording notes and doctor's answers in, 100
  qualities affecting choice, 91–92, 182
  questioning, 91, 98, 100
  second opinions, 4, 11, 59, 91–92, 95–98, 181
  surgeons, 179–80
Dressler, June, and uterine cancer, 15, 40, 321–22
Drucker, Abby, and mother's uterine cancer, 15, 98–99, 310
Ducksworth, Frederick, Jr., and

soft-tissue sarcoma, 15, 194–96

Dunne, Jerry, and non-Hodgkin's lymphoma, 15–16, 112–13, 285–86

Dwin, Betty Marx, and throat cancer, 16, 366, 389

E

Eastman, Laura, 16

Eldrid, Kathleen (primitive neural ectodermal tumor), 16–17, 95–96

Encore National Board, 208

encouragement, 80

Epstein, Fred, 59

esophagus, cancer of, 10, 56–57, 182–83, 184–85, 187–88

experimental protocols, 31, 104–5

F

faith healers, 267–68

family, 293–311
  children of a parent with cancer, 302–6
  extended, 310–11
  fears of, 79–80
  parents, 297–301
  parents' perspective, 301–2
  sharing diagnosis with, 70–71
  siblings, 306–8
  spouses, from patient's point of view, 294–96
  spouses, supporting, 296–97
  as support group, 78, 298, 318–20
  talking to cancer veterans for you, 78

fear, 44, 49, 51, 77–89
  and communication, 98
  and meditation, 113
  moving from, to peace, 84–85
  post-treatment, 362–63
  and radiation therapy, 159

feelings. *See also* anger; depression; fear; grief; sense of loss
  acknowledging, 81, 82
  post-treatment reactions, 362–63

Feldenkrais, Moshe, 211

Fellowship Community, Spring Valley, NY, 264

fertility concerns
  choosing and using a sperm bank, 132–33
  conception information, 365
  frozen sperm taken before treatments, 3, 128–32, 134
  making babies after cancer, 373–77
  and radiation, 159

fibrous histiocytoma, 34, 48–49, 190

financial concerns. *See also* insurance companies
  assistance from hospital social worker, 353–55
  assistance from organizations, 347–48
  bill collectors, dealing with, 348, 356
  documentation/paperwork, 348–49
  and Medicaid, 353

First You Cry (Rollin), 208

Fischer, Susan, and breast cancer, 17, 80, 159, 162, 284, 300, 362–63, 367–68

Fisher, Stanley, 260

Flax Oil as a True Aid Against Arthritis, Heart Infarction, Cancer, and Other Diseases (Budwig), 265

Fortunes of War, The (O'Brian), 82

Fox, Michele, and acute monocytic leukemia, 17, 45–46, 112, 121, 146–47, 175, 176–77, 256–57, 314–15, 329, 384

Frank, Jacqueline, and Hodgkin's disease, 17, 316–17, 363–64, 385–86

Freundlich, Jerry, and non-Hodgkin's lymphoma, 17–18, 98, 234, 390

friends, as support system, 312–25

  things to ask of them, 318–19

G

Georgetown University Hospital, 329

Gilda's Club, 3, 15, 28

Goss, Bill, and melanoma, 18, 105, 294

grief. *See also* sense of loss

  at diagnosis, 50, 66

Gunter, Ivy!, and bone cancer, 18, 156–57, 190, 237–38, 313

H

hair loss, 18, 145, 153, 157, 220–32

  looking your best, tips, 228–30

Hall, John, and Hodgkin's disease, 18–19, 103, 118–19, 153, 156, 253

Handler, Enid, and leukemia of her son, 19, 205–6, 301–2, 348, 351–52, 355–56

Handler, Evan, and acute myelogenous leukemia, 19, 130–32, 172–73, 177–78, 203–4, 242–43, 251–52, 348–49

Handzo, George, 339–40, 342

Havazelet, Tali, and ovarian cancer, 19–20, 151, 226, 313–14, 368

Higginbotham, Ginnie, and ovarian cancer, 20, 96, 155, 180–81

Hill Burton Free Hospital Care, 348

Hodgkin's disease, 1–4, 10, 12, 13, 14–15, 17, 18–19, 21, 24, 26–27, 29, 33, 40–44, 82, 93–94, 101, 110–11, 118–19, 120–31, 149–50, 337–38, 372, 376–77

  bone marrow transplant, 24, 26–27, 271–72

  causes, 365

  financial assistance, 347

  post-recovery depression, 363–64

  recurrence, 271–74

Hollingsworth, Lisa Eubanks, and leukemia, 20, 46–48, 155, 157, 240, 284, 295, 374

Horsley, John Shelton, M.D., 7

hospital stays, 169–78

  billing problems, 188, 353, 355–56

  control, taking, 172–74

  good experiences, 203–4

  rooms, changing/decorating, 170–71

social worker, help with fees/
charges, 348, 353
*How to Get Pregnant with the
New Technology* (Silber), 375
humor, 86, 112, 175, 177–78,
224–25, 240–41, 309–10,
379–81
hypnosis, 258–60

I
Indiana University Medical
Center, 25
information on cancer, 117–27
on-line, 117–18, 122–26
insomnia, 147
insurance companies. *See also*
financial concerns
claims forms, 355–56
difference between companies,
357
disputed charges, 347–48, 357
experimental procedures, 356–
57
getting the most from, 349–51
items not covered, 352
limitation of coverage, 353–54
National Association of Claims
Assistance Professionals, 351
refusal to pay, 352–53, 357–
58
student policy, 353–54
International Myeloma
Foundation, 334
Iscador, 264–65

J
Jackson Memorial Hospital,
Miami, FL, 15
Johns Hopkins Hospital, 19,
203–4, 205–6, 209
Johnson, Danny, and synovial

sarcoma, 20–21, 239, 278–
79, 370–71, 376
Jubb, Betsy, 124

K
Kaplan Cancer Center, NYU
Medical Center, NY, 10
Kaplan, Jill, 171
Kaul, Leslie, and Hodgkin's
disease, 21, 40–41, 93–94,
114–15, 162, 245–46, 307–
8, 331–32, 337
Kaul, Rachel, and cervical
cancer, 21, 53–56, 100–101,
181–82, 185, 244, 274,
307–8, 327, 365–66, 373–
74, 386–87
Keeper of the Moon, The
(McLaurin), 86, 279
King, Dean, and Hodgkin's
disease, 21–22
and blood tests, 108
and CAT scan, 110–11
and chemotherapy, 138, 151
and fear, 82
having children after cancer, 3,
374–77
and hospital gowns, 167–68
and radiation therapy, 160–61
and rectal exams, 113–14
and sperm bank, 134, 374–
75
sports after cancer, 369–70
and steroids, 287
waiting room time, 107
and writing of book, 2
King, Jessica, 21–22
and care/support of cancer
patient, 289, 296
and children, after cancer, 374–
76, 377

King, Jessica (*continued*)
  coping, 79–80, 120–21, 364–
    65
  and Dean's chemotherapy, 289,
    296
  and Dean's radiation, 160–61
  hearing the news, 1–2, 79–80
  and information on Hodgkin's
    disease, 120–21
  and insurance company, 356
  and second opinions, 160–61
  and sperm bank, 365
  and support systems, 315
  writing the book, 3
Ko, Monica, and non-Hodgkin's
  lymphoma, 22, 71, 152,
  175–76, 225, 264
Kogel, Joe, and melanoma, 22,
  103–4
Kruk, John, and testicular
  cancer, 22–23, 61–64,
  166
Kubel, Gloria, 285

L
Laggner, Susan, and
  medulloblastoma, 23, 85
laparotomy, 17, 162
LaPorte, Madeleine, and ovarian
  cancer, 23, 104
laryngectomy, 366
larynx, cancer of the, 14, 100,
  286–87, 366
Lawrence, Karen, and breast
  cancer, 23, 70, 327–28,
  366
Lawrence, Walter, Jr., 7, 391–
  93
Lebow, Fred, 330, 372
Lenox Hill Hospital, 10
leukemia (all types), 10, 14, 17,
    19, 20, 25, 33, 34, 45–48,
    112, 121, 146–48
  financial assistance, 347
  and hospital stays, 172–73
Leukemia Society of America,
  334, 347
Levy, Jodi, and non-Hodgkin's
  lymphoma, 23–24, 68, 79,
  126, 139–40, 162, 222–23,
  225–26, 230, 299, 322–24
  financial assistance, 347
Life on the Line (Nelson), 27
lifestyle after cancer, 155–57,
  233–48, 318–19
Listening to the Body (Houston
  and Masters), 211
Livingston Foundation Medical
  Center, San Diego, CA, 12,
  266–67
Long Island Jewish Medical
  Center, 35
Love, Meditation, and Miracles
  (Siegel), 252
lung cancer, 12, 13, 93, 99
  non-small cell, 29, 81
  pneumonectomy, 12
  treatability of, 12, 95
lymphangiogram, 166
lymphoma. *See* Hodgkin's
  disease; non-Hodgkin's
  lymphoma

M
M-BACOD, 119
macrobiotic diet, 22, 103
Magnetic Resonance Imaging
  (MRI), 111–12
Maharishi Ayurveda Health
  Center, 257, 265
Maine Medical Center, Portland,
  ME, 16

Malen, Josh, and Hodgkin's disease, 24, 234, 301, 322, 335–36

Manheimer, Karen, non-Hodgkin's lymphoma, 24, 81, 110, 140, 152, 154–55, 172, 221–22, 239

Mannheim, Harriet, 319

marijuana, for nausea, 151, 260–61

Martin, Elizabeth, and breast cancer, 8, 24, 86, 139, 152, 212, 217–19, 324, 364, 389–90

Masinelli, Theresa A., 230

Matsch, Kristina, and breast cancer, 25, 96–97, 213–14, 221, 223–24

Matus, Catherine, and ovarian cancer, 9

McConnell, Karla (AML), 25, 72–73, 170–71, 176, 231–32, 294–96, 306, 315, 319–20, 340

McElhinny, Melanie, and osteogenic sarcoma, 25–26, 177, 188–90, 192–94, 317–18, 388–89

McElveen, Leland J., 94

McGehee, Eleanor, 88

McLaurin, Tim, and multiple myeloma, 26, 85–86, 199, 279, 290, 356–57, 380, 387–88

M. D. Anderson Cancer Center, Houston, TX, 20, 96, 147, 238

Medicaid, 353, 358

Medical College of Virginia, Richmond, VA, 25, 34, 392

medical records, keeping own file, 100–101

medical team, 391–93. *See also* doctors; nurses

meditation, 250–58
and fear, 113
mindfulness, 87–88

melanoma, 18, 22, 30, 51, 103–4, 105, 118, 185–87

Memorial Sloan-Kettering Cancer Center, 3, 10, 11, 12, 14, 15, 17, 18, 19, 21, 22, 23, 27, 31, 32, 339

Mobile Infirmary Medical Center, Mobile, Alabama, 9

monoclonal antibodies, 24

Moosnick, Marcia, and breast cancer, 26, 109, 140

Mount Sinai Medical Center, NY, 16, 19, 24

mouth sores, 151–52, 162, 227

multi-targeted treatment approach, 4

My Breast (film), 212

myeloma, multiple, 4, 26, 30–31, 85–86, 387–88
bone marrow transplant, 356–57, 387–88
vaccine program, 31

N

Narcisco, Frank, and Hodgkin's disease, 26–27, 140, 271–72

National Association of Claims Assistance Professionals, 351

National Brain Tumor Foundation, 334

National Cancer Institute (NCI)
death rate statistics, 4
-designated cancer centers, 90

radiation therapy, 159
toll-free number, 90, 117
National Coalition for Cancer
  Survivorship, 334
nausea. *See* chemotherapy;
  radiation therapy; Zofran
Nelson, Karl, and Hodgkin's
  disease, 27, 109, 145–46,
  148, 149–50, 152, 162–63,
  272–74, 288
New York Hospital, 12, 31
New York Road Runners Club,
  NYC, 330, 372
New York University Medical
  Center, 11, 32
non-Hodgkin's lymphoma, 3, 12,
  15–16, 17–18, 24, 28, 31,
  51–53, 79, 81, 83, 88–89, 98,
  100, 111–13, 121–22
  bone-marrow transplant for, 3,
    12, 22, 33, 198, 199–202,
    275–76
  chemotherapy protocol, 119
  follicular nodular lymphoma,
    33
  recurrence, 274–76
Noonan, Claire, and breast
  cancer, 27, 49–51, 68, 69–
  70, 143, 172, 174, 176, 184,
  212–13, 214, 386
Noyes, Diane, and ovarian
  cancer, 27–28, 81, 230–31,
  232, 239
nurses, 92, 93–94, 109, 148–
  49, 160, 176–77
nutrition and diet, 265–66,
  283–92
  soy as a cancer-fighting
    supplement, 285
  vitamin supplements, 261–62,
    266–67

O
O'Brian, Patrick, 82
orchiectomy, 13, 31
oropharynx, cancer of, 16
osteogenic sarcoma, 25, 188–90
osteosarcoma, 10, 89
ovarian cancer, 9, 19–20, 23,
  27–28, 35, 81, 96, 104,
  180–81
Owen, Kathy, and brain tumor,
  28, 59–60, 185

P
pain
  art, as relief, 255–56
  and chemotherapy, 144
  coping with, 258–61
  and hypnosis, 258–60
  and mindfulness meditation,
    88
  post-surgical, 184–85
pancreatic cancer, 12, 92–93,
  126–27
  complementary medicine for,
    264–65
  islet cell carcinoma, 35
  Whipple procedure, 12
Paoli Memorial Hospital, PA,
  25
PDQ (Physician Data Query),
  117
Pearlroth, Ariana, 7
Pearlroth, Jonathan, and non-
  Hodgkin's lymphoma, 28
  attitude, 71–72, 83, 88–89,
    174, 344–45
  bone marrow transplant, 3, 28,
    198–202, 352–53
  breaking the news, 66–68
  chemotherapy, 28, 88, 101,
    119, 128–30, 154, 226–27

control over treatment, 83, 101, 119
financial concerns, 352–53
nutrition and diet, 154
philosophy, 28, 344–45
recurrence, 3, 198
scheduling testing, 115
self-image/hair loss, 226–27
sperm bank, 128–30
support systems, 174, 320–21, 324–25
surgery, 28
total body radiation, 28
volunteerism, 3, 28
Pennington, Charlene, 310
perspectives, new, after cancer, 191, 328–29, 336, 367–68, 369–70, 378–90
transcendental moments, 379–84
volunteering, 388–90
Phinney, Damon, and prostate cancer, 28–29, 254, 269–71, 280
Phinney, Davis, 29
Piedmont Hospital, Atlanta, 18
pneumonectomy, 11
Polk, Melanie, 292
Porter, Elsa, and breast cancer, 29, 99, 211, 217
prayer, 339, 340, 344. *See also* religious beliefs, as support
prednisone, 145–46, 185
primitive neuroectodermal tumor, 16, 95–96
Princess Margaret Hospital, Toronto, 29
prostate cancer, 28, 269–71
psychotherapy, 334–38

Q
Quantum Healing (Chopra), 257

R
radiation therapy, 158–68
dental care, 159, 163–65
and infertility, 159
information on, 159
lifestyle during treatment, 233–48
for sarcoma, 11
second opinions, 160
side effects (including nausea), 158–59, 163–67, 331–32
tattooing, 159–60, 161, 162
total body, 14, 28
"Radiation Therapy and You: A Guide to Self-Help During Treatment," 159
Rakoff, David, and Hodgkin's disease, 29, 130, 337–38
Ravan, Genya Zelkowitz, and non-small cell lung cancer, 29–30, 81, 252
reactions of others to cancer, 320–24
recovery and re-entering life, 361–77
and depression, 363–64
fears of recurrence, 363
getting back in physical shape, 368–73
new beginnings, 366–68
post-treatment emotions, 362–63
rectal exams, 113–14
recurrence, dealing with, 271–77
Rein, Ilana, 7
Rein, Jody, 7
relaxation and calming techniques, 79, 80, 87–88, 150, 257, 335. *See also* meditation; visualization
religious beliefs, as support, 85, 339–46

Ritchfield, Blythe, and squamous cell cancer, 30, 85, 139, 250, 286
Road Runners Club. *See* New York Road Runners Club
Roberts, Linda, 45
Rogue Valley Medical Center, Medford, OR
Russian tea, 265
Russo, Virginia, 343

S

Sabatier, Lou Ann, 30, 91–92, 296–97, 306–7
Sabatier, Mike, and throat cancer, 30
Sacré Coeur Hospital, Montreal, 23
St. Agnes Hospital, Westchester County, NY, 24
St. John, Ruth, and melanoma, 30, 51
Samuel Waxman Cancer Research Foundation, 21
sarcoma, 11, 83
  brachytherapy for, 11
Schmidt, Brian, and multiple myeloma, 4, 30–31, 149, 150, 265, 344
Schmidt, Peggy, 4, 31, 73–74, 122, 238–39, 302–4, 343–44
Schover, Leslie R., 248
second opinions. *See* doctors; treatment
self-image, 176, 220–32. *See also* hair loss
  looking your best, tips, 228–30
sense of loss. *See also* hair loss
  feelings associated with, 44
  and mastectomy, 216

minimizing, what to do, 44–45
  post-surgical, 185–87
  sexual, 243–44
sex, love, and sexuality, 212–13, 234, 235–36, 242–48, 314–15, 366
Sheiner, Alan, 165
Sheridan, Frank, and non-Hodgkin's lymphoma, 31, 51–53, 100, 111–12, 121–22, 143–44, 148–49, 246, 340–41, 372, 381–82
Shulman, Kevin, and testicular cancer, 31, 157, 297–98, 320, 321, 345
Silverman, Rhoda, and breast cancer, 31–32, 70, 95, 210–11, 343
Simonton Cancer Center, 251
Sims, Charles A., 133
skin ulcers, from radiation, 165–66
Sloane, Charlene, and breast cancer, 32, 216, 224, 284, 336
Smith, Jeffrey J., 183
Sobrato, Sheri, and brain tumor, 32, 83–84, 108, 140, 252, 328–29, 366–67
Social Security Disability, 349
soft-tissue sarcoma, 15
soy as a cancer-fighting supplement, 285
sperm bank, 132–33, 374–75
  and insurance coverage, 352
spirituality, 339–46
  God at the head of the bed, 345–46
splenectomy, 162
squamous cell cancer of the sphincter muscle, 30

Steiner, Rudolf, 264
stem cell transplant, 11, 33, 78,
    141, 197
steroids, 149, 238, 287. *See also*
    prednisone
Stone, Elsie, and non-Hodgkin's
    follicular nodular lymphoma,
    33, 170, 299–300, 304
stress, 82
  center, 257
  combating, 79
  and emotional release, 81, 82
  and guided imagery, 150
  mindfulness meditation, 87–88
support systems
  cancer veterans, 78, 81
  chaplain, role of, 342
  co-workers, 69–70, 71, 72
  family, 70–71, 78, 222, 293–
    311
  friends, 312–25
  groups, 328–34
  in hospital, 170, 174
  psychological, 334–38
  religion, 85, 339–46
  social workers, hospital, 348,
    354–55
surgery, 179–96, 321–22. *See
    also* amputation
  preparing for, 183
synovial sarcoma, 20

T

tamoxifen, 25, 285, 336
Taxol, 8, 209
testicular cancer, 11, 12–13, 22–
    23, 31, 60–64, 80
  children after, 13
  recurrence, 276–77
testing
  blood, 108–9

bone marrow, 112–13
CAT scans, 110–11
and control of results, 109
enduring the waiting, 106–7,
    114–16
Magnetic Resonance Imaging
    (MRI), 111–12
scheduling, best times, 115
veins, asking for competent
    bloodtaker, 107, 108–9
Thomas, Bill, and Hodgkin's
    disease, 8, 33, 166
Thomas, Janice, and acute
    lymphatic leukemia, 33, 238,
    314, 385
throat cancer, 30, 286–87, 296–
    97, 366, 389
Totty, Dale, and fibrous
    histiocytoma, 34, 48–49,
    190, 190–92, 195, 277–78,
    279–80, 354
Traber, Wendy, 256
transcendental moments, 379–
    84
treatment. *See also*
    chemotherapy; radiation
    therapy
  alternative or complementary
    medicine, 13, 16, 18, 249–
    68
  control over, 83, 101, 102,
    111, 126–27
  progress in, 391–93
  second opinions, 4, 11, 91, 95–
    98, 160, 181
Trusty, Clara, and leukemia, 34,
    157, 175

U
UCLA, 30
United Ostomy Association, 334

University of Michigan Hospital, 24
University of Pennsylvania Medical Center, 25
University of Washington Hospital, Seattle, 28
uterine cancer, 15, 40, 98–99, 321–22

V
Veterans Administration hospitals, 357
visualization or guided imagery, 83–84, 138, 139, 250–57
volunteering, 3, 9, 10, 12, 13, 15, 16, 18, 19–20, 21, 22, 25–26, 28, 31, 32, 33, 34, 35, 330, 372, 388–90

W
Wadler, Joyce, 212
waiting rooms, 107–8
Ward, Logan, 7
Waxman, Samuel, M.D., 2–3, 7, 160
Weiner, Judy (AML), 34, 147–48

Weintraub, Samuel H., 346
Wells, Charlotte, and breast cancer, 34–35, 74, 97–98, 153, 208–9, 210, 211–12, 287, 316
Whipple procedure, 12
Whitworth, Jery, 263
Winard, Sue, and mother's ovarian cancer, 35, 70–71

Y
Yaffe, Bev, and pancreatic cancer, 35, 92–93, 111, 126–27, 227–28, 261, 268, 279–80
Yale-New Haven Hospital, 10
Y-ME National Organization for Breast Cancer Information and Support, 207

Z
Zavistovski, Toni Rapport, and breast cancer, 35, 75–76, 92, 119–20, 141–42, 208, 225, 237, 261–62, 284, 298, 363, 385
Zofran, 2, 33, 78, 138, 143–44, 155, 260

ABOUT THE AUTHORS

A husband-and-wife team, **Dean** and **Jessica King** have been writing and editing together since the mid-1980s. Jessica is a former senior editor at American Express Publishing. Dean, who overcame Hodgkin's disease in 1991, is the series editor of Heart of Oak Sea Classics (Henry Holt). He is the author of several companion books to Patrick O'Brian's Aubrey-Maturin novels and most recently the editor of *Every Man Will Do His Duty: An Anthology of Firsthand Accounts from the Age of Nelson*. The Kings have collaborated on eight books. Their articles have appeared in many publications, including *Esquire, Food & Wine, Men's Journal, The New York Times,* and *Travel & Leisure*. They recently moved from New York City to Richmond, Virginia, where they live in Dean's childhood home with their three daughters, Hazel, Grace, and Willa.

Jonathan Pearlroth is an author and an attorney. He conducts orientations for prospective bone marrow patients at Memorial Sloan-Kettering and works with people who have cancer and their families at Gilda's Club. He was diagnosed with lymphoma in 1985, had a bone marrow transplant in 1986, and has been cancer-free since then.